Paging God

Paging God

RELIGION IN THE HALLS OF MEDICINE

Wendy Cadge

The University of Chicago Press   CHICAGO & LONDON

WENDY CADGE is associate professor of sociology at Brandeis University. She is author of *Heartwood: The First Generation of Theravada Buddhism in America*, also published by the University of Chicago Press.

The University of Chicago Press, Chicago 60637
The University of Chicago Press, Ltd., London
© 2012 by The University of Chicago
All rights reserved. Published 2012
Printed in the United States of America

21 20 19 18 17 16 15 14 13 12   1 2 3 4 5

ISBN-13: 978-0-226-92210-2 (cloth)
ISBN-10: 0-226-92210-3 (cloth)
ISBN-13: 978-0-226-92211-9 (paper)
ISBN-10: 0-226-92211-1(paper)
ISBN-13: 978-0-226-92213-3 (e-book)
ISBN-10: 0-226-92213-8 (e-book)

Library of Congress Cataloging-in-Publication Data
Cadge, Wendy, author.
Paging God : religion in the halls of medicine / Wendy Cadge.
pages cm
Includes bibliographical references and index.
ISBN 978-0-226-92210-2 (cloth : alkaline paper) — ISBN 0-226-92210-3
(cloth : alkaline paper) — ISBN 978-0-226-92211-9 (paperback :
alkaline paper) — ISBN 0-226-92211-1 (paperback : alkaline paper) —
ISBN 978-0-226-92213-3 (e-book) — ISBN 0-226-92213-8 (e-book)
1. Medicine—Religious aspects. 2. Chaplains, Hospital—United
States. 3. Hospitals—Sociological aspects. I. Title.
R725.55.C33   2012
362.11—dc23
2012021906

CONTENTS

On a Sunday afternoon in 2002, I visited Thai Buddhist monk Taan Čhaokuhn Rattanamēthē at a hospital outside of Philadelphia. Born outside Bangkok in 1938, Taan Čhaokuhn came to Philadelphia in 1984 to help start Wat Mong-koltepmunee, a Thai Buddhist temple. I met him at the temple in 2000 while conducting research for my first book, *Heartwood: The First Generation of Theravada Buddhism in America* (University of Chicago Press, 2005). Shortly after I began the research, I learned that Taan Čhaokuhn had liver cancer. He traveled regularly to Texas, where he received treatments from Thai-born physicians. When he returned, laypeople offered Ensure protein drinks and money for airfare in addition to their usual donations.

A few days before he died, Taan Čhaokuhn was admitted to a local hospital. He was sleeping when I arrived—a small man in a large hospital bed, clad in the bright-orange robes of a Buddhist monk. I sat down at the foot of his bed, careful to keep the top of my head below the top of his head, Thai etiquette for laypeople in the presence of a monk. He was on oxygen and intravenous pain medication and was surrounded by monks and laypeople speaking in hushed voices.

As I watched Taan Čhaokuhn sleep, I thought about the hospital staff caring for him and wondered if they knew the norms for interacting with Buddhist monks. While he was hard to miss in his orange robes, I thought about other patients whose religious and spiritual beliefs were not immediately evident and wondered how hospital staff members interacted with them. I wondered whether this hospital had a chaplain who might visit Taan Čhaokuhn, and how a chaplain would spend time with a monk who spoke little English.

Thinking about hospital chapels, I wondered how American medical centers located in religiously and ethnically diverse cities negotiated that diversity in their chapel spaces, in questions about religion or spirituality on admissions forms, and in the work of hospital chaplains. I wondered if religious and spiritual concerns were strictly the job of the chaplain or were taken up by physicians and nurses, especially in end-of-life situations like this one.

Much of my scholarly work considers how people from different religious and spiritual backgrounds live together in the contemporary United States, and it struck me that hospitals are microcosms for such questions—likely made more intense by the life-and-death issues that arise within them. Patients, families, and staff might have religious or spiritual beliefs that influence their experiences in hospitals, and hospital administrators have to make decisions about how to accommodate or ignore those beliefs in their physical spaces, policies, and staffing.

Taan Čhaokuhn woke up as I sat at his bedside, and I put my hands together in prayer position, bowing slightly toward him. My Thai friends donated money and protein shakes—which joined several cases already stacked under his bed—and we talked briefly. Taan Čhaokuhn told us about his pain and the upcoming Thai New Year. He sipped from a straw in a white plastic cup and told me to keep attending the temple and practicing my Thai language skills. When he fell asleep again, we quietly left his room.

Taan Čhaokuhn died in this hospital's hospice unit several days later—at an auspicious time, on an auspicious day: 9:30 p.m. on the night of the full moon. He did not see a chaplain or visit the hospital chapel before he died, but the time I spent with him at the hospital motivates this book's central questions: How are American health-care organizations responding to people's religious and spiritual beliefs and practices? How do chaplains and other health-care professionals, sometimes themselves people of faith, engage these beliefs and practices? How do hospitals negotiate religious and spiritual diversity, and what do their explicit and more implicit negotiations tell us about religion in the contemporary United States?

While my experiences with Taan Čhaokuhn as a patient motivate these questions, the book is based primarily on the words and observations of hospital staff. While I regret not being able to gather the stories of patients myself—and hope someone else will write such a book—my focus on staff helps me see how hospitals respond to religion and spirituality as organizations and what this suggests about religion in the contemporary United States more broadly. Keeping the late Taan Čhaokuhn in mind, I approach this project aware of America's Christian majority as well as the experiences of Buddhist, Muslim, Jewish, and Hindu patients and health-care providers and the growing numbers of Americans who claim no religious beliefs or affiliation.

A fellowship from the Robert Wood Johnson Foundation Scholars in Health Policy Research Program nurtured this project and made possible the fieldwork that is at the core of the book. In the National Program Office, Alan Cohen, Eileen Connor, Nora Zelizer, and others ran the program smoothly and supported me during my time as a fellow and beyond. At the Harvard University site, Kathy Swartz, Nicholas Christakis, Dan Carpenter, Paul Cleary, Mary-Jo Good, Gary King, Joe Newhouse, Peter Marsden, Mary Ruggie, and fellow scholars taught me—a sociologist of religion—about health care and health-care policy. Others in the program, particularly Paula Lantz, Hal Luft, and participants in the annual meetings, asked critical questions and encouraged me along the way. Shortly after I arrived at Harvard, Nicholas Christakis introduced me to his mentor, Renée Fox, Annenberg Professor Emerita of the Social Sciences at the University of Pennsylvania. Renée provided foundational guidance throughout this project. Without her ongoing support, consistent insights, and steady mentorship, this book would never have come to fruition.

A fellowship from the Radcliffe Institute for Advanced Study at Harvard University provided the time and space I needed to complete much of the manuscript. Judy Vichniac expertly directed the fellowship program; Dean Barbara Grosz created a stimulating intellectual environment; administrator Melissa Synnott kept track of many details; and fellow scholars educated me about a wide range of topics. Academic leaves from Bowdoin College and Brandeis University made fieldwork and writing possible. I am grateful to Deans Craig McEwen (Bowdoin College) and Adam Jaffe (Brandeis University), who granted me leave, and Pam Endo, Judy Hanley, Cheryl Hansen, and others at Brandeis University who helped organize and administrate many related details. At Brandeis, Laura Gardner helped me find my voice as she taught me to write some of my first op-ed pieces on these topics. For her patience and her curiosity—especially about prayer—I am grateful.

Additional financial support for this and related projects came from a General Grant and a Religious Institutions Grant from the Louisville Institute, an Individual Research Grant from the American Academy of Religion, funding from the Cognitive and Textual Methods Project at Princeton University, the Research Partnership Program at the Radcliffe Institute for Advanced Study, the Theodore and Jane Norman Fund for Faculty Research at Brandeis University, and Student-Scholar Partnerships at the Women's Studies Resource Center at Brandeis University.

Social scientists, medical professionals, religious leaders, and friends read drafts of this work, offered field contacts, and provided advice that helped it take shape. I am especially grateful to Debbie Beecher, Peter Cahn, David Cunningham, Joshua Dubler, Elaine Howard Ecklund, John Evans, George Fitchett, Marla Frederick, Renée Fox, Sharon Ghamari-Tabrizi, Nicholas Guyatt, Lance Laird, Bonnie McDougall Olson, Sara Shostak, Despina Stratigakos, Wilson Will, and Robert Wuthnow, who read chapters—sometimes more than once—or a full draft of the manuscript and provided detailed feedback. M. Daglian expertly transcribed all the interviews. For conversations, contacts, and more, additional thanks to Betsy Armstrong, Linda Barnes, Susan Bell, Courtney Bender, Chuck Bosk, Carol Caronna, Dan Chambliss, Joy Charlton, Mark Chaves, Sarah Coakley, Peter Conrad, Lynn Davidman, Helen Rose Ebaugh, Penny Edgell, Chris Ellison, Kathleen Garces-Foley, Don Grant, Grove Harris, Kieran Healey, Jonathan Imber, Debra Jarvis, Taryn Kudler, Jackson Kytle, Peggy Levitt, Jim Lewis, Diana Long, Keith Meador, Laurie Meneades, Margo McLoughlin, Frances Norwood, Paul Numrich, Abraham Nussbaum, Laura Olson, Katie Pakos, Stephanie Paulsell, Nina Paynter, Sarah Pinto, Stephen Prothero, Jen'nan Read, Susan Reverbe, Dudley Rose, Charles Rosenberg, Susan Sered, Katrina Scott, Laura Stark, Winnifred Sullivan, Robert Tabak, Mary Martha Thiel, Stefan Timmermans, R. Stephen Warner, Fred Wherry, and members of the 2004–2005 Younger Scholars in American Religion Program at the Center for the Study of Religion and American Culture at Indiana University–Purdue University, Indianapolis. Thank you to Elizabeth Alford, Megan Eyre, Bob Day, Mindy Day, Wesley Shaw, and Craig Williams for help with research photographs.

Questions from audiences at the annual meetings of the American Academy of Religion and the American Sociological Association, the annual meeting of the Association of Professional Chaplains, Boston University, Brandeis University, the Center for the Study of Religion and Society at the University of Notre Dame, Duke University, the annual meeting of the Eastern Sociological Society, Harvard University, the Hospital of the University of Pennsylvania, the Institute for Pastoral Supervision, Loyola University of Chicago, Lutheran Healthcare, Massachusetts General Hospital, Princeton University, the Radcliffe Institute for Advanced Study, the annual meetings of the Robert Wood Johnson Foundation Scholars in Health Policy Research Program and the Society for the Scientific Study of Religion, the Spiritual Care Collaborative Meeting, Smith College, and the University of Washington sharpened and challenged my thinking.

In the final stages of the project, the manuscript was the focus of a program at the Religion and Public Life Program at Rice University. Elaine Howard Ecklund kindly organized the event with the assistance of Katherine Sorrell. Elizabeth Armstrong, Farr Curlin, and Helen Rose Ebaugh reviewed the entire manuscript at the event and provided valuable feedback.

Collaborations on related projects with Nancy Berlinger, Katherine Calle, Elizabeth A. Catlin, Nicholas Christakis, Farr Curlin, M. Daglian, Raymond DeVries, Jennifer Dillinger, Elaine Howard Ecklund, Brian Fair, George Fitchett, Jeremy Freese, Nicole Fox, Elizabeth Gage, Clare Hammonds, Lance Laird, Qiong Li, Kenneth Rasinski, Emily Sigalow, Nicholas Short, and Angelika Zollfrank improved my thinking on this one. Research assistants Lynda Bachman, Shevy Baskin, Angelica Colon, Casey Clevenger, Scott Frost, Daniel Garcia, Clare Hammonds, Sarah Kinsler, Joy Lee, Dennis Lorusso, Madison Lyleroehr, Kathryn Lyndes, Aylin Mentesh, and Marisa Tashman were a tremendous help. And librarians, archivists, and staff at the American Hospital Association, American Medical Association, Joint Commission, Association for Professional Chaplains, National Association of Catholic Chaplains, National Association of Jewish Chaplains, Harvard University Libraries, and Pitts Theological Library were invaluable. Doug Mitchell, Tim McGovern, Ruth Goring, and Nicholas Murray at the University of Chicago Press patiently guided the book through the publication process—for which I am grateful.

This book is built around the words and experiences of more than one hundred and fifty hospital chaplains, physicians, respiratory therapists, social workers, and nurses. I am deeply grateful for their frankness, the time they took to talk with me, and their willingness to let me shadow them and learn about their work lives. I am sorry that our agreements about confidentiality do not allow me to thank each by name. The staff of the Chaplaincy Department at Overbrook Hospital and the neonatal and medical intensive care units at City Hospital welcomed me as a sociologist in their midst; they deserve special thanks. The directors of each took a risk when they invited me in, and I hope some of what I write helps them better care for themselves, each other, and the patients and families they work with daily.

I was sustained through this project by the love of family and friends. My parents and sisters Amy, Barbara, Donald, and Laura Cadge, and Nancy and David Walls were a source of strength, as were my grandparents. Friends Anjali Avadhani, Linda Callahan, Katie Klingensmith, Dana Lehman, Estelle McCartney, Sara Shostak, and Despina Stratigakos were my circle of support. With integrity, patience, and a lot of laughter, Deborah Elliott taught me new ways to love and to care during the second half of this project. For Deborah, our son Nate, the household pet zoo of Harley, Graham, Gus, and Max, and all of those named here, I am grateful. Writing about the pain and suffering I witnessed while conducting fieldwork for this project would have been even more difficult without each of you.

A NOTE ON THE PHOTOS

The photos in this book come from various sources and do not contain images of the hospitals I visited or people I interviewed in the course of the research. The historical photos in chapter 2 are from the Boisen Paper Collection at the Chicago Theological Seminary and the Chaplaincy Department at Massachusetts General Hospital respectively. Chaplains offered the images of chapel spaces and chaplains in chapters 3–5. I selected images of chapel, prayer, and meditation rooms that had features in common with those I write about in chapter 3. I aimed to show a diverse set of chaplains in chapters 4 and 5 doing a range of tasks. All of the chaplains and patients who appear in these images gave consent for their photos to be published. Practical and ethical considerations prohibited my photographing staff in intensive care units. I purchased the two photos included in chapter 6 and print them here with permission.

CHAPTER 1

In the Beginning—A Tour

Meg's day at Overbrook Hospital begins early when she is coming off overnight call.[1] I meet staff chaplain Meg, in her sixties, wearing street clothes and serious shoes, and carrying a binder overflowing with papers, and Daniel, a Clinical Pastoral Education (CPE) student, at 6:30 a.m. on a summer morning in the chaplaincy staff room. Looking remarkably rested for having slept on a hospital cot, Meg says good morning to me before finding scissors to cut today's Communion list into sections. Spending the night at the hospital is like being on a red-eye, she tells me as she cuts. The night was quiet, though. She was not paged to any deaths or code blues—called when a person's heart stops—and actually got some sleep. "I think this is the only hospital in the city that has in-house 24/7 chaplain coverage," she says as she files the lists for the Eucharistic ministers who will deliver Communion to Catholic patients later in the day. Gathering up her binder, she gestures for Daniel and me to follow her to the preoperative surgery unit, where she will begin her morning rounds.

Patients coming into the hospital for same-day surgeries, Meg explains on the way, wait here until their operating rooms are ready. We go through double doors and into a large, open room divided into cubicles with curtains. Everything—hospital gurneys, chart racks, machines—is on wheels. About twenty patients in hospital gowns, many with family members nearby, sit or lie in their curtained spaces. Physicians and nurses in scrubs move quickly through the unit. Stopping in front of a whiteboard by the nurses' station, Meg turns to Daniel. "I don't know how other chaplains do this," she says pointing to the board, "but I like to know the name of the patient first, so why don't you take that column and I'll take this column." Medical staff members are often with patients, so the idea is to quickly meet patients and their families before they are wheeled into surgery and not to interrupt any medical staff in the process.

Daniel begins his rounds, and I follow Meg to the first curtained cubicle. She knocks in the air, saying, "Knock knock," and then enters slowly, greeting the patient by name. "My name is Meg, and I am here from the chaplain's office," she begins. "We are coming around this morning to wish people well and see if there is anything we can do for you." A few people respond quickly, indicating in words or by tone of voice that they do not want a visit, and Meg moves on. Most invite her into their tiny, curtained areas, where she asks about their surgery, their family members, or the anxieties that are often palpable in the small space.

After they chat for a few minutes, she asks patients if they have a religious affiliation they feel comfortable sharing. If the answer is Catholic, as it is most frequently here, she asks patients if they would like to be on the Communion list. She offers kosher food and electric Shabbat candles to Jewish patients. Meg generally closes her short visits by saying, "I would be happy to say a prayer for you if you would like." Most accept, and she moves in closer, taking the patient and family members by the hand. Standing with an elderly Catholic patient and his family this morning, she prays, "I put my hands on you in the name of God the Father, his Son Jesus, and in the name of the Holy Spirit. Thank you for this day. . . . We ask you to guide the hands of the surgical team and give them the wisdom and resources they need. . . . We seek your healing in body, mind, and spirit." Later, when I ask more directly about these prayers, Meg tells me that she mentions Jesus more often when praying with African American and evangelical Christian patients. She rarely prays with Jewish patients, both because they do not have a strong tradition of public prayer and because some feel uncomfortable, thinking she is trying to convert them—something her professional code of ethics strictly forbids.[2]

I think of the visible ways that Chaplain Meg prays with patients a few weeks later as I sit in a conference room by the neonatal intensive care unit (NICU) at nearby City Hospital. Christina, a young NICU nurse, is talking with me about prayer. In her twenties, Christina wears scrub pants and an NICU sweatshirt, and seems to exude positive energy. Like Meg, she prays publicly with patients and families, though usually only if the unit chaplain is not available. "Different times in the middle of the night," she explains, "when the chaplain had not gotten here yet and the baby is dying—we've [the nurses] been told that we are instruments of healing, and we've actually taken water and blessed it, and blessed the baby ourselves at four o'clock in the morning when a baby has passed away." Thinking of a specific situation, she continues, "One time in the middle of the night I remember a couple of the [Catholic] nurses, three of us, just started saying the 'Our Father,' 'Hail Mary,' and the 'Glory Be,' and we just prayed over the water and did the sign of the cross and just put it on the baby—you know, head, heart, side, side." She gestures, crossing herself as she speaks.

In addition to the visible ways that Christina prays in the intensive care unit, she also prays for her patients in less visible ways. While commuting home after a tough day, she talks to her mother, who, in turn, calls Christina's grandmother. "My grandmother has this religious candle in her kitchen that has pieces of tape with pieces of paper with every person that she's praying for. And at the bottom of the candle there is a paper for all of the babies in the NICU, . . . and it is lit most times during the day but specific times when babies are not doing really well at all, I'll call mom and say, 'Have Nana light the candle,' and she will." When caring for a particular long-term patient, Christina started a prayer circle with a few other nurses and their families: "We told the family [of this patient] that not only us but our relatives, our families, are praying for the baby as well, because our families are as much a part of this as we are." When her family members ask how they can help with her work, Christina tells them to "say a prayer" just as she does privately for all of her patients—regardless of how they are doing—every day.

*

Prayers offered—visibly and invisibly—by Meg, her chaplain colleagues, Christina, and other intensive care nurses are one way that religion and spirituality are present at Overbrook and City Hospitals. The hospital chapel, prayer book, questions asked at admissions, and conversations among patients, family members, nurses, and doctors—especially around end-of-life issues—are others, not just at Overbrook and City Hospitals but in large academic medical centers across the country. This book is about how religion and spirituality are present in formally secular hospitals.[3] It is about the public and not so public forms religion and spirituality take in medical settings, the reasons they take these forms, and the ways staff members act around them in their daily work.[4]

The questions I address here are just one aspect of growing public attention to religion, spirituality, prayer, health, and medicine. *Time* magazine's February 23, 2009 cover story, "How Faith Can Heal," reflects other questions and is the most recent in a string of magazine covers with headlines like "The God Gene," "The Power of Prayer," and "God and Health: Is Religion Good Medicine? Why Science Is Starting to Believe."[5] Related news articles are on the rise, including recent reports about parents withholding children's medical treatment on religious grounds, religiously infused debates about abortion in national health-care reform, and public discussions of stem cells and the rights of conscience for health-care providers.[6]

Academic research about the relationship between religion and health is also increasing, especially since 1990. The number of scholarly articles about religion/spirituality and prayer catalogued in PubMed, the main biomedical research database, increased significantly between 1990 and the present, as shown in figures 1.1 and 1.2.[7] Many of these studies ask whether personal religion or spirituality—measured in terms of beliefs, affiliations, and behaviors—influences health. The press picks up positive findings and spreads them under headlines like "Is Religion Good for Health? Researchers Say Amen" and "Dose of Religion Tied to Good Health in North Carolina."[8]

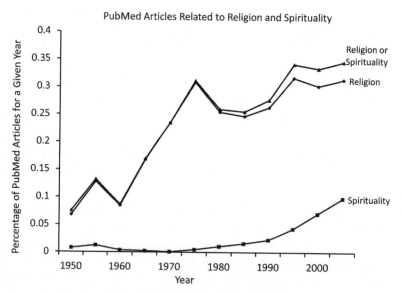

FIGURE 1.1 Fraction of all articles catalogued in PubMed that have derivations of the terms *religion* or *spirituality* in any search field, over time.

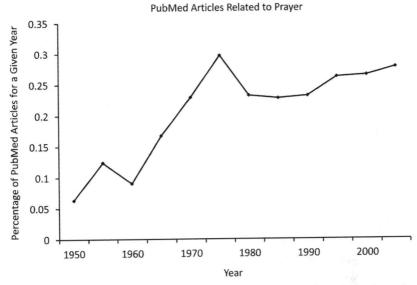

FIGURE 1.2 Fraction of all articles catalogued in PubMed that have derivations of the word *prayer* in any search field, over time.

Also in recent years, university centers like the George Washington Institute for Spirituality and Health (GWish) and the Center for Spirituality, Theology, and Health at Duke University opened to support research and help new generations of health-care providers be more aware of religious and spiritual issues.[9] For the past several years the Department of Continuing Education at Harvard University has cosponsored courses with titles like "Spirituality and Healing in Health and Medicine" (2002) and "Spirituality and Healing in Medicine: Including New Intercessory Prayer Findings and the Concept of Emergence" (2006). Growing numbers of medical schools offer related elective courses as part of their regular curriculum.[10] Books with titles like *Is Faith Delusion? Why Religion Is Good for Your Health* (2009), *How God Changes Your Brain* (2009), and *The Healing Power of Faith: How Belief and Prayer Can Help You Triumph over Disease* (2001) are being published alongside more academic books like *The Handbook of Religion and Health* (2001) and popular books for people struggling with specific health conditions, such as *Everyday Strength: A Cancer Patient's Guide to Spiritual Survival* (2006) and *The Bible Cure for Heart Disease* (1999).

Some health-care providers, scholars, and journalists praise growing relationships between religion, spirituality, and medicine. Others are more skeptical. Columbia University's Richard Sloan is among the skeptics. Studies that show positive relationships between religion and health, he argues in his book *Blind Faith: The Unholy Alliance of Religion and Medicine*, are frequently flawed and may harm patients.[11] In that book and on op-ed pages and in news magazines, Sloan frequently spars with Harold Koenig, a physician who directs the Center for Spirituality, Theology, and Health at Duke University, as well as other prominent advocates of positive relationships between religion and health. They argue about what roles religion and spirituality should play in health care through interactions between patients, physicians, and other staff. Such questions are no less complex than those about the appropriate place of religion and spirituality in public education or politics and may provoke even more controversy, given the life-and-death issues potentially at stake.

Despite the prevalence of research about religion's effects on health and the veracity of related debates in health care, participants rarely pay much attention to how religion and spirituality are *actually* present in the day-to-day workings of health-care organizations. Physicians and pundits spend more time arguing about whether patients want their physicians to inquire about their religious and spiritual backgrounds or pray with them than they do actually listening to how the topics come up in physicians' offices.[12] People argue about the morality of public funding for abortion or euthanasia more than they visit health-care organizations or hospices to observe how religion or spirituality actually influences the work of staff and the decisions made by patients and families.

Overshadowed in heated public debates about religion, spirituality, and health—in other words—are the voices of Chaplain Meg, Christina the intensive care nurse, and other health-care workers across the country who see religion and spirituality in their daily work. I take you inside large academic hospitals in this book to show how these people understand religion and spirituality and how they see them *actually* present in day-to-day events at these hospitals. Unlike the flashy, romantically infused hospital scenes in *ER*, *Grey's Anatomy*, and other popular television shows, this book focuses on the ways religion and spirituality are evident in the architecture of hospital buildings and in the daily routines of hospital life.

This "on-the-ground" approach to religion and spirituality in hospitals is essential for historical and contemporary reasons. Religion has played an important role in the history of American hospitals. Many of the nation's first hospitals were started by religious organizations, and religion shaped hospital expansion in the nineteenth and twentieth centuries. While scholars have written about Catholic and Jewish hospitals, some of which have closed or become secularized in recent years, almost nothing is known about how religion informs daily work in secularized hospitals or others founded as secular organizations.

Such questions are especially important, given that the Joint Commission, which sets policies for health-care organizations, has called on all hospitals to address the religious and spiritual needs of patients since 1969. The 2010 guidelines stipulate that hospitals are to respect "the patient's cultural and personal values, beliefs, and preferences" and accommodate "the patient's right to religious and other spiritual services."[13] The Joint Commission singles out particular groups of patients for spiritual assessment, including those dealing with the end of life, alcohol and drug abuse, and emotional and behavioral disorders. The commission also says that hospitals are also to consider spiritual issues when making decisions about food, education, and training for staff.

While stipulating that hospitals must respect, accommodate, and in some cases gather information about spirituality from patients, Joint Commission guidelines have never stipulated how hospitals are to do so. Little is known about how these guidelines evolved and how hospitals try to meet them in the context of America's religious diversity. According to the 2008 American Religious Identification Survey (ARIS), 25.1% of Americans are Catholic, 49.5% are Protestant or non-denominational Christians (including 3.5% Pentecostal/Charismatic), 1.4% are Mormon, 1.2% are Jewish, and less than 1% are Buddhist or other eastern religions or Muslim. Just over 1% reported being members of other religions. Fifteen percent said they were not religious, and 5% did not respond to the survey question.[14] More recent surveys conducted by the Pew Forum show that many people combine ideas from a range of religious and spiritual traditions.[15] Scholars and health-care providers have yet to understand how hospitals respond to such diverse beliefs and practices as they strive to meet Joint Commission guidelines.

In addition to historical and policy motivations, it is important to understand how religion and spirituality are present in hospitals because the topics are important to many in hospitals—patients and staff alike—who do not check their beliefs at the door. Recent surveys report that 80% of Americans think personal religious/spiritual practices, including prayer, can help with medical treatments, and close to 25% say they have been cured of an illness through prayer or another religious/spiritual practice.[16] Seventy percent regularly pray for their own health or that of a family member.[17] And close to 75% believe God can cure people who are given no chance of survival by medical science.[18] A 2008 article in *Archives of Surgery* reported that 60% of the public and 20% of medical professionals believe that it is possible for an individual in a persistent vegetative state (a coma) to be saved by a miracle.[19] Such beliefs may help explain why religious patients receive more life-sustaining treatments in hospitals than others at the end of their lives, which sometimes leads to conflict with medical teams.[20]

Like Americans generally, hospital staff also have religious and spiritual beliefs that influence health and health care. Such influences are often more subtle than in public debates about whether physicians can refuse patients medical care on religiously related grounds of conscience.[21] Just over half of physicians in a nationally representative survey conducted in 2005 reported that their religious beliefs influenced their practice of medicine. They were more likely than the general public to be members of minority religious traditions, including Judaism, Hinduism, Islam, Orthodox Christianity, and Mormonism. They were twice as likely as members of the public to consider themselves spiritual but not religious. Close to two-thirds (61%) said they cope with major problems in life without relying on God in comparison to less than one-third (29%) of the public.[22] While more research is needed, these findings suggest that physicians may draw on different religious traditions and sources of authority than do members of the general public when making decisions, a fact that is especially important in light of research suggesting that religion influences how physicians make decisions.[23]

Nurses and social workers tend to be more personally religious than physicians and more open and aware of the influence that religion and spirituality may have on patients. One study conducted at a large academic medical center found that 91% of nurses considered themselves spiritual, and 80% thought there was something spiritual about the care they provided. Almost none believed that promoting spirituality was at odds with medicine.[24] National data that would allow for comparisons among the religious demographics of nurses, medical social workers, and the American public has not yet been gathered.

Given the religious histories of many hospitals, the religious demographics of staff and patients, and the existential issues so often addressed inside them, hospitals provide a unique vantage point for thinking analytically about religion in contemporary American life. As microcosms, Overbrook, City, and other large academic hospitals located in religiously diverse geographic regions provide insights about secularization, medicalization, and the ways religious and spiritual diversity are explicitly and implicitly negotiated in daily life.

APPROACHING HOSPITALS: EARLY DECISIONS

I begin, given the complexity of the American health-care system, by focusing on just one set of health-care institutions: hospitals. The close to six thousand hospitals in the United States range from small community hospitals with just a few beds to large academic medical centers with more than one thousand. I focus on large, secular, academic medical centers here that, in addition to providing cutting edge health care, train generations of health-care workers. As centers of science developing new technologies and treatments for disease, these were the hospitals where—despite some of their religious histories—I least expected to see religion and spirituality present.

I focus on seventeen top hospitals as ranked by *U.S. News and World Report.*[25] At each hospital, I interviewed the director of chaplaincy and a staff chaplain, and moved throughout the public areas of the hospital. I visited hospital chapels, prayer and meditation rooms, and attended religious services in the hospital. I also became part of the Chaplaincy Department at Overbrook Hospital, one of these seventeen hospitals, for one year. In addition to shadowing Meg and her chaplain colleagues, attending staff meetings, and attending meetings across the hospital, I interviewed most of the staff, students, and volunteers in the department.

Aware that religion and spirituality are present in hospitals when chaplains are not around, I also focused on a neonatal and medical intensive care unit where medical staff care for acutely ill newborns and adults. While medical advances and reductions in the length of patient stays in the hospital make many units of large academic hospitals like intensive care units of the past, I focused on a neonatal and medical intensive care unit as two (of many) places in hospitals where religion and spirituality might be present, especially given the intense beginning- and end-of-life issues they bring into focus. Ideally these two units would have been at Overbrook, but the challenges of getting permission, as explained in the appendix, led me to City Hospital, another of the seventeen large academic medical centers. I shadowed Christina and other nurses in each ICU and interviewed physicians, nurses, social workers, and chaplains about how religion and spirituality come up in their work and how they respond professionally and personally.

This book is based primarily on the words and observations of hospital staff. As in physician/sociologist Nicholas Christakis's book *Death Foretold: Prophecy and Prognosis in Medical Care,* the experiences of patients and families come through only in the stories that nurses, chaplains, physicians, and social workers tell about them.[26] While I regret not being able to gather the stories of patients myself, my focus on staff helps me to see better how secular academic medical centers prepare for and respond to religion and spirituality as organizations—in their physical spaces, decisions to employ chaplains, ways of integrating chaplains into the institution, and norms around religion and spirituality in intensive care.[27]

As I made my way through long hallways and around the construction projects in progress at many hospitals, I thought about how to conceptualize religion and spirituality.[28] The terms *religion* and *spirituality* are themselves contested in academic and public debates about religion, spirituality, and health.[29] In the past ten years, many seeking to more fully integrate these issues in health care have shifted from the term *religion* to the term *spirituality*, viewing it as a more universal or inclusive, less baggage-laden, term.[30] A physician who is a proponent of connections between spirituality and health chided me early in this research for using the word *religion*. "There is so much more than religion going on," she explained, telling me that the word *religion* is a stumbling block to having work about religion in health care accepted— especially in medicine—because in her view people hear the term *religion* and think about right-wing religious groups and radical religious acts.

Sociologists and religious studies scholars view the division this physician makes between the concepts of religion and spirituality as a recent idea, as is the notion that the spiritual is more inclusive or somehow better than the religious.[31] Sociologist Courtney Bender argues that spirituality, as a concept, is embedded in the contexts in which it is produced and must be understood there. "Most definitions" of spirituality, she argues, "have served to protect, defend, debunk, or claim certain territory for the spiritual; these definitions confound more than they illuminate."[32] Bender calls on scholars to investigate how the concept of spirituality is used. Doing just that, medical anthropologist Simon Lee argues that the term *spirituality* is being "strategically deployed" by hospital chaplains to extend their work and "realm of relevance to any patient's 'belief system,' regardless of his or her religious affiliation."[33] Winifred Sullivan, a scholar of religious studies and law, makes a similar argument, seeing proponents using and defining *spirituality* as something that is intrinsic to all people, whether we recognize it as such or not.[34]

Following the leads of Bender, Lee, and Sullivan, I approach the terms *religion* and *spirituality* inductively and empirically here, listening to how hospitals and hospital staff use them, asking what they mean, and considering how they are understood and strategically deployed.[35] I pay particular attention to what these hospitals and the people who work in them describe as religious, spiritual, or pertaining to the chapel or chaplaincy as the historical holder of religion and spirituality in the institution. While prayer, one aspect of religion and spirituality, is sometimes included in studies of complementary and alternative medicine (CAM), I do not focus specifically on CAM here. Neither do I focus directly on hospitals' bioethics committees, which are often informed historically by religious and spiritual people and ideas.[36] I try to situate the concepts of religion and spirituality historically, particularly in the next chapter, aware that separation between them is a contemporary idea and that tensions between the terms in use and the boundaries they demarcate are an important part of the story I tell.

STEPPING INSIDE

Much as Meg brought me into the pre-operative surgery unit at Overbrook Hospital and Christina allowed me to shadow her in the neonatal intensive care unit, I bring you inside hospitals in the rest of the book to highlight in different chapters the locations where I learned about aspects of religion and spirituality. Readers primarily interested in particular locations or specific groups of staff are advised to skip directly to those chapters.

Many patients first encounter a question about religion or spirituality at the admissions/registration desk. At City Hospital, hospital rules required me to pass health tests before I could be granted formal permission to do research. Like any other patient, I stopped first at the admissions desk to register. An older staff member led me to his cubicle, where he typed my full name, address, date of birth, and insurance information into his computer. He asked several more questions before looking up and asking, "What is your religion?" Surprised, I responded by asking if he asks that question of everyone. Yes, he told me, so the hospital knows who to call when people pass away. "I don't think it is any of the hospital's business," he continued, explaining that he stopped asking the question for awhile but had to start again after getting in trouble with his boss. People give a wide range of answers, and some get upset or suspicious, especially Jewish people ("Who can blame them," he sighed). Not sure I would want anyone, other than my partner, called if I died at the hospital I replied "None," though I belong to a musical ensemble at a local Protestant church and have spent significant amounts of time doing research in Buddhist organizations.

City Hospital is not alone in asking patients about their religious or spiritual backgrounds, either during admission/registration or in nursing assessments. This information is often shared with chaplains, who told me, almost uniformly, that it is wildly inaccurate, perhaps because—like me—patients are surprised by the question, not sure what the information will be used for and, therefore, not sure how to respond. Staff members, like the man I interacted with at City Hospital, may also be uncomfortable asking the question. "We need to work with our admitting folks to do a better job with it," the Chaplaincy Department director at University Hospital told me, "because they really, I think, feel uncomfortable asking, and it has been an issue for awhile now." The director of the Chaplaincy Department at Eastern Hospital told me that people are asked about their faith during the registration process, "but I discourage chaplains from paying much attention to it."

Once in their rooms, patients at a few of these hospitals find materials about religion and spirituality.[37] One Chaplaincy Department supplies every room with a book of psalms, a New Testament, and a booklet entitled "Prayers for Comfort and Healing" that they compiled from across religious traditions. They note that materials from other religious traditions are available in the Pastoral Care Office, including Bibles, Qur'ans, and other religious texts often donated by local or national organizations such as the Gideons; electric Shabbat candles; and Muslim prayer rugs. Pamphlets about the department and about responding to trauma, dealing with bad news, coping with illness, and other topics are also frequently available.[38]

Outside their rooms, patients, families, and staff may see references to religion and spirituality in a range of public spaces. All seventeen hospitals have chapels and prayer or meditation rooms that I describe in chapter 3. A number have memorial quilts hanging in their lobbies that include mention of angels, God, and heaven. Several have concrete reminders of patients' religious backgrounds in the trinkets and books for sale in hospital gift shops and in Shabbat elevators that allow observant Jews to move between floors on the Sabbath without initiating the use of electricity. "We block out one of the elevators," a Jewish chaplain explained, "and for twenty-four hours it is just set to run automatically floor by floor. It stops on each floor automatically and holds the door open for exactly ten seconds and then closes it." This hospital, located in a city with a large Orthodox Jewish population, also has an *eruv*, which marks the area within which observant Jews can carry objects on the Sabbath.[39] While some hospitals used to announce prayers and ceremonies over their PA systems, none do now—choosing instead to make recorded prayers available on Chaplaincy Department telephone lines.

In their hospital rooms, some patients and families not only see related literature but meet chaplains, like Meg, who usually wear street clothes and hospital ID badges rather than clerical collars or white coats.[40] I describe who chaplains are, what they see themselves bringing to hospitals, and how they frame their work as religious professionals in hospitals in chapter 4. At half of the hospitals, chaplains are assigned to specific units—like medical ICUs or emergency rooms—where they work as part of patient-care teams. They are responsible for all the patients on their teams, regardless of the match between their own religious or spiritual backgrounds and those of their patients. "I have the medical-oncology unit [and] the stem cell bone marrow transplant unit," one chaplain explained to me. "I try to meet everybody. That's our goal. . . . I go in, introduce myself, let them know that I'm here, that I'm the chaplain on that particular unit, . . . do a certain amount of chit-chat, and then see where it goes." If a patient needs a particular chaplain, like a Catholic priest, for a ritual, this chaplain pages that person after assessing the need. At the other half of the hospitals, some chaplains are assigned to specific units, while others, especially Catholic priests and rabbis, move throughout the hospital, seeing only patients and families in their own traditions. "Regular chaplains are basically the beat cops," a Catholic priest working in this model explained. "They're working their neighborhoods [units]. I'm the SWAT team. I go in for the Catholics. . . . I'm the sacramental SWAT team." These staffing decisions influence how chaplains are integrated into hospital units, as do decisions about whether chaplains are automatically included in protocols. There are significant variations among hospitals in how chaplains are integrated institutionally, which I describe in chapter 5.

Shifting from chaplains who move freely through hospitals, I visit intensive care units in chapters 6 and 7. I describe how medical staff members in a neonatal and medical ICU see and respond to religion in their work in chapter 6. I then shift from the visible to the more invisible ways that religion and spirituality influence how ICU staff members like Christina personally approach their work. I explore the personal beliefs and practices they bring in chapter 7, asking how they make sense of the suffering and death they witness as part of their jobs.[41]

I begin to conclude in chapter 8 by showing how religion and spirituality are present in hospitals with regard to certain topics, primarily death. In some hospitals this association is evident historically in their architecture, as mortuary chapels were built next to morgues—usually in the basement—so that families could view the bodies of their deceased loved ones. Currently, this association is evident as hospital staff, over and over in conversations with me, equated religion and spirituality with concerns about death. I move from patient rooms to morgues and memorial services, with chaplains showing how they name death, facilitate conversations about death, and help to manage death not just for families but for staff and hospitals as organizations.

THE BIGGER PICTURE

The story I tell in this book is a messy story. The ways in which religion and spirituality are present on the ground in large academic hospitals are messy. I do not conclude with a grand synthesis or neat way of explaining all the variation that I document.[42] While it would be analytically tidy to find that secular hospitals with chapels that reflect particular religious traditions hire particular types of chaplains and have ICU staff who speak and act about religion in particular ways, that is not the case. American health-care organizations respond to people's religious and spiritual beliefs and practices in ways that are in fact fragmented, inconsistent, and very different in different hospitals.

Much of this messiness is driven by the different—professionally informed—languages that chaplains and ICU staff use to think and talk about religion and spirituality. Chaplains are increasingly framing their work in terms of spirituality, which functions, I argue, as a strategically vague frame. While Chaplain Meg and colleagues do administer religious rituals like baptism and communion, they speak broad languages of presence, healing, and hope more than they speak of or frame their work in the categories of one or a series of religious traditions. Their approach is part of what Winifred Sullivan calls "areligious secularism"—which "denominates a still emerging post-Christian space where religion is honored as a human universal and religious pluralism can be creatively negotiated in sites of cultural exchange."[43]

Just as I find that hospitals increasingly remove religious symbols from chapels rather than combine those from different religious traditions in the space, chaplains are jettisoning tradition-specific religious language in favor of seemingly neutral—what I call least-common-denominator—approaches to spirituality, at least in the ways they describe their work to others. This is happening even as Chaplaincy Departments retain religiously specific volunteer programs—like those involving Catholic Eucharistic ministers—and make items like Bibles and Qur'ans available through their offices.

Physicians and nurses, in contrast to chaplains, do not always pay attention to spirituality and religion. When they do, however, they speak of patients' religious beliefs and practices in terms of traditional religious affiliations—primarily Catholicism at City Hospital. Nurses pay more attention to these topics than do physicians, and all medical staff members think about them most often when a patient is dying. While some medical staff members are responsive to chaplains' broad approach and language of spirituality, neither they nor chaplains recognize the differences in their languages and approaches or translate easily between them. On the ground, their differences lead to misunderstandings, because chaplains conceive of their work more broadly than do staff in ICUs.

Paradoxically, religion and spirituality seem to be most present in these hospitals when they are visibly absent and most absent when they are visibly present. It is chaplains, in other words, who are the visible, present, professional carriers of religion and spirituality in hospitals. Rather than filling their chapels, prayer, and meditation rooms with the widest possible range of religious and spiritual symbols and visibly naming religion in its multiple forms, chaplains seem to be doing the opposite. Seemingly neutral, symbol-free chapels, interfaith prayer services that one chaplain in training described as "so watered down you could find it in the phone book," and descriptions of their work that emphasize hope and wholeness make the visible ways that religion and spirituality are present in hospitals seem almost devoid of content and conspicuously absent. By sometimes relying on silence, for example, as a rhetorical and tactical means to invoke religion and spirituality, chaplains downplay the images, symbols, and rituals that have traditionally been used to transmit religion among and between people and make their own visible role in the hospital paradoxically more invisible.

It is when religion and spirituality seem to be visibly absent, in contrast, that they seem most present, particularly in the ICUs. While a visitor to the neonatal or medical ICU at City Hospital will not often see Christina or other nurses publicly praying, they will see medical staff making space for patients' religious and spiritual beliefs and practices—up to a point—if they watch and listen carefully. ICU staff members understand religion primarily in terms of its institutional manifestations and make space, for example, for Catholic Eucharistic ministers, religious rituals, and, in cases like Christina's, their own private prayers that are quite different from chaplains' broadly framed spiritual approaches. These seemingly invisible ways that religion and spirituality are present in hospital units are rarely mentioned, however, in social scientific or popular depictions of hospital life and work. It is ironic that chaplains, whose social role in hospitals focuses on religion and spirituality, are at times—it seems—less likely to invoke God or religious symbols or rituals than are ICU staff, whose social roles focus primarily on the provision of medical care.

Some of this paradox results from the development of chaplaincy as a profession, while other aspects of it—particularly the broad ways in which chaplains frame their work—reflect chaplains as professionals and hospitals as secular organizations in the contemporary United States that are trying to accommodate religious diversity in their midst. It is not only in hospitals but in public schools, workplaces, prisons, the military, and other formally secular institutions that leaders have to make decisions about excluding or accommodating people from different religious backgrounds. First amendment jurisprudence influences some of these decisions—especially in public schools and prisons—while other issues are negotiated informally.[44]

In *A New Religious America*, religious studies scholar Diana Eck considers how such negotiations took place historically as she narrates an American religious and cultural history of a movement "from many to one." She uses the concepts of exclusion, assimilation, and pluralism to describe the different ways that people in the United States have responded to religion and increasing religious diversity over time. While exclusionists did not welcome new participants in the American religious conversation, people who favored assimilation invited newcomers, telling them to "to come but leave your differences behind as quickly as possible."[45] For the pluralists, in Eck's words, "the American promise was to come as you are, with all your differences, pledged only to the common civic demands of citizenship. In other words, come and be yourselves."[46]

The academic hospitals described here are microcosms in which leaders decided how to respond as their patients and staff became more religiously diverse over time. Many Americans experience religious diversity on a personal scale, as Robert Putnam and David Campbell argue in their recent *American Grace*, but little is known about how that diversity is managed in workplaces, hospitals, and other secular organizations.[47] While some hospitals historically catered to people within single religious traditions, their formal secularization and the increasing religious diversity of the American population makes providing religious services to only one religious group almost unthinkable in urban areas today. As they have acted as assimilating organizations or as religious pluralists, these hospitals illustrate the tensions of trying to welcome and make space for people from various religious backgrounds, including none.[48]

Chaplaincy directors generally see themselves as religious pluralists and increasingly see spirituality as the broad umbrella concept under which people of all religious and spiritual backgrounds—including none—may cluster on their own terms. Whether spirituality as a frame actually works this way in hospitals is one of the central questions that I explore empirically. Whether it does or not has implications for other hospitals and broader sets of secular institutions that I outline in the conclusion.

It is not only in hospitals, after all, that decisions must be made about whether to place Christmas trees in public areas and whether to celebrate Christmas or other December holidays. In *Heaven's Kitchen*, Courtney Bender analyzes a secular AIDS service organization in New York City and describes the December "holiday feast," which is similar to the "holiday" parties many businesses and public schools now host. Six months after I first shadowed Meg at Overbrook, the December holiday question came up as the director of chaplaincy rushed into a staff meeting with several boxes of holiday cards in her arms. She opened them quickly, and asked everyone present to write a few before a representative from an area organ-procurement organization would arrive for an educational session. Chaplains assigned to particular units were to write cards for their units, while others, like me, could write cards to staff groups in the hospital, such as those for dining and environmental services.

Eager to help, I selected a few cards, but when I opened the first, I did not know what to write inside. The chaplains around me started to ask each other the same question. One said he writes, "Blessings to all in this holiday season," while a chaplain in training expressed frustration, almost under his breath, at the task, wondering if the department sends cards for Eid and other non-Christian "holidays." The conversation was cut short as the speaker arrived, but not before I quickly and uncertainly wrote "Thanks for all you do all year. Wishing you all the best in the new year" in one card and signed it "Your friends in the Chaplaincy Department." I quietly put the rest back in the box, wondering not just about how hospitals historically celebrated religious holidays, but how they currently negotiate religious symbols, rituals, conversations, and holiday greetings in light of their religious diversity—formally and informally, visibly and invisibly, in their daily practices.

I begin to answer these questions in the next chapter by introducing Overbrook Hospital, tracing the professional history of hospital chaplaincy, and providing some general background about how religion and spirituality have been present in secular American hospitals since 1920.

Looking Back: Glimpses of Religion and Spirituality in the History of Academic Medical Centers

Overbrook Hospital, like many of today's large, academic medical centers, was founded as several different hospitals that eventually merged into one. Annual reports from the early twentieth century described clergy making weekly visits to at least one of these early hospitals, giving sermons to patients, and sitting on the Board of Trustees. A few predecessor hospitals had chaplains who were volunteers or paid by local churches or women's auxiliary groups. Designated as "trustee appointments," they were Protestant, Catholic, and Jewish and saw patients in their own religious traditions. Before the first full-time chaplain, an Episcopal minister paid by a local Episcopal diocese, started work in the 1970s, chaplains were affiliated with nursing departments. Nurses "also deal with the spiritual problems of the patient," in addition to the chaplains, according to annual reports.

Since the 1970s, Chaplaincy Department directors at Overbrook have aimed to provide what they called "non-denominational" and later "spiritual" care for all patients, families, and staff. "I feel the message the chaplaincy brings to patients," Rev. Cook, the first full-time chaplain and department director, said at a graduation ceremony for newly trained chaplaincy volunteers in the early 1980s, "is that they are important, inestimably important. Everyone that passes through the doors of a hospital is made in the image and likeness of God." What makes a chaplain different from other visitors, he explained, "is in the effort to reflect the wholeness of the patient—to try and see this person as he is seen in the eyes of God, to help a person strike a balance of acceptance between what he can manage in his life and what he cannot control." Chaplains help patients to, "recognize the hallowedness of their lives, to help them celebrate what has been joyful, to help them work through the pain, and to bring them with wholeness to the point where they may depart in peace."

While Rev. Cook aimed to make the message of chaplaincy accessible to people from all religious backgrounds, early chaplaincy leaders at Overbrook—and nationally—were Protestant, and their underlying theologies were often evident in their descriptions of their work. Overbrook's department directors consistently emphasized chaplains' accessibility and interfaith orientation. As a director in the late 1980s explained, reflecting strands of liberal Protestant theology, "We try to bring that other dimension—what I call God and others might call something else—into that room. We say to the patient, 'You're loved, you're important.' But that message might come across while we're talking about sports, the weather, or the patient's favorite place on earth. It doesn't have to be in a specifically religious context." In this director's words, "I believe we are called upon to be representatives of the love of God. . . . How we express that love depends on the needs of the particular patient." Similarly, a department director in the 1990s explained, "We see a patient or family whether or not they have a religious affiliation and work with them to access the resources which help them to cope with the crisis. For some, this means traditional resources of prayer and ritual. For others, it means supportive conversation, . . . [or] teaching guided relaxation, or exploring options about their medical treatment."

Today, Overbrook—like many academic hospitals—employs individuals from Protestant, Catholic, Jewish, Muslim, and Unitarian Universalist faith traditions as interfaith chaplains who are assigned to specific units in the hospital.[1] They visit about 60% of admitted patients and close to everyone who dies in the hospital. "The hospital has chaplains," Chaplain Meg told nursing assistants at a new staff orientation, "because the hospital believes people are whole bodies with minds and spirits. . . . Doctors, nurses and others take care of the physical and sometimes emotional parts of people. Chaplains have specialized training . . . to provide spiritual and emotional services." By visiting people from all religious backgrounds, chaplains support "many people who are in the hospital who have never been sick before and are scared," she explained. "Chaplains help people use their inner resources to cope with crises." After describing how chaplains are trained and listing reasons to call a chaplain, she told the nursing assistants that chaplains are there for them too. "We are also your chaplains, so if you have a concern or spiritual need, feel free to come and talk with us, and we will help you in whatever way we can."[2]

Sitting in Overbrook's library on a cold spring morning with Joy, the hospital librarian, I tried to piece together the history of chaplaincy at Overbrook and how religious people, organizations, and beliefs have influenced the hospital more generally. Historical materials have not been kept in any systematic fashion, Joy told me, thumbing through a set of books and old annual reports on her desk. As our conversation turned from chaplaincy to the hospital chapel, Joy picked up the phone and called Agnes, "a crusty old soul" who has worked in one of the medical staff areas for sixty years, to see if she remembered anything. Agnes was sure there was a chapel in an earlier building but could not remember much more, so she told Joy to call Arthur, a burly older man in the facilities department to test his memory. After several more phone calls and a lot of digging through filing cabinets, Joy and I pieced together materials that show how religion was formally present at Overbrook Hospital through the work of hospital chaplains and the physical space of the chapel. While religion and spirituality have also been present in conversations between staff and patients and in the personal lives of staff, patients, and families, this informal presence was more difficult to document.

This chapter provides historical background by showing how religion has been formally present at Overbrook, City, and other American hospitals since 1920.[3] While multiple histories of American hospitals, both religious and secular, have been written, I focus primarily on the formal ways in which religion—and, increasingly, spirituality—have been present in secular general hospitals through the development of professional chaplaincy and the evolution of related Joint Commission policies.[4] I incorporate what I could learn about religion and spirituality in the professional lives of medical staff, although such historical materials are more limited. Readers primarily interested in the current experiences of medical staff members are advised to skim this chapter and skip to chapter 6. I also pay limited attention to how religion and spirituality influenced the historical development of bioethics, because that story has been well told by others.[5]

I detail here how chaplaincy emerged in the last century, and how chaplains—as formal carriers of religion and spirituality in hospitals—professionalized, medicalized, and responded to secularization and religious diversity over time. This development took place in stages as hospitals shifted from having retired clergy volunteers handle religion and spirituality to hosting specially trained Protestant clergy as chaplains and employing interfaith chaplains, as most do now. While chaplains across time periods spoke of providing spiritual support, the meaning of the term *spiritual* shifted from describing aspects of people's experiences within specific religious traditions to describing how people find meaning in any part of their lives. Chaplains today see themselves as providing spiritual support not only when they pray with patients, as they would have in the past, but as they speak with them about pets, family members, favorite places, and anything else that provides meaning and purpose. These transitions took place slowly at first and then intensified, especially in the last several decades with the involvement of some nurses and physicians in what I call a broader spirituality in health care movement.

At the broadest level, the transitions I document were fueled by demographic changes resulting from immigration, the country's shifting racial and ethnic composition, and religious shifts in the past century. Especially since the 1960s, increasing numbers of people have become seekers who combine aspects of multiple religious traditions with nature, exercise, and practices like meditation and yoga in their sense of what is personally meaningful.[6] Such demographic changes coupled with the cultural decline of mainline Protestantism and increasing religious and ethnic diversity created by post-1965 immigration brought wider ranges of people with broader meaning-making systems into hospitals.[7] There they encountered Protestant and later Catholic and Jewish chaplains who were grappling with their own senses of professional identity as they struggled to stake consistent professional claims and collaborate with other health-care professionals. Some of these struggles reflected chaplains' internal struggles to professionalize—which included efforts to medicalize—as they valued their identities as Protestant, Catholic, and Jewish over a shared identity as professional chaplains. They also reflect Protestant chaplains increasing efforts to make their work relevant in light of the numeric and cultural decline of mainline Protestantism, especially since the 1950s. Growing attention to spirituality in nursing and medicine over time resulted from similar demographic factors as well as from the advocacy of groups of physicians, nurses, and centers like the George Washington Institute for Spirituality and Health (GWish) that cohered into what I call a spirituality in health care movement beginning in the 1990s.[8] Before outlining the stages of these developments, I briefly describe the history of American hospitals before 1920.

AMERICAN HOSPITALS BEFORE 1920: A SHORT HISTORY

Sharing an etymology with the words *hostel* and *hotel*, hospitals in the early American colonies developed from precursors that provided lodging for the homeless, the poor, and travelers. Like the Jewish, Christian, and Muslim hospitals of previous centuries, early American hospitals provided more shelter than specialized medical care.[9] They were charity institutions for the poor, gravely ill, and desperate; everyone else was cared for in their homes. Little could be offered medically in hospitals that could not be provided at home, and admission, granted by committee, was defined primarily by social need. Stays were long, and patients and their caregivers were socially and ethnically distinct from hospital's trustees and medical staff.[10] While some hospitals were founded by city and state organizations, others were started by religious organizations where, as historian Charles Rosenberg argues, "Christianity and the imperatives of traditional stewardship, not the values of the medical profession, often determined particular hospital policies."[11] Moral as well as physical healing was part of many early hospital's orientations: Bibles were available, patients at some hospitals were required to attend religious services on Sundays, and card-playing and other vices were forbidden.[12]

Demographic and economic growth led to the founding of increasing numbers of hospitals after the Civil War, including many Catholic and Jewish ones. Advocates argued that existing hospitals were Protestant, regardless of their formal affiliations, and sought places where growing numbers of immigrants could be treated without possibly being proselytized. By 1885 there were more than a hundred and fifty Catholic hospitals in the United States which, according to historian Bernadette McCauley, offered not only a sense of ethnic identity but also the dignity of being treated as a paying patient rather than a charity case.[13] Jewish hospitals first opened in the 1850s with a second wave in the 1890s following the arrival of immigrants from Eastern Europe. These hospitals met Jewish patients' needs for kosher food and familiar organization while providing for the training of Jewish physicians.[14] Catholic and Jewish hospitals—like all hospitals after the Civil War—were open to everyone and primarily housed poor and working-class people.[15]

It was not until the early twentieth century that hospitals moved from the periphery to the center of American health care as they began offering therapies not available in private homes. New scientific ideas and instruments like X-ray machines and clinical laboratories allowed physicians to look into the body and informed developing clinical understandings of disease. Reforms to medical and university education more broadly brought science and clinical practice together in hospitals where medical education increasingly took place. The Flexner Report, published in 1910, marked the culmination of these reforms as medical schools and large hospitals increasingly worked together, and medicine professionalized and standardized.[16] Formal training for nurses also began in the late nineteenth century, though it was not until the 1930s that more skilled nurses than nursing students worked on hospital floors.[17]

By 1920, changes in medical care and education had brought hospitals closer to how we think about them today. They were, in Charles Rosenberg's words, a "national institution, no longer a refuge for the urban poor alone."[18] Founded as charity institutions, they had transitioned to scientific biomedical facilities now offering a range of biomedical services.[19] Initially slow to use them, middle-class patients came into hospitals in greater numbers during the 1920s as paying patients seeking obstetric services and surgeries, such as having their tonsils, appendixes, or adenoids removed.[20] Physicians were in charge on hospital floors and, like nurses, especially into the 1930s, were increasingly likely to have specialized training.[21] Critics of these hospitals, as in more recent years, charged that they were bureaucratic, impersonal, and not focused on care of the whole person. Science was the arbiter in medical decisions, as were bureaucratic accreditation processes in administrative ones.[22]

While religion has long been present in hospitals—it is not for nothing that they were known as "hotel Dieu" in early modern France—chaplains became the formal carriers of religion and spirituality in American hospitals in the 1920s, if not before. In secular American hospitals at this time, chaplains were retired or volunteer clergy with no special training who visited patients in their own religious traditions alongside other volunteers frequently organized through women's auxiliaries.[23] At Creekside Hospital, one of the hospitals described in this book that was founded before 1920, Protestant clergy held services and regularly visited patients. Area religious organizations donated flowers, Bibles, and hymnals to hospital wards, and a private donor gave funds to build a mortuary chapel that held up to twelve dead bodies on ice.[24] Special meals, decorated Christmas trees, and small gifts for patients and nursing students were delivered at Christmas and Easter, reflecting the Christian—specifically Protestant—orientation of the volunteers. At many so-called secular hospitals, Protestant volunteers and staff did not understand the experiences of Catholic and Jewish patients, which presented a formidable barrier and led Catholics and Jews to seek care at Catholic and Jewish hospitals that typically had priests or rabbis assigned.[25] It is widely believed, but not documented, that positions for religious leaders in all hospitals were seen as low status, outpost assignments suitable for retired clergy and those who could not tolerate the rigors of parish ministry.

Outside of hospitals in the 1920s, changes to the way future hospital chaplains would be trained and work were emerging, as Protestant clergy—drawing from the writings of William James—were incorporating ideas about psychology and self-development into their understandings of religion, personality development, and pastoral care.[26] Clergy had been losing the broad jurisdiction they held over personal problems as psychological and psychiatric ideas increasingly gained cultural power.[27] This led Protestant churches and seminaries to engage with psychology inside and outside of the classroom, including in new field-education programs. They emphasized psychological aspects of religious experience as a pastoral psychology movement also began to develop.[28]

It was in this context, buttressed by the social gospel movement, that Episcopal priest William S. Keller began a summer school in Cincinnati designed to enrich the education of Protestant theological students by having them work in social service agencies in the city.[29] His impulse to get Protestant theological students out of their classrooms and into real-life situations was the same impulse that led to the development of hospital-based training programs that influenced the development of hospital chaplaincy in subsequent decades. The initial goal was not to create a group of specially trained hospital chaplains but to jolt theological education and ultimately to transform Protestant churches.

THE EMERGENCE OF CPE-TRAINED PROTESTANT CHAPLAINS, 1925–1950

Nurses—the staff most frequently at the bedsides of patients—offered some religious care in secular (and religious) hospitals in the early decades of the twentieth century, probably especially if they shared a religious background with the patients. Florence Nightingale saw patients' spiritual needs as intricately related to their physical needs, and such ideas trickled into some nursing curricula.[30] Nurses and retired clergy working as chaplains were slowly joined by Protestant hospital chaplains after 1925, newly trained in Clinical Pastoral Education (CPE). At some hospitals, CPE-trained chaplains worked alongside chaplains with no such training, visiting patients and offering conversation, prayers, and rituals. It was not until the 1940s that CPE-trained Protestant chaplains began to organize as a distinct profession, following the institutionalization of CPE as a training process, the creation of professional organizations to certify hospital chaplains, and growing public awareness of chaplains through the presence of military chaplains in World War II.[31] Whether positions for CPE-trained chaplains were new at hospitals or slowly replaced those held by retired clergy or others without CPE training is an open question. No systematic data has been gathered.

Clinical Pastoral Education as a training process for hospital chaplains developed from an article published by Richard Cabot, a prominent Harvard physician, in 1925. Entitled "A Clinical Year for Theological Students," the article argued—much as William S. Keller had done in Cincinnati—that

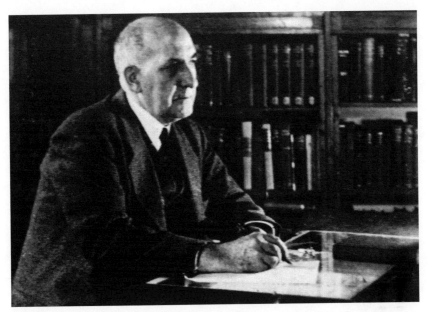

FIGURE 2.1 Anton Boisen, founder of Clinical Pastoral Education. Photo courtesy of Chicago Theological Seminary.

theological students would benefit from a year of clinical training.[32] In addition to attempting to influence theological education, Cabot—also known as the father of medical social work—had recently introduced case conferences in medical education and was encouraging his medical colleagues to look beyond the physical body in making diagnoses and caring for patients. In Boston, Cabot collaborated with Anton T. Boisen (fig. 2.1), a Presbyterian pastor with training in pastoral counseling and psychology, as influenced by William James. Born in 1876 and trained as a Presbyterian minister, Boisen explored several career possibilities, including serving as the pastor of two rural churches, before being hospitalized in a Massachusetts state psychiatric hospital with what he and others at the time believed was schizophrenia. He emerged from his hospitalization convinced both that he had gone through a profound religious experience and that Protestant churches neglected their ministries to the mentally ill.[33]

In 1924, Anton Boisen was appointed chaplain of Worcester State Hospital in Massachusetts, where he started a program to bring seminary students into contact with patients, whom he called "living human documents," in the summer of 1925.[34] The goal was to supplement their classroom training and encourage them to think theologically. Boisen often taught through case stud-

ies he wrote about patients. As CPE developed in later years, students themselves wrote case studies called *verbatims*—reports of conversations between
themselves and patients that were then discussed by the group of students
and their instructor, a CPE supervisor.

Richard Cabot and Anton Boisen parted ways in the early 1930s, but CPE
and positions for CPE-trained chaplains in hospitals developed from their
collaborations.[35] As the late chaplain and chaplain historian John Thomas
explained, training in CPE teaches an individual to "understand one's self in
terms of motivations and one's patterns in human relationships, and thus is
given a new understanding of one's 'call' to ministry and one's relationship
with The Transcendent."[36] It has often focused on psychology as much as
theology and helped Protestant students—and later those in other religious
traditions—to develop identities as pastoral caregivers and to experience caring for those in need.

Cabot invested in CPE training at Massachusetts General Hospital, where
students worked primarily with patients who had physical illnesses. With
Cabot's financial support, Massachusetts General Hospital appointed the
first CPE-trained chaplain, Austin P. Guiles, in 1930, who was followed in
1933 by Russell Dicks (fig. 2.2), whom Cabot met while Dicks was hospitalized there. The hospital also allowed theological students to enroll in CPE ,
where they visited with patients and worked as orderlies under the guidance
of supervisors. Dicks and Cabot continued to work together, and in 1936 they
wrote *The Art of Ministering to the Sick*, which shifted attention from the education of theological students to the care of patients.[37]

In the 1930s and 1940s, a number of formal programs were created to in-
stitutionalize and support CPE. Leaders drew insights from theological liber-
alism, philosophic pragmatism, Freudian psychology, and religious existen-
tialism.[38] Most of the people who completed a unit of CPE in these years
were Protestant seminary students who did so to develop theologically and
fulfill requirements for ordination.[39] By the end of the 1950s, CPE programs
were offered in 117 hospitals or other training centers and supported by forty
theological schools. By 1955 more than four thousand Protestant students had
completed some form of CPE, and the National Council of Churches was
providing scholarships for Protestant clergy who wanted to take a unit.[40] The
first formal CPE organization, the Council for Clinical Training of Theological Students, started in 1930 in Boston and later moved to New York.[41] In 1944,
theological educators and chaplains in the Boston area founded a second organization, the Institute of Pastoral Care, initially at Andover-Newton Theological Seminary and closely connected to Massachusetts General Hospital.[42] In

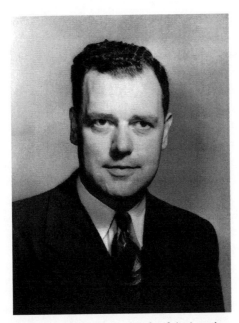

FIGURE 2.2 Russell Dicks, early leader in the chaplains' section of the American Protestant Hospital Chaplains, which developed over time into the Association of Professional Chaplains. Photo courtesy of Massachusetts General Hospital.

1967 the two groups merged with the Lutheran Advisory Council on Pastoral Care, founded in 1950, and the Southern Baptist Association of Clinical Pastoral Education, founded in 1957, to form the Association for Clinical Pastoral Education (ACPE). A US Department of Education accrediting organization, the ACPE today continues to establish standards for CPE, provide accreditation for CPE training centers, and certify program faculty.[43]

While most people who completed courses, called units, of CPE in the decades after 1925 did not go on to become chaplains, a few did. Their presence raised questions among hospital staff and religious leaders about how CPE-trained chaplains differed from other chaplains not so trained. Russell Dicks addressed this question in his 1939 lecture, "The Work of the Chaplain in a General Hospital," delivered at a meeting of the American Protestant Hospital Association. Dicks laid out four requirements for an effective hospital chaplain that were connected to training in CPE.[44] First, he said, chaplains must be in touch with other hospital staff caring for patients. Second, chaplains must have a plan, based on the severity of a patient's illness, referrals, or information shared at admission, that determines which patients they see. As a chaplain gets to know the staff, staff referrals should determine most of the patients he sees. Third, chaplains must be responsible to someone in the hospital, even if they are appointed and paid by someone outside of the hospital. Finally, chaplains should keep written records of their visits. More broadly, Dicks defined the CPE-trained chaplain not as someone who conducts religious rituals, as chaplains traditionally did, but as a person interested in patients' physical recoveries and their "spiritual growth." In Dicks's words, a chaplain, "knows that in suffering and stress, people are either thrown back or else they gain confidence in the fundamental nature of things, and it is the chaplain's hope to steady them in any way he can during such stress."[45] CPE brought attention to aspects of human experiences beyond the physical and to ways of being present and "steadying" people through difficult times.[46]

In the 1940s, hospital chaplains who had been trained in the early years of CPE (all white, Protestant men) began to organize and professionalize. They formed the first professional organization of hospital chaplains in 1946 at the Annual Meeting of the American Protestant Hospital Association (APHA). Russell Dicks issued an invitation, and the nineteen who gathered created a chaplain's section of the APHA named the Association of Protestant Hospital Chaplains. About a third of the hospitals described in this book had chaplains who were early members. The group changed its name to the Chaplains' Division of the American Protestant Hospital Association in 1962 and then to the College of Chaplains in 1967, remaining affiliated with the American Protestant Hospital Association until 1990, when it separated and later formed the more interfaith Association of Professional Chaplains.[47] A second group of chaplains working in mental hospitals formed a separate organization in 1948, the Association of Mental Health Clergy, which welcomed non-Protestants from the start. They changed their name to the Association of Mental Health Chaplains in the early 1960s and merged with the College of Chaplains in 1998 to form the Association of Professional Chaplains.[48]

From 1925 to the present, hospitals employed chaplains—trained through CPE or not—by choice. With the exception of veterans' hospitals, which have been required to have chaplains since 1945, regulatory agencies have never required hospitals to have chaplains.[49] When they do hire chaplains, hospitals have not been required to hire people trained in CPE. Chaplains, unlike nurses and physicians, have never had professional licenses regulated by the state. As a result, CPE-trained chaplains have tried, from the start, to convince hospital administrators and staff of their potential value—as chaplains and as CPE-trained chaplains—to institutions. Unlike those in professions created to meet a new demand, CPE-trained chaplains provided a new supply of workers for whom they aimed to create a demand in hospitals. Professional

CPE-trained chaplains tended not to argue, as they worked to professionalize, that patients had new religious or spiritual problems that they could address. Rather, they argued that they, as professional chaplains, had new or unique skills, learned through CPE and evident in their commitment not to proselytize, that would help them support patients better than chaplains without such training and commitment.

People in hospitals and religious organizations alike have often viewed hospital chaplains as individuals walking between the worlds of religion and medicine, pastor and clinician, and religious organizations and medical centers.[50] Because of this ambivalent role, many people before World War II—as today—did not know who hospital chaplains were or what they did. The war helped with this a bit, as almost eight thousand chaplains, including three hundred rabbis, served as military chaplains and did a lot of counseling for servicemen and women.[51] In the process, they familiarized many with what chaplains generally did, which helped CPE-trained hospital chaplains to develop their profession in the United States in the 1940s. At individual hospitals, however, the role of the chaplain before 1950 included a broad range of responsibilities that varied by institution. At Massachusetts General Hospital, for example, chaplains did not have office space or telephones until the late 1940s, and then only by a resolution of the Board of Trustees. At most hospitals, chaplains' specific work varied by unit and department director as well as the amount of funding available to pay them.[52] Protestant chaplains tended to see patients in their own and other Protestant denominations, while Catholic and Jewish chaplains saw patients in their own traditions.[53] While some chaplains worked with physicians and even more with nurses, little is known about what physicians learned about religion and spirituality in training between 1925 and 1950.[54]

TEMPORARY PROFESSIONAL COLLABORATION AND SLOW RELIGIOUS DIVERSIFICATION, 1950–1975

Following the 1946 passage of the Hospital Survey and Construction Act (the Hill-Burton Act), the number of hospitals increased across the United States on the federal government's dime. Splits between community and teaching hospitals became more pronounced as physicians at teaching hospitals, in subsequent decades, increasingly concentrated on research with the support of federal research and training grants. Hospital costs also continued to rise, which presented challenges to chaplains paid by hospitals, because the costs of their services, like those of other auxiliary services, were not reimbursed by insurance companies.[55]

Despite financial challenges, the number of CPE-trained, professionally certified chaplains continued to expand after 1950 and slowly diversified religiously. Collaboration around religion in health care also increased more generally during this period through the work of the American Hospital Association, the American Medical Association, and professional chaplaincy organizations. In 1969, the Joint Commission made their first related statement. In the *Standards for Accreditation of Hospitals* published in 1969, the Joint Commission interpreted a standard as including patients' spiritual needs. The standard read, "The governing body, through the chief executive officer, shall provide appropriate physical resources and personnel required to meet the needs of patients and shall participate in planning to meet the health needs of the community." The interpretation included the sentence, "Patients' spiritual needs may be met through hospital resources and/or through an arrangement with appropriate individuals from the community."[56] While asserting that patients had "spiritual needs," the Joint Commission's interpretation—which remained unchanged until 1978—did not say what they were or who in the hospital or community was responsible for meeting them. Attention to religion and spirituality also grew in the nursing literature during this period, especially in the 1960s, with growing attention to holistic care.[57]

Collaborations around religion in medicine and health care after 1950 were evident in the 1955 founding of the Institute of Religion at the University of Texas Medical Center in Houston. As sociologist Renée Fox and historian Judith Swazey explain, the institute was founded to "bring a spiritual presence to health care delivery," in part through educational programs for "religious and medical caregivers."[58] In the 1960s such efforts expanded to professional medical organizations, notably the American Medical Association (AMA). The AMA founded a Department of Medicine and Religion in the 1960s to facilitate greater understanding about religion among physicians and mostly Protestant clergymen.[59] As Paul Rhoads wrote in the *Journal of the American Medical Association*, "The primary purpose was to create a climate in which doctors and their clergymen colleagues . . . could work together most effectively."[60] The director, Paul McCleave, a physician and clergyman, explained in a 1965 talk,

> Throughout all America, there is a new recognition on the part of many of the concept that man is a whole being. He is physical, he is spiritual, he is mortal, and he is social in his total health. It is widely recognized that a weakness in any one of the four factors of his health can and does militate toward ill health in any one or all three of the other factors. . . . The faith of

the individual patient is a vital factor in total health. The patient must be treated and cared for within the scope of that faith. . . . There needs to be greater understanding between the physicians and all faith groups as to the requirements of those faiths relative to patient care.[61]

The department sponsored local gatherings of clergy and physicians through county medical societies. It also supported the development of educational materials in medical, nursing, and theological schools, assisted with the development of hospital chaplaincy, and facilitated the publication of related articles in the *Journal of the American Medical Association*. By the time the department closed in the 1970s, programs had been held in local community hospitals, with seminarians, and in medical schools, and planning had begun for a textbook about religious values in medical education.[62] The films and exhibits that the department sponsored were among the most popular of the AMA materials at the time.

While the AMA addressed religion more directly in the 1960s than it had in the past, attention to such issues did not quickly spread to the textbooks used to train medical students.[63] Not until 1975 did the *Cecil Textbook of Medicine*, a prominent general medical text, first talk about religion, and then only under a heading about patients with terminal illnesses. In a chapter entitled "The Care of the Patient with Terminal Illness," the author, W. P. L. Myers, encouraged physicians to "enlist the help of a clergyman or rabbi, preferably the patient's or, if he doesn't have one, the hospital chaplain or rabbi." "Patients may seek assurances from a clergyman that death is imminent," Myers wrote, "believing that the physician will not provide such assurances because doing so would be a denial of his role in preserving life."[64] Similarly, Harrison's well-known *Principles of Internal Medicine* did not mention religion or spirituality until 1974, and then also in relation to "incurability and death."[65] The extent to which such information in textbooks informed physicians' actions on the ground is an open question. Some medical schools also had clergy who worked through campus ministry groups, but little is known about their influence on physicians in training.[66]

Hospital chaplains benefited after 1950 from the work of the American Hospital Association and their own advocacy efforts. As hospital Chaplaincy Departments slowly grew across the country, the American Hospital Association convened a committee and in 1961 published a pamphlet entitled, "Essentials of a Hospital Chaplaincy Program." The committee, made up of representatives of Protestant, Catholic, and Jewish traditions, emphasized the importance of providing "ministry" to "all patients in conformance with their faith and expressed desire for counseling," of having clergy coordinate with health teams, and of facilitating "close working relationships with all religious groups in the community and the hospital."[67] In 1967 the American Hospital Association published a "Statement on Hospital Chaplaincy," which called chaplaincy programs a "necessary part of the hospital's provision for total patient care" and asserted that qualified chaplains, adequate facilities, and the support of other staff were "essential in carrying out an effective ministry for patients." It said that hospitals should "accept the responsibility to participate in the appropriate development of these elements of Clinical Pastoral Education," while recognizing that "only religious bodies have the qualifications and responsibility for the religious aspects of the training of clergymen as hospital chaplains."[68]

Chaplains also continued to revise the educational and certification requirements for Protestant hospital chaplains that would certify them as professional chaplains, distinct from chaplains who were retired clergy. The formal requirements for certification as a chaplain in 1961, for example, were a college and seminary degree or their equivalent, ordination or ecclesiastical endorsement, twenty-four weeks of full-time CPE, three years of pastoral experience or its equivalent, two recommendation letters from accredited chaplains, one recommendation letter from another professional, a letter of recognition from an employing institution, and membership in good standing in the American Protestant Hospital Association and the Chaplains' Association of the APHA.[69] Prospective chaplains also had to complete an application, including a verbatim or case example of their work and an interview with already certified chaplains. All applicants had to be Protestant, because the Chaplains' Association, which became the College of Chaplains in 1967, required membership in the American Protestant Hospital Association (the association explicitly rejected a Unitarian applicant in 1957).[70]

Certified, CPE-trained chaplains continued to explain and make a case for their work in the 1960s, increasingly emphasizing the personal relationships they could form with patients from a range of religious traditions, regardless of their personal backgrounds. In a 1966 address to the American Hospital Association, "Why Chaplaincies?" Harold Nelson, the director of a Department of Pastoral Care at a Chicago hospital, declared that he was not in favor of all chaplaincies. "I am not in favor of those chaplaincies where emphasis is placed on fitting the chaplain into a stereotyped religious role. I am in favor of those chaplaincies that place emphasis on internal values such as the quality of personal relationship developed with patients." He described chaplains as members of the health-care team who provide more counseling and psychological support than ritual support, echoing lessons from CPE about meeting patients where they are, being present, and valuing relationships.[71] Such language reflects how certified chaplains continued to negotiate between their own theologies and what they gradually came to see as patients' universal existential or spiritual needs.[72]

While the precise number of people working as hospital chaplains—certified or not—during this period is not known, the American Hospital Association collected information about chaplains in their affiliated hospitals in 1954. Two-thirds of these hospitals had a chaplain, as shown in table 2.1.

The chaplain was full-time in 1,125 (20%) of hospitals, part-time in 764 (13%) of hospitals, and on call in 2,028 (34%) of hospitals.[73] In 1972 the American Hospital Association reported that 3,038 (43%) of all hospitals had chaplaincy services—fewer than in 1954 for reasons that are not clear.[74] These hospitals included a total of 9,394 chaplains. Three-quarters worked part-time, and one-quarter full-time. The majority were Protestant (74%) but there were also Catholic chaplains (20%), Jewish chaplains (5%), and other chaplains (less than 1%). Just over half of the chaplains were paid by the hospital, religious groups, or community organizations. The rest were volunteers. Approximately 1,700 (24%) of the hospitals surveyed had a chaplaincy program organized by and administratively accountable to the hospital.[75] These hospitals tended to have separate Chaplaincy Departments through which chaplains worked with hospital inpatients, community clergy, and other hospital staff. Chaplains served as liaisons with local clergy, visited patients at the time of death, conducted religious services, counseled families, and visited with patients when admitted and before surgery.[76] They also frequently worked with staff and provided counseling, public relations, and other services for the hospital.

The ranks of certified chaplains slowly began to diversify religiously in the 1960s through the creation of new chaplaincy organizations, as shown in table 2.2.[77] The impetus came first from Catholic priests working in the Veterans Administration after Vatican II. They sought training programs that were federally recognized and would draw participants from a national pool and increase their professional status. Looking to their Protestant counterparts, these priests called for training beyond seminary education and began to develop programs for chaplain-priests, first in Catholic hospitals and then more generally. They formed the National Association of Catholic Chaplains (NACC) to accredit, certify, and train Catholic chaplains in 1965 under the auspices of the Catholic Bureau of Health and Hospitals of the National Catholic Welfare Conference.[78] While nuns had served as "sister visitors" in hospitals for many years, membership in the NACC soon opened up to include not

TABLE 2.1 Chaplaincy service in US hospitals

Year	Total hospitals	Reporting hospitals	Hospitals reporting chaplaincy service	Reporting hospitals with chaplaincy (%)
1954		6,049	4,036	66.7
1966			2,914	41.0
1972	7,097		3,038	43.0
1980	6,965	6,277	3,643	58.0
1981*	6,933	6,276	3,371	53.7
1982	6,915	6,277	3,499	55.7
1983	6,888	6,353	3,670	57.8
1984	6,872	6,302	3,817	60.6
1985	6,872	6,304	4,000	63.5
1992	6,539	5,916	3,175	53.7
1993		5,789	3,398	58.7
2002	5,794	4,876	2,581	52.9
2003	5,764	4,946	2,934	59.3
2004	5,759	4,854	2,954	60.8
2005	5,756	4,852	2,999	61.8
2006	5,747	4,836	3,076	63.6
2007	5,708	4,899	3,102	63.3
2008	5,815	4,862	3,136	64.5
2009	5,795	4,759	3,089	64.9

Sources: For 1954 data: *Journal of the American Hospital Association* 29, no. 8 (1955): 96, table F. For 1966 and 1972 data, see Kuby and Begole 1974. For fiscal years 1980–1985, 1992, and 2002: *AHA Annual Survey* (Chicago: Health Forum, LLC, an American Hospital Association company). For 1993 and 2003–2009: *AHA Hospital Statistics* (Chicago: Health Forum, LLC, an American Hospital Association company).

* The 1981 survey distinguished between hospital-based/staffed and hospital-based/contracted. When the two hospital-based categories are combined, the total is 3,371. The number in this table is for hospital-based/staffed only. This was the only year in which the question was asked in this way.

only priests but nuns, brothers, deacons, and laypeople certified as chaplains in the reforms following Vatican II. The fraction of NACC members who are not priests has increased steadily since then.

Drawing on Jewish traditions of *bikur cholim* and *mitvah*s for visiting the sick, many rabbis visited hospitalized Jewish patients under the auspices of

Jewish Chaplaincy Councils or local boards of rabbis in the 1960s. Jewish Hospitals appointed rabbis as chaplains in the 1950s to lead worship and certify kosher food. Jewish hospital chaplains did not form a professional organization until 1990 when the National Association of Jewish Chaplains began. An orthodox rabbi, Fred Hollander, was certified as the first Jewish Clinical Pastoral Education supervisor in 1958, but it was not until thirty years later that a second Jewish supervisor, Rabbi Jeffrey Silberman, was certified, reflecting both lack of interest—many people interested in Jewish chaplaincy

TABLE 2.2 Membership in professional chaplaincy organizations and percentage of members certified as professional chaplains over time

Year	AMHC	APHA/ College of Chaplains	APC	NACC	NAJC
1945			n/a	n/a	n/a
1950			n/a	n/a	n/a
1955		341	n/a	n/a	n/a
1960		390	n/a	n/a	n/a
1965	551	566	n/a		n/a
1970		781	n/a	784 (53%)	n/a
1975	558 (46%)		n/a	1,630 (69%)	n/a
1980		1,470 (61%)	n/a	2,267	n/a
1985		1,682	n/a	3,222 (69%)	n/a
1990	239 (35%)	1,899 (67%)	n/a	3,520 (62%)	
1995	176 (44%)	2,617 (63%)	n/a	3,547 (70%)	211 (38%)
2000	n/a	n/a	3,472 (59%)	3,455 (69%)	410 (20%)
2005	n/a	n/a	3,782 (71%)	3,154 (74%)	584 (16%)
2010	n/a	n/a	4,072 (75%)	2,625 (73%)	601 (18%)

Sources: Data about the Association of Mental Health Clergy from Emory University, Pitts Theological Library Archives; see also Aist 1996. Data about the College of Chaplains from Emory University, Pitts Theological Library Archives, as well as the archives of the Association of Professional Chaplains, Schaumburg, IL. Data about the Association of Professional Chaplains from Beth Stalec, APC. Data about the National Association of Catholic Chaplains from *The National Association of Catholic Chaplains: Fortieth Anniversary Reflections, 1965–2005* (Milwaukee: National Association of Catholic Chaplains). Data for 2010 provided by David Lichter, NACC. Data about the National Association of Jewish Chaplains from Cecille Asekoff, NAJC.

Notes: The AMHC is the Association of Mental Health Clergy. The APHA is the American Protestant Hospital Association, which housed the College of Chaplains. The APC is the Association of Professional Chaplains; the NACC is the National Association of Catholic Chaplains; and the NAJC is the National Association of Jewish Chaplains. Blank cells indicate missing data, and n/a indicates that the organization did not exist in the year in question.

got social work degrees—and the dominant Protestant assumptions of CPE that did not suit the experiences of Jews.[79]

The work of the American Hospital Association, the expansion of professional chaplaincy organizations, and broader interest in religious aspects of health care, led representatives from a range of organizations to begin to work together in the 1960s. These included representatives from the American Protestant Healthcare Association (APHA), the Chaplain's Division of the APHA, the American Hospital Association, the American Medical Association (AMA), the Chicago Board of Rabbis, and the United States Catholic Conference.[80] These inter-organizational meetings, convened in Chicago at the headquarters of the AMA, were sponsored by the AMA's Department of Medicine and Religion and included discussion of more cooperative ways to provide hospitalized patients with religious and spiritual care. Joint projects included the American Hospital Association's publications about chaplaincy and the promotion of better understanding among all concerned about their respective responsibilities. In 1967 the group affirmed the importance of chaplaincy with the statement, "No healing institution's staff complement is complete unless a staff and department for meeting the spiritual needs of the patient are provided. We endorse the principle that a chaplaincy position should be filled only by that clergyman endorsed, nominated and accredited by the proper respective faith organization."[81]

Most of the hospitals described in this book had some kind of a chaplaincy department by 1975. Some were staffed by traditional chaplains, who mostly offered religious rituals, and others had CPE-trained chaplains, who also did guest lectures or collaborated with faculty in schools of medicine and divinity schools. As in earlier years, hospitals varied in the ways chaplains worked. At Brookfield Hospital, for example, a current director remembered that chaplains were given little more than "a desk and a chair . . . either in the waiting room or in the hallway outside of one of the wards," while at others they were more integrated into hospital life. Funding for chaplains' salaries also remained challenging as some hospitals decided to pay the salary of a CPE supervisor, who trained CPE students, who in turn provided care to hospitalized patients for free. Other hospitals funded more staff chaplain positions or had positions supported by outside organizations, believing that chaplaincy care was best provided by trained chaplains, not students. While it may have been different in religious hospitals, several chaplaincy directors working in secular hospitals described the histories of their own departments during this period, and more generally, as challenging: "There wasn't that much interest from the administration," one explained. "And that's the way the history has been. It's been kind of a slugging, uphill battle."

By the mid-1970s, collaborations among national organizations around religion and medicine had ended, and chaplains were struggling with identity issues concerning their status as professionals and with how to serve increasingly religiously diverse patient populations.[82] Professional Protestant and Catholic chaplaincy organizations continued to certify chaplains in their traditions. Representatives of the College of Chaplains considered—and rejected—the possibility of certified Jewish chaplains, though some recognized that change was coming as a result of increasing religious and ethnic diversity. These individuals began to ask whether the College of Chaplains should be interfaith or multifaith, a question that preoccupied some for the next twenty years.[83] The question of whether certified chaplains were clergy or health-care professionals was also much debated. Some held on to their identity as clergy, and others sought recognition as "allied health professionals," which would facilitate their becoming members of health-care teams, though at the cost, opponents argued, of medicalizing their profession in name and content.[84]

A RISING SPIRITUALITY IN HEALTH CARE MOVEMENT, 1975–2000

Hospitals, including teaching hospitals, faced multiple challenges in the 1980s and 1990s as financial pressures led to system mergers and closings, and inpatient stays were shortened in efforts to cut costs.[85] Technological developments led to new ethical dilemmas in patient care, and demographic changes meant that more religiously and ethnically diverse patients were being seen in hospitals. Chaplains continued to struggle to define themselves professionally and to professionalize as growing numbers of nurses and physicians advocated for religion, increasingly framed in terms of the broad, meaning-making concept of *spirituality*, at least at the national level. By the 1990s, a loosely organized "spirituality in health care" movement had emerged, led more by physicians, nurses, and researchers than by chaplains.

The Joint Commission drew increasing attention to religion (and then spirituality) in hospitals after 1975 through a series of related statements. In the late 1970s, in a chapter entitled "Rights and Responsibilities of Patients" in the *Accreditation Manual for Hospitals*, the commission said that religion—like race, creed, sex, national origin, and course of payment—was not to influence whether individuals were "accorded impartial access to treatment or accommodations that are available or medically indicated." Patients were also seen as having "the right, within the law, to personal and informational privacy, as manifest by the right . . . to wear appropriate personal clothing and religious or other symbolic items, as long as they do not interfere with diagnostic procedures or treatment."[86] In addition to saying that patients' spiritual needs should be met, such statements expanded in the late 1980s to say that hospitals were to assess the spirituality of patients treated for alcoholism or other drug dependencies.[87] The Joint Commission increasingly brought attention to religion and spirituality at the bedside, but whether chaplains were what historian David Rothman would call "strangers at the bedside" who were gathering this information is an open question.[88]

By the 1990s the Joint Commission had mostly replaced the word *religion* with the word *spirituality* in its standards and interpretations. Hospitals were to assess spirituality in patients being treated for alcoholism and other drug dependencies, as well as in patients and families facing end-of-life situations and grief.[89] In the section on alcohol and drug dependence, the commission explained the intent of standard AL.2.4.8: "Spiritual orientation may relate to the dependence in terms of how the patient views himself/herself as an individual of value and worth. The patient's spiritual orientation should not be considered synonymous with his/her relationship with an organized religion."[90] In subsequent years, the commission added attention to spirituality in discussions of patient education (1994), end-of-life care (1995), food (1995), rehabilitation services (1996), and mental and behavioral disorders (1997). In the 1995 guidelines, the commission also recognized the rights of hospital staff by directing hospitals to address conflicts between staff members' "cultural values, ethics and religious beliefs" and their work. Their use of the word *religious* rather than *spiritual* here is notable because the commission seemed to refer to beliefs connected to religious traditions rather than broader meaning-making systems.[91]

Despite years of lobbying by chaplaincy organizations on behalf of certified professional chaplains, the Joint Commission has never established specific guidelines about who can or should provide spiritual care in hospitals. They mentioned pastoral services departments and pastoral personnel from outside of the facility in the late 1990s, suggesting that small hospitals should "maintain a list of clergy who have consented to be available to the hospital's patients in addition to visiting their own parishioners," while larger hospitals should "employ qualified clinical chaplains who have graduated from an accredited master of divinity degree program."[92] The commission did not use the word *chaplain* until 1999, then stating that "clinical chaplains assess and treat patients using individual and group interventions to restore or rehabilitate spiritual well-being." They also "counsel individuals who are experiencing spiritual distress, as well as their families, caregivers, and other service providers about their spiritual dysfunction or the management of spiritual care."[93]

Use of the concepts "spiritual well-being," "spiritual distress," and "spiritual dysfunction" in Joint Commission statements in 1999 reflect related developments in nursing diagnoses that developed alongside "spiritual assessment" tools. All of these concepts served to assess and medicalize spirituality, increasingly bringing it within a biomedical frame. In the more recent words of the Joint Commission's associate director of standards interpretation, spiritual assessments "determine how a patient's religion or spiritual outlook might affect the care he or she receives. . . . At [a] minimum, the spiritual assessment should determine the patient's religious denomination, beliefs, and what spiritual practices are important to the patient."[94] In the late 1970s, nurses and, later, physicians began to develop questionnaires designed to assess people spiritually, which chaplains had often used, at least informally. The North American Nursing Diagnostic Association (NANDA) approved spiritual concerns, spiritual distress, and spiritual despair as nursing diagnoses in 1978 and then combined them into one category of spiritual distress.[95] Related diagnoses have been added since then. *Spiritual distress* is today defined as "impaired ability to experience and integrate meaning and purpose in life through connectedness with self, others, art, music, literature, nature and/or a power greater than oneself."[96] Religious studies scholar Sophie Gilliat-Ray argues that nurses created such broad concepts in an effort to expand their professional jurisdiction following the rise of the holistic health movement, but actually succeeded in excluding many people, particularly members of minority religious traditions for whom this concept and the questions asked in spiritual assessments make little sense.[97]

Physicians also developed spiritual history and assessment tools between 1980 and the present, seeing spirituality as something that could be assessed as an aspect of all people.[98] To align with medical norms, founders gave these tools acronyms formed with the first letters of the questions to be asked in the assessment—names like SPIRITual History, FICA, FAITH, and HOPE. The latter, for example, asked questions about sources of *H*ope, *O*rganized religion, *P*ersonal spirituality and practices, and *E*ffects on medical care and end-of-life issues.[99] Theoretically, such tools encouraged a broader range of physicians to gather information about spirituality from patients and represent efforts to standardize and medicalize the information gathered. In addition to developing new tools, physician leaders also tried to expand related medical training. Physicians David Larson and Christina Puchalski were leaders:

Larson founded the National Institute for Healthcare Research, and Puchalski later founded the George Washington Institute for Spirituality and Health (GWish) with the financial support of the John Templeton Foundation. They encouraged medical schools to offer courses about spirituality and medicine, and between 1990 and 2000 the fraction that did so grew. With the support of the National Institute for Healthcare Research and the John Templeton Foundation, the American Association of Medical Colleges also published a report in 1999 detailing the importance of spiritual and cultural concerns in medical education.[100]

How spiritual assessment tools, new curricula, and broader education concerning religion and spirituality led nurses and physicians to engage with patients and families about such topics in their daily work before 2000 remains an open question. Prominent medical textbooks, including the *Cecil Textbook of Medicine* and Harrison's *Principles of Internal Medicine*, expanded their focus on religion and spirituality during these years but still said little, mostly focusing on patient beliefs, organizations, and religious professionals who provided support with regard to death and dying.[101] Specialized medical textbooks addressed the issue in more detail. Studies of nurses reported that many felt spiritual care was important, but they were not always sure what it included or how to provide it. Results varied by specialization and background.[102]

Certified chaplains continued to professionalize, justify their work, and attempt to articulate their contributions to health care in the 1980s and 1990s. Slightly less than 60% of hospitals have had chaplains since the early 1980s, but the fraction that were certified, paid by the hospital, and were from particular religious backgrounds is not known.[103] In the early 1980s, changes in hospital financing threatened chaplains' already weak financial bases, leading the president of the College of Chaplains to write, "*Survival* may be the key issue facing chaplaincy at this point in time. . . . The problem is not centered on the competency of chaplains or in the pastoral care needs of institutions. It is centered in the area of available finances. . . . As financial pressures increase on private institutions, non-revenue producing departments are subject to increased jeopardy."[104]

In response, professional chaplaincy organizations again tried to articulate their value to hospitals, even as they continued to struggle with their own internal identity issues. They tried to regulate internally the training of chaplains, whom hospitals could hire, and how chaplains did their work—difficult tasks in the absence of state licensing or formal guidelines about how chaplains spend time in hospitals. At City Hospital, a chaplain remembered:

When I was here in the 1980s, chaplaincy was no more integrated into any health-care team than anything. Talk about being lone rangers—we would be called to the emergency room to go in and pray for someone who was having a heart attack, and it was like—you would walk in and you could see people looking at you as if to say, "Who are you and what do you think you're doing here." And I remember I had one doctor come out after me after I said a prayer at the family's request, and he said, "What was that?" So we were tolerated at best and, frankly, looked at with suspicion at worst.

At other secular hospitals things were different: supportive administrators found ways to pay chaplains directly, helping them become more integrated and accountable to hospitals.

With financial support directly from hospitals and the proliferation of ideas about spirituality—broadly conceived—as an aspect of all people, certified chaplains increasingly transitioned to interfaith staffing models, in which chaplains were assigned to units where they were responsible for all of the patients on the unit, regardless of the match between their and the patients' religious backgrounds.[105] One such hospital, for example, employed traditional chaplains who conducted rituals until, as the director remembered, the hospital "assumed the financial burden for all full-time positions, including the director, Catholic priests, and Protestant chaplains in 1980 because it wanted control over who was hired." After a few years, the hospital shifted to an interfaith staffing model. Another hospital did not have paid chaplains before the early 1990s, but medical staff increasingly saw a need for more formal spiritual care. The hospital was concerned about church-state issues in figuring out how to provide such care, so it formed an administrative team that went through a study process and later hired their first chaplain.

Nationally, and in local hospitals, chaplains continued to struggle during these years with questions of professional identity and with challenges related to religious diversity. These tensions came to a head in discussions about whether chaplains were health-care professionals expected to act as members of health-care teams or clergy who maintained confidentiality in their relationships with patients as they would with parishioners. At issue was whether chaplains should document their visits in patients' charts, sharing information with the health-care team as other professionals do. Financial pressures on hospitals in the early 1980s led some chaplains to chart their visits as a way of documenting their contributions to patient care.[106] National chaplaincy leaders encouraged chaplains to chart both because of their history—Russell

Dicks had urged as much in 1939—and because of a desire to show the Joint Commission that they were the ones providing such care. Some did, but others were hesitant and uncomfortable with this medicalization of their work; they clung instead to the confidential nature of clergy-parishioner relationships. By the mid-1990s more chaplains had started to chart, but even then some just noted that they had been there, while others included information that might be relevant for the health-care team. Spiritual assessment tools could, theoretically, have helped chaplains communicate with the health-care team in chart notes, though I rarely heard about this being the case in my interviews with chaplains.[107]

Increasing religious diversity also remained a challenge for chaplains on other levels. Internally, the demographics of chaplains themselves were expanding to include not just white Protestant men but Catholics, Jews, women, and people of color. Such transitions, taking place in the aftermath of the feminist and civil rights movements, were challenging: new chaplains had new ideas about what chaplaincy was or could become. Directors of chaplaincy (still usually Protestant) and the leaders of professional organizations also struggled with how departments should be staffed and on what basis chaplains, who were increasingly working with people from a range of religious backgrounds (including those with no such background), did their work. For its part, the College of Chaplains argued that chaplains served all people on the basis of their "academic learning experience provided by formal theological education," and their "theological understanding of people as people rather than as denominational people."[108]

Despite increased discussion of spirituality by the Joint Commission, nurses, and physicians, the main professional chaplaincy organizations remained religiously segregated into the 1990s. The College of Chaplains (Protestant), the National Association of Catholic Chaplains, and the National Association of Jewish Chaplains certified their own chaplains. Some members belonged to multiple organizations or tried to develop partnerships across organizations, but these were slow to develop. The first national joint meeting of chaplaincy organizations did not take place until the 1980s.[109] Such efforts started in the late 1970s when a new group, the Council on Ministry in Specialized Settings (COMISS), began trying to develop working relationships among different professional chaplaincy organizations through joint projects like Pastoral Care Week, which started in the mid-1980s.[110] While some relationships were built, others were hindered by the absence of a sense of common purpose across organizations, strong commitments to faith traditions, internal debates within faith traditions, and by leaders who focused on their own organizations rather than on developing awareness of the goals and potential of hospital chaplaincy as a broader profession.

While the Protestant College of Chaplains did not merge with the Catholic or Jewish chaplaincy organizations in the 1990s, it did shed its formal Protestant identity in 1990 and merged with the Association of Mental Health Chaplains (AMHC) in 1998.[111] Together they started the Association of Professional Chaplains (APC), a "multifaith association established to certify and serve its membership and to promote professional chaplaincy."[112] The APC is the largest professional chaplaincy organization in the United States today.[113] This transition from a Protestant to an interfaith organization was considered for many years before it happened, and the College of Chaplains was assisted by outside consultants along the way. These consultants spelled out some of the issues around professional identity in a report prepared before the merger took place. Professional identity was the College of Chaplains' "single most important issue," the consultants argued.

> The fundamental issue is where is identity rooted? As an organization, is the College primarily a collegial fellowship of people of faith called to minister in specialized settings or a professional body existing for the primary purpose of certifying the technical competence of its members? Are chaplains first of all ministers called by God, therapists trained by experts, or theoreticians proficient in dialogue? As chaplains, which relationship is (or should be) of greater importance: the relationship with the church that sets them apart to minister or the relationship with a professional organization that certifies technical competency? Is the key to carrying out the chaplain's stated mission proficiency in therapeutic technique or spiritual commitment or both? What is more basic to identity for a chaplain: the pastoral/spiritual calling or clinical/therapeutic competence?[114]

At issue in the decision to separate from the American Protestant Hospital Association and merge with the AMHC was whether the College of Chaplains should remain Protestant, should become an interfaith organization seeking a "least common denominator" theology, or should cultivate a multifaith approach in which people from different religious traditions were "granted the particularity of [their] own faith and worship while agreeing to certain common principles" as outlined by the consultants.[115] These were the same questions that Chaplaincy Departments at many large academic hospitals faced in the 1990s—and continue to face—as they slowly moved toward interfaith organizational models, framing their work in terms of spirituality.[116]

By the end of the twentieth century, religion and spirituality occupied a much different place in American hospitals than they had one hundred years before. Formally, many religious hospitals had secularized or merged, especially for financial reasons. Chaplains, initially retired clergy or volunteers, had been replaced in many hospitals by those with CPE training and the certification of a professional chaplaincy organization. While certified chaplains initially saw people from their own religious backgrounds, over time they saw a broader range of people, especially into the 1990s, offering support not just around religion but around spirituality, understood to encompass all the ways people make meaning. Nurses and physicians, perhaps motivated religiously in earlier decades, increasingly learned about spirituality—broadly conceived—in nursing and medical schools and through medical diagnostic categories and spiritual assessment tools. Supported by research showing positive relationships between religion/spirituality and health, a growing number of national leaders—physicians, nurses, and social workers—were working together by 2000 in a loosely organized "spirituality in health care" movement. They focused on improving the provision of religious and spiritual care in hospitals as well as providing better education for physicians and nurses.[117] Despite their long histories in hospitals, chaplains were involved in this movement only on the periphery.

SPIRITUALITY IN HEALTH CARE: THE CONTEXT SINCE 2000

Since 2000, hospitals—especially large academic ones—have been caring for individuals who are sicker, older, and facing more complex medical problems, including chronic diseases, than in the past. People with more minor medical concerns are treated as outpatients in efforts to keep lengths of stay short and reduce hospital costs. Medical interventions continue to extend people's lives while sometimes creating complex ethical decisions for patients and their families. As patient stays get shorter and the medical care provided becomes more technologically sophisticated, concerns voiced decades ago about hospitals as bureaucratic machines not focused on the care of whole people are more frequently repeated. While patients and families might experience questions about religion and spirituality—as one aspect of their broader lived experiences—as a way of focusing on whole people in hospitals, they might also see them as invasive or not relevant to their experiences. Staff might also have no time to ask about such issues as they struggle to care for patients who are sicker than in the past and hospitalized for shorter periods of time.

The Joint Commission has continued to say that spirituality—now the dominant frame—should be respected among hospitalized patients. The 2010 guidelines stipulate that hospitals are to respect "the patient's cultural and personal values, beliefs, and preferences" and accommodate "the patient's right to religious and other spiritual services."[118] Hospitals are to single out particular groups of patients, including those dealing with end-of-life situations, alcohol and drug issues, and emotional and behavioral disorders, for spiritual assessment just as spiritual issues are to be considered with regard to food, education, and training for hospital staff. Joint Commission language concerning "spiritual assessments" and psychosocial diagnostic tests that help gauge individuals' "spiritual outlook" is increasingly common.[119]

At the national level, some nurses and physicians continue to advocate for more training involving spirituality. Many nursing programs include spiritual dimensions of care in their curricula, and related issues are discussed in textbooks. The growing body of research by nurses that focuses on spiritual aspects of care though studies of practicing nurses also shows a fair amount of confusion about what spirituality is and how such care should be provided. Many nurses report feeling unprepared to offer spiritual care and, when they do offer it, say they learned how to do so from patients and families.[120] That said, the research shows that nurses more than other medical staff most often refer patients to chaplains.[121]

Such findings are interesting in comparison to information about the personal spiritual experiences of nurses. In a survey conducted at a large academic medical center, sociologist Don Grant and colleagues found that 91% of the nurses they surveyed considered themselves spiritual people, and more than 80% thought there was something spiritual about the care they provided. Close to 60% reported that their job provided opportunities to put their spiritual beliefs into practice, especially when working in intensive care units. Such conversations came up much more with patients, however, than with coworkers.[122] These findings point to a gap both between nurses' personal experiences of spirituality and their work—especially with coworkers—and between the experiences of nursing researchers and those of nurses working in hospitals.

Similar gaps are also likely evident for physicians. National leaders have expanded medical school courses about spirituality, and textbooks say more about the subject than in the past, though what they say still primarily concerns death.[123] In the 2004 *Cecil Textbook of Medicine*, for example, physician J. Andrew Billings explains in a chapter entitled "Care of Dying Patients" that "the physician's role is not to answer unanswerable questions or to provide premature reassurance, but rather to help the dying person explore spiritual issues and find supportive resources (e.g., the hospital chaplain) while clarifying how spirituality influences decision making and coping."[124] Related discussion is included in the critical care and oncology sections as well as in *Harrison's Principles of Internal Medicine*. Specialized textbooks focused on oncology, palliative care, and other topics likely say much more about spirituality, just as related professional associations have addressed the issue in their standards of practice.[125]

National surveys suggest that significant numbers of physicians are aware of spirituality and religion among patients, though evidence about how often they inquire about them is mixed.[126] Many of these studies focus on what physicians say they will do rather than on what they actually do around religion and spirituality. Smaller qualitative studies suggest that it is patients and families, not physicians, who most often bring up issues related to spirituality or religion, and that physicians often see such issues as important in helping patients connect with their families and communities rather than with medical teams.[127]

Chaplains who work in close to two-thirds of American hospitals, including all of the hospitals described in this book, situate their work firmly within the broad realm of spirituality, at least at the national level.[128] In 2001 the professional chaplaincy organizations came together to publish a professional manifesto, "Professional Chaplaincy: Its Role and Importance in Healthcare," outlining who they are and what they do.[129] Adopting the language of spirituality as a way of bridging religious differences and articulating a common professional purpose, the document states that "persons are not merely physical bodies that require mechanical care" but individuals in need of "time-tested spiritual resources." By helping people "focus on transcendent meaning, purpose and value," chaplains provide spiritual resources that benefit patients, families, and staff members in health-care organizations. Assuming that everyone has a spirituality or some "transcendent meaning, purpose and value," the authors argue that chaplains respond to challenges in health care "in unique ways, drawing on historic traditions of spirituality that contribute to the healing of the body, mind, heart and soul."

After publishing this manifesto, professional chaplaincy organizations continued working together, formally approving common standards in training, education, ethics, and ways of registering complaints. The common standards for board-certified professional chaplains across these organizations include endorsement of a faith tradition, an undergraduate degree and graduate-level theological degree, four units of Clinical Pastoral Education (1,600 hours) or its equivalent, and payment of dues to a professional chaplaincy association. Prospective chaplains must demonstrate competence in a written application and certification interview in four areas focused on theories of pastoral care; identity and conduct; pastoral skills; and professional skills, and must also participate in continuing education and peer review every five years. Several of the North American organizations contributed to the formation of a new organization, the Spiritual Care Collaborative, as "an international group of professional organizations actively collaborating to advance excellence in professional pastoral and spiritual care, counseling, education and research." They aim to provide "a collective voice to promote the highest standards of professional practice" and to advance "the field of professional spiritual care."[130] The Association of Professional Chaplains, however, recently discontinued its participation.

The fact that board-certified chaplains must have the endorsement of a faith tradition but increasingly work across religious traditions, including with people who have no religious affiliation, to support people spiritually—understood broadly—points to the complexities of chaplaincy training and work today.[131] While the profession increasingly argues that board certification is required before chaplains can be hired by hospitals, hospitals continue to hire a range of people as chaplains. Few employ only board-certified chaplains, and most divide the work of chaplain among board-certified staff chaplains, CPE students, volunteers, and others.

Numerous studies have outlined what chaplains do as they work with patients, families, staff members, and sometimes local clergy in hospitals. Studies suggest that directors of nursing, social service, and medicine, as well as hospital administrators especially value the end-of-life care that chaplains provide, as well as the prayer and emotional support they offer.[132] In keeping with the norms of other health professions, chaplaincy leaders recently released "standards of practice" to outline and attempt to standardize their work and help them communicate about it with each other and other health-care professionals.[133] National chaplaincy leaders have also focused on best practices, quality improvement, collaborations with other professional groups, and research in recent years that might develop an evidence base for their work.[134] Chaplains have struggled not just to articulate their contributions but to measure them; relatively few studies empirically demonstrate a connection between the work of chaplains and patient or family outcomes.[135]

Many of the changes promoted by chaplain leaders rely on the willingness of individual chaplains, the directors of Chaplaincy Departments, and hospital administrators to share their vision. While they would like hospitals—for example—to hire and pay only board-certified chaplains trained to offer spiritual support based on current standards of practice as members of healthcare teams, institutional inertia and other factors—such as demographics and finances—limit these possibilities. As a workforce, the average age of members of the Association of Professional Chaplains is 55, and in the National Association of Catholic Chaplains, it is 63. About 60% of the members of the APC are men in comparison to one-third of NACC members.[136] Many became chaplains as a second career and are more mainline Protestant, Catholic, and Jewish than national averages, as shown in table 2.3. Hospitals with large populations of Catholic patients often need priests to administer sacraments,

TABLE 2.3   Religious distribution of members in the Association of Professional Chaplains, National Association of Catholic Chaplains, and National Association of Jewish Chaplains compared to the religious distribution of the US population

Religion	Percentage of US population	Percentage of combined APC, NACC, and NAJC members
Evangelical Protestant	26.3	12.5
Mainline Protestant	18.1	31.8
Catholic	23.9	43.2
Historically black churches	6.9	1.1
Mormon	1.7	<1
Orthodox	.6	<1
Jewish	1.7	9.7
Muslim	.6	<1
Buddhist	.7	<1
Hindu	.4	<1
Jehovah's Witness	.7	<1
Other faiths	<1.8	<1
Unaffiliated	16.1	0
Don't know	.8	0

Sources: US Religious Landscape Survey (http://pewforum.org/), 2007; Association of Professional Chaplains (2010); National Association of Catholic Chaplains (2009); National Association of Jewish Chaplains (2009).

Note: To construct this table, I combined the data from the APC, NACC, and NAJC, assuming that all members of the NACC were Catholic, and all members of the NAJC were Jewish. While some of the 129 Catholic members of the APC in 2010 might also be members of the NACC, and some of the 34 Jewish members of the APC in 2010 might also be members of the NAJC, I double-counted them for purposes of this table. I then classified all the members of the APC, NACC, and NAJC according to the religious affiliation categories used in the US Religious Landscape Survey. Percentages do not sum to 100 due to rounding.

so Roman Catholic priests, especially in light of national priest shortages, are much in demand. Hospitals often hire immigrant priests from Africa and Asia with minimal training in CPE to meet this need. Similarly, hospitals with large populations of Muslims or members of other minority religious traditions seek chaplains from those backgrounds who may not be trained as chaplains or share the visions of chaplaincy leaders.[137] Finances also remain a factor, as some hospitals pay their chaplains directly, while others continue to rely on outside organizations that influence not only who they can hire but which patients those chaplains will see. Salaries are low in comparison to those of other professionals in health care.[138]

CONCLUSIONS

At Overbrook Hospital, community clergy still visit their parishioners as they did before 1950, but they no longer give sermons or sit on the board of directors, nor are they invited to visit anyone—following patient privacy laws passed in 1996—while they are there. When they stop at the Chaplaincy Department office on the way out to have their parking tickets validated, they are likely to have seen sicker patients than in the past and to have talked about more complex ethical issues. Many patients do not have religious leaders visiting, either because they are not involved with religious organizations or because they have come to Overbrook for treatments not available closer to home. It is with these individuals that Overbrook's interfaith chaplains, CPE students, and volunteers most often spend time.

Conversations with these patients and their families focus not just on religion but on spirituality in general—how they find and create meaning in their lives. While Father William, the Catholic priest at Overbrook, is paged if a Catholic patient requests the Sacrament of the Sick, interfaith chaplains care for all of the patients on their assigned units, regardless of the match between their backgrounds and those of the patient. As I sat with Judy, a lay Catholic woman spending a year as a chaplain resident at Overbrook in preparation for board certification, our conversation focused not just on the religious rituals and prayers she sometimes offers patients, but on songs and birds. Before our conversation, I saw a colleague hand Judy an obituary. The woman who died was a patient who liked a particular song. Not known for her singing, Judy had convinced Father William and another colleague to join her at this woman's bedside to sing the song. The woman seemed to enjoy it and later asked for them to come back. Describing how she interacted with another, older female patient, Judy explained, "There was one woman who loved birds, so I went on the web . . . and found and printed a picture of these macaws." Judy spent time talking with the woman and then gave her the photo. "I said [to the woman] something like, 'Here are your birds watching over you.' . . . That is sort of how God comes into play sometimes. It's just through things that speak to each of us individually. I don't know if for her [the woman] it meant the same thing as it meant to me, but it was a way of my being able to reverence what was meaningful to her."

Fueled by the cultural decline of mainline Protestantism, within which hospital chaplaincy largely emerged, and by changes in immigration, growing racial and ethnic diversity, and changing religious demographics that have brought patients with a wider range of backgrounds into hospitals, hospital chaplaincy as a profession continues to evolve. It is not just through religious rituals and prayers but in singing and conversation about birds that chaplains in training at Overbrook are taught to tap into the spirit or sense of meaning that they believe is present in all people. While religion may be too divisive or not relevant for some patients, figuring out what patients care about and supporting them in those matters is another way chaplains continue to try to stake their professional claim around spirituality—broadly conceived—in hospitals. As professional chaplaincy continues to evolve, chaplains increasingly encounter nurses and physicians involved in a loosely organized "spirituality in health care" movement, some of whom may engage with patients concerning spirituality by using a growing number of spiritual assessment tools and diagnostic categories. Fueled by dissatisfaction with contemporary medicine and supported financially by groups like the John Templeton Foundation, members of this movement also seek to support patients and families in their spirituality, defined by physician Christina Puchalski and researcher Anna Romer as that "which allows a person to experience transcendent meaning in life. This is often expressed as a relationship with God, but it can also focus on nature, art, music, family, or community—whatever beliefs and values give a person a sense of meaning and purpose in life."[139]

Within this historical context, the ways in which spirituality and religion are present in the daily work of hospitals today are largely unknown. I explore those ways in the rest of this book as I watch chaplains, physicians, and nurses differently engage with patients and families around such issues. Their different trainings and orientations lead them to ask different questions and sometimes to understand and engage spirituality and religion in different ways. Before saying more about how the chaplains and ICU staff I spent time with see religion and spirituality in their work, I focus in the next chapter on the chapels located in the lobbies of many of these large academic hospitals.

CHAPTER 3

From Symbols to Silence: The Design and Use of Hospital Chapels

The chapel at Overbrook Hospital sits just inside the main entrance. Overhead signs and three panels of interwoven blue, green, and purple stained glass by the double doors draw visitors into the quiet, dimly lit space, mostly devoid of religious or spiritual objects. Twenty chairs are arranged in rows opposite a light-colored wooden lectern, a table holding cut flowers, and a few artificial plants. A book where visitors write their prayers sits on a table near two electric candles—no open flames are allowed in the hospital. Several Muslim prayer rugs are on a shelf to one side, and copies of the Bible, Hebrew Scriptures, Qur'an, prayer cards, and pamphlets about bereavement support groups and hospital fund-raising are on a shelf in the rear.[1] A piano sits under a tapestry hung by one of the chaplains in an effort to make the space warmer and more welcoming. At the back of the room, a shiny gold tabernacle holds consecrated hosts that Father William, the chaplain-priest, keeps stocked for Catholic communion.[2] Light wood finishes, a few additional panels of stained glass, and strategically designed lighting almost disguise the fact that the chapel has no windows.

Physical space for a chapel was part of the original plans for this building when it was designed more than twenty years ago. Ten years before that, the hospital's first chaplain, Episcopal minister Rev. Cook, began calling for an "interdenominational chapel," describing his vision as an "aesthetically attractive building" that would provide "the ground for private meditation, comfort, and beauty-in-the-midst of chaos." "What we are trying to accomplish in a rather small room located next to one of the busiest areas in this large teaching hospital," Chaplain Cook later wrote, "is to create a room with a feeling of depth, tranquility, and serenity that transcends any denominational purpose and reaches out to all patients, visitors, and staff as a room for prayer, meditation, and thought."[3] He hoped the chapel would welcome people from all religious traditions by seating fifty and including a place for an organ, choir, eight instrumentalists, altar, font, robing room, and sacristy.[4]

His vision was scaled back significantly when the building was designed; the first chapel was a small, fifteen-by-fifteen-foot room with an altar/communion table and a few chairs decorated in red and gold located near the main hospital entrance. Chaplain Cook raised funds for the interior of this chapel from local donors, a federal grant, and a friend of the hospital who paid a local artist to design the stained glass.[5] He described the first chapel as "interdenominational, and not exclusively Christian" even though it centered on an altar/communion table and members of other religious traditions were not involved in its design or opening. The chapel was consecrated by an Episcopal bishop and, even before the consecration, Rev. Cook held the first service there, blessing Bibles donated by the Gideon Society for all patient beds in the hospital.

The chapel has moved twice since its original opening. Chaplaincy directors successfully lobbied each time to keep the chapel near the main lobby. "There were many fights over the location of the chapel with various high-powered physicians," a former chaplaincy director remembered, "because it was on the first floor. . . . 'Why were we wasting the space on the chapel?' was the language on some occasions." It stayed there, the former director explained, because its location made it accessible to patients and families as "a place of calm amidst this chaos."[6] In these renovations, the chapel also shifted from having some Christian religious symbols to having few. "In an attempt to become interfaith and respectful," Pat, the current director of the Chaplaincy Department, explained, "we became neutral." What Pat describes as the interfaith orientation of the chapel is signified by a series of interlocking circles on paper signs displayed in a glass case outside the door. The middle circle says "Interfaith," and the words *Islam, Hinduism, Buddhism, Christianity, Unitarianism,* and *Judaism* are in circles with pictures of tradition-specific symbols around them.

Traditional Protestant services and Catholic masses that took place in the chapel in the past were replaced in the 1990s by short interfaith prayer services designed to welcome everyone. Staff chaplains and residents lead these sparsely attended services at noon on weekdays. In addition to commenting on the poor attendance, some chaplains are unhappy that as interfaith services—in the words of Marty, an individual completing a year-long chaplain residency at the hospital to prepare for future work as a chaplain—their language has to be theologically "so watered down . . . you could find it in the telephone book." "It is nice to love nature," he explained, referring to the nature symbolism that often dominates, "but I want to include my faith tradition as well. It is who I am and I'm willing to share it."[7]

A few other staff chaplains and residents share Marty's frustration with these services and with the chapel's current appearance, especially its mostly blank walls.[8] Some are aware of the Christian atmosphere in the supposedly neutral space, which is evident in the Advent wreath placed there at Christmas, the lilies at Easter, and the services for Catholic holy days that sometimes take place. Despite the sign pointing toward Mecca for Muslim prayer in the chapel, some wonder whether it is really a space for Christian worship. With its seemingly generic decor and daily interfaith prayer services, the chapel at Overbrook is open to staff, families, and patients twenty-four hours a day, seven days a week. During the day, there are usually two or three people inside sitting, sleeping, quietly praying, or reading in the dim light. Apart from seeking any spiritual or religious significance, many people, especially family members, come to the chapel for its quiet and for the centrally located space it provides to sit behind closed doors listening to nothing more than air moving through the heating and cooling vents of the hospital.

*

This chapter focuses on the physical spaces that Overbrook Hospital and the sixteen other secular academic medical centers described in this book allocate as chapels, prayer, and meditation rooms.[9] Some of these spaces were part of hospital buildings when they were constructed, while others were built or renovated more recently. I describe where these spaces are located in hospitals, what they are called, and how they are designed, furnished, and used. The appearance and use of these spaces has shifted over time as chapels designed primarily for Christian and Jewish worship—even if they were called interfaith—were slowly replaced or renovated so they could, at least theoretically, be utilized by people from a range of spiritual and religious backgrounds, including those with no such beliefs or affiliations.

I briefly discuss the history of chapels in American hospitals before describing the spaces in these hospitals along a continuum that ranges from those that remain tradition-specific to those expanded to be multifaith, which include objects from many religious traditions, and those, like the one at Overbrook, which are what Pat, the chaplaincy director, described as "neutral" and include few religious or spiritual symbols or objects.[10] While some of these spaces are truly neutral—they include no explicit religious or spiritual symbols and look like art galleries or fancy waiting rooms—others maintain religious, usually Christian, undertones, reflecting their histories and the disproportionate number of Christian, usually Protestant, chaplains who maintain them.[11] Seemingly neutral spaces are increasingly the norm, however, as is evident in new construction and recent renovations.

Despite the movement toward neutral physical spaces, variation in what the spaces look like today persists, and all of these hospitals continue to hold formal religious services either in their chapels or in larger conference rooms or auditoriums. Some services, like Catholic mass and Muslim prayers on Fridays, are tradition-specific and others, like those at Overbrook, are interfaith. Memorial services are also common. Aside from memorial services, other formal services seem like historical remnants, as their frequency has declined over time. Chapels are more commonly used for private reflection and contemplation today. Families and staff especially use the spaces, as most in-patients well enough to visit a chapel have already been discharged, given declining lengths of hospital stays.

I view chapel, prayer, and meditation spaces in this chapter as indicators of how chaplaincy directors, and hospitals more generally, imagine the boundaries of religious and spiritual inclusivity, not just in their work but in their physical spaces. The shift from traditional to more neutral chapel spaces mirrors the transition from religion to spirituality in health care broadly and in the self-understandings of chaplains. While seemingly inclusive chapel spaces could be multifaith and include objects from a range of religious and spiritual traditions, it is notable that they increasingly do not. Instead, these generic, often blank-walled rooms point to a particular response to religious diversity that is less about recognizing and naming various religious or spiritual beliefs and practices, and more about efforts to remove such symbols and create generic spaces intended to accommodate people and not offend. Perhaps this reflects Americans' discomfort at mixing and matching religious objects and symbols in seemingly secular organizations, or perhaps it suggests an approach that emphasizes similarities—like the need for space—rather than differences in how people assemble personal meanings.[12] Regardless, the variation in the hospital chapels described here shows that the shift toward seemingly neutral spaces is not uniform or complete, just as the art glass, nature symbolism, and running water in these seemingly neutral spaces do not necessarily encourage everyone to "come as you are," as religious studies scholar Diana Eck writes but are instead seen as unfamiliar by some and are, in some cases, rarely used.[13]

Relatively little is known about chapels, prayer, or meditation rooms in modern hospitals.[14] The term *chapel* was first used in the twelfth century and comes from the word *capella*, "cloak." According to the etymology in the *Oxford English Dictionary*, the cloak of St. Martin "preserved by the Frankish kings as a sacred relic" was "borne before them in battle and used to give sanctity to oaths." The term was then "applied to the sanctuary in which this was preserved under the care of its *cappellani* or 'chaplains,' and thence generally to a sanctuary containing holy relics, attached to a palace, etc., and so to any private sanctuary or holy place, and finally to any apartment or building for orisons or worship, not being a church." Initially a chapel was consecrated and had an altar, though the originally Christian term *chapel* has now come to describe "a room or building for private worship in or attached to a palace, nobleman's house, castle, garrison, embassy, prison, monastery, college, school, or other institution."[15] Two-thirds of the spaces I describe here continue to be called chapels; the remaining one-third are called meditation rooms (the majority) or prayer rooms.

Hospital chapels have shrunk in size and been secularized in purpose since the twelfth century. Before the hospital as an institution separated from its religious forebearers, hospitals and chapels were, in a sense, one. In *The Hospital: A Social and Architectural History*, John Thompson and Grace Goldin write of the important relationships between open wards and chapels in the twelfth century, specifically whether patients could see the altar from their beds and how the chapel was oriented in the building.[16] The Byloke Hospital in Ghent (1234), they explain, had a chapel that paralleled the ward, making it possible for patients to hear, if not see, masses taking place. With the closing in of open hospital wards, the beginning of private rooms, and the shifting contributions of religious organizations to the care of the sick in later centuries, hospital chapels changed—often becoming smaller if not less centrally located.[17]

Little is known about the history of chapels in American hospitals. Some hospitals—for example, Pennsylvania Hospital (1751), New York Hospital (1771), and Massachusetts General Hospital (1811)—founded in the eighteenth and early nineteenth centuries do not appear to have had chapels.[18] Others, like New Haven Hospital (1826), did, at least according to historical records suggesting that the hospital's Gifford Chapel temporarily housed some of the two hundred soldiers sick with typhoid who were sent there during the Spanish-American War.[19] Hospitals started by religious groups in the nineteenth and twentieth centuries were probably more likely than secular hospitals to have chapels.[20] Thompson and Goldin describe the central chapel of St. Luke's Hospital in New York City (1857) as an "immense reservoir of pure air for the wards."[21] Catholic and Jewish hospitals also frequently had Catholic and Jewish chapels and offered related services as part of their daily routines.[22] Reflecting the rise of religiously run hospitals, architect Edward Stevens wrote in *The American Hospital of the Twentieth Century* that "as a large part of the smaller hospitals today are being maintained by one or another religious society, it very often follows that the provision for a chapel must be incorporated into the plans of the institution."[23] Larger hospitals, Stevens noted, often had chapels set away from the main buildings, clustered with laboratories, classrooms, rooms for autopsies, and the morgue.[24]

In the United States, as in Britain, some hospitals linked religion and death structurally by building mortuary chapels next to morgues where relatives could view the bodies of recently deceased loved ones. A British Ministry of Health circular in the 1960s recommended that every hospital have "a chapel or room set apart to serve as a chapel" to be made "available by mutual arrangement for the services of the denominations who wish to use it." The space was to be centrally located and attractively designed: "The chapel should be architecturally and decoratively lit and bright, symbolizing life, hope, and healing." It was to be open day and night, with enough space for beds and wheelchairs in the aisles.[25] In addition, this circular called on the chaplain to regularly visit the mortuary chapel "and see that it is properly and reverently maintained." Far too often, the author commented, "such chapels seem to be neglected, and it should be one of the main concerns of the chaplain to liaise with the mortician and the hospital authorities and see that everything is done to keep the chapel in good and decent order."[26]

At least two of the seventeen hospitals I describe here used to have mortuary chapels. Funded by a donor, the mortuary chapel at one was built in the 1930s so that wealthy families would have spaces to view the bodies of their loved ones. "It backed up on the morgue so that a body could be wheeled in the back of the room and hidden behind a decorative wooden screen," a chaplain who has researched its history explained to me. "You could enter the chapel, see the screen ahead of you, and not know there was a body in the room, if you didn't go behind the screen." Centered on an alter holding a large gilded cross, the chapel was also used for baptisms and funerals. After years of chaplains' complaints that it was too small and did not meet the needs of patients, the hospital replaced the mortuary chapel with a much larger chapel, with the support of another wealthy donor. The mortuary chapel has since been put to other uses and currently serves as the office of the hospital's executive chef.[27]

With time, architects Stephen Verderber and David Fine argue, chapel spaces "in most hospitals" were "gradually being downsized to a waiting room off a bleak corridor," through there is no systematic historical evidence of this transition.[28] A 1970 *Manual on Hospital Chaplaincy* published by the American Hospital Association stipulated that "space for religious services for inpatients is one of the most important requirements in facilities for a chaplaincy program." The space could be a single chapel, several chapels, or a multipurpose room, and should "demonstrate the hospital's appreciation for various religious faiths." The authors encouraged chaplains and hospital administrators to work with "consultants from major religious groups in the community" in determining the "symbols to be used in designing the furnishings" and to aim for "harmony and better understanding among all faith groups."[29]

Little is known about how hospitals followed these guidelines, if at all, though in 1974 the American Hospital Association reported that of the 3,038 hospitals with chaplain services (43% of all hospitals), 98% provided some kind of worship space or office facility for chaplains. The survey reported that 55% had a chapel for use by all denominations, 19% had a chapel for use by one denomination, 22% had an additional prayer chapel or meditation room, and 13% had a prayer chapel or meditation room only.[30] Researchers did not gather any additional information about these spaces, and no systematic information about hospital chapels in the United States has been collected since.[31] Several recent media reports describe hospitals' efforts either to turn Christian chapels into interfaith spaces for prayer and meditation or to create new spaces.[32] Beyond such reports, little is known about the current design and use of these spaces.[33]

CURRENT DESIGN

All the hospitals I studied had chapels or meditation rooms in their buildings. More than half had more than one such space, often because the hospital was the result of merging two earlier hospitals, each of which had a chapel.[34] Most are small, with space to seat six or eight, though a few are very large, with seating for several hundred. Like academic hospitals nationally, these seventeen hospitals are large, covering multiple campuses or city blocks. "It's not a real warm, fuzzy place" one of the chaplains said dryly, describing the hospital where she works and the many buildings it owns in the city. "I think at last count we had 555,000 square feet [in the building she works in], . . . the largest footprint of any of the other buildings on the campus, I believe I was told."

Most chapels are in the lobby or near the main entrance to the hospital, perhaps suggesting that they were intended from the start to be used by families, staff, and visitors more than by hospital in-patients cared for in other areas of the buildings. A few hospitals have separate chapel spaces in pediatric wings or built into the design of recently opened cancer centers.[35] "There is a small, twelve-by-twelve room" in the Cancer Center, one chaplaincy director explained. When outpatients come in for treatment, they or their family members "can go in there for some quiet time and some privacy. . . . People are free to use it at will." Most chapels are open twenty-four hours a day, seven days a week, and are called "chapels." With renovation and new construction, some are now called "Interfaith Chapels," or their names have been changed to "Meditation Room" or, less often, "Prayer Room," especially on the West Coast. About half bear the names of hospital donors, and most include plaques recognizing the individuals and organizations that contributed to their construction or renovation.[36]

As they were at Overbrook, chapel spaces were part of the original architectural plans at several hospitals. "The hospital always had a chapel or prayer room," the chaplaincy director at Lakeview Hospital explained. Hospitals formed through mergers almost always have multiple chapel spaces—one in each of the original hospital buildings. Speaking of the two chapels his hospital has as the result of such a merger, the chaplaincy director at Streamside explained, "I don't think they [the chapels] have moved an inch in decades. . . . One has been radically remodeled and the other adapted a bit, again in the direction of being welcoming of many faiths and more oriented to meditation than worship." While some hospitals have renovated spaces built as Catholic or Jewish chapels, others have not, and the spaces retain tradition-specific names like Saint Anne's Chapel.

Some hospitals added chapels to existing buildings in the mid-twentieth century, often after hiring their first chaplain. Perhaps in an effort to legitimize his position in the hospital, an Episcopal minister paid by a local diocese to work in one hospital began to raise money for a hospital chapel shortly after he arrived. He sent more than 1,500 handwritten letters to friends of the hospital, asking for their support. Foreshadowing later attempts to make chapel spaces welcoming to all people, he wrote as follows to describe the chapel built a few years later: "The simple fact that it, with its beauty, its traditions, its suggestions of mystery and spiritual presence, is in the center of a great Hospital for the healing of men's bodies [*sic*], creates an atmosphere throughout the wards, and all who pass by the doors feel it and carry its silent message."

While this chapel originally had a Christian cross, hospital trustees voted to remove it several years after the chapel opened, fulfilling the chaplain's initial desire that "there should be no permanent religious symbols in the chapel, thereby making it truly available for the 'spiritual refreshment of all, regardless of race or creed,'" according to a committee report. The Christian-themed stained-glass windows, vaulted ceilings, and pews that were part of the original design remained, and the possibility that they might make some non-Christian visitors uncomfortable in the chapel, even absent the cross, was not acknowledged in historical documents or by the current chaplains I interviewed. The chaplains at this hospital see the absent cross and versatility of the altar space—which also includes a Protestant lectern, Roman Catholic altar, and portable Jewish ark—as what makes the space not tradition-specific and open to all. What "spiritual refreshment," "mystery," or "silent message" visitors access in the space remains undefined.

While some current chapel spaces were designed with original hospital buildings or added in the mid-twentieth century, others were constructed more recently. Oceanview Hospital did not have a chapel until it hired its first professional chaplain in the last twenty years. "The staff was saying we need a space" the current director remembered, so the first director worked to find a small room. It currently holds several rows of chairs facing a stained-glass window with an abstract design. At Eastern Hospital, Muslim staff looking for a place to pray recently persuaded the hospital to set aside a patient room as what they call a "meditation prayer room." The director of chaplaincy is raising funds to create a larger space that he hopes will meet the needs of everyone in the hospital for, in his words, a "sacred space" as a "place of respite." At Forest Hills Hospital, a new cancer center was built in the late 1990s, and a chaplain explained, "They built the meditation room then at the same time . . . right at the entrance." At this same time, the hospital hired its first chaplain dedicated exclusively to working with cancer patients and their families, and built an office for that person right next to the meditation room. Decorated in soft shades of purple and gray, the meditation room holds information about an intensive prayer program in the hospital, materials for cancer patients and their families, and a small set of tinkling wind chimes.

Most hospital chapels twenty years old or older have been renovated since they were constructed. As at Overbrook, these spaces, without exception, transitioned from being spaces built to serve single religious traditions to ones that chaplains now describe as more inclusive and flexible. At Grace Hospital the first chapel was built largely by Episcopalians in the mid-1950s and looked to "all the world like a Protestant chapel," according to the current chaplaincy director. Since then, it has been renovated every twenty years. The original stained-glass Rose window, common in Christian churches, remains, but the permanent altar was replaced with one that is "movable depending on the service." Also, the director explained, the "cabinetry was structured" in the most recent renovation, "so it was neutral, so it took away the feeling of being in a more intentional Christian church. . . . We certainly tried to be responsive." A shift to movable altars is common across hospitals in these renovations. "There are religious symbols only when there is a worship event going on" in the chapel, one director explained. "So if it's a Catholic mass, they'll be Catholic religious symbols. At the end of the mass, the chapel becomes generic again." Furniture on wheels is also common. "The lectern, the podium . . . used to be anchored into cement, but I took that out, and it is on wheels now, so it can be pushed aside." Using Muslims as an example, the director of chaplaincy at Lakeview Hospital explained, "Muslim employees who know the story behind this can come in, go behind the altar, pull open a drawer . . . take out prayer rugs, have their Muslim prayers, and put the prayer rugs back. So it is a very flexible space."

At other hospitals, chaplaincy directors and hospital administrators made more radical changes during renovations by replacing stained-glass windows and Christian symbols with nature imagery, waterfalls, and artfully designed decor. "When I came here," one director told me, "they had the ugliest depressing chapel that I'd ever seen." Rather than renovating it in its existing space, he convinced the hospital to close the older chapel and create a new space, twice as large, in another area of the hospital. This chaplaincy director negotiated carefully, leaving the stained glass window from the old chapel behind so that the new chapel would be an "interfaith space," complete with plants, comfortable chairs, a nature scene made from stained glass, and a constantly flowing indoor waterfall. Signs with names of different religious traditions hang on one wall of this chapel, and the room is otherwise devoid of religious symbols. While this renovation went smoothly, others have not. At Streamside, a traditionally Christian chapel was renovated, turning what the director described as a "very Christian space with pews facing front and a large picture of Jesus" to a space that would be "flexible, inviting, and supportive

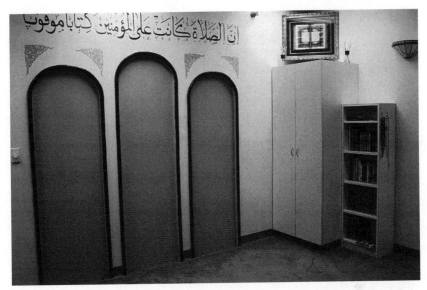

FIGURE 3.1 The mosque (or *masjed*) opened in 2005 at the Lutheran Medical Center in Brooklyn, New York. Photo courtesy of the Lutheran Medical Center.

to people from a range of faith traditions." The chaplaincy director at the time took "a lot of heat" through this process as Christian staff and visitors accused him of "driving Christ out of the hospital," the current director recalled.

In addition to renovating chapels to make them more inclusive, several hospitals have added Muslim prayer rooms in recent years or created and explicitly named spaces where Muslims pray (fig. 3.1). Muslims, like Orthodox Jews, traditionally understand their faith to forbid prayer in the presence of religious symbols, gods, or images of living beings. To pray, they need open rooms with furniture that can be stacked or removed to make space for prayer and with easy access to sinks where they can wash before prayer. Janice Neumann, a reporter for the *Washington Post*, reported in 2006 that about a dozen hospitals have opened Muslim prayer rooms nationwide.[37] Two of the seventeen hospitals I studied have opened Muslim prayer rooms in the last ten years. One includes a carefully designed mihrab with a quotation in Arabic from the Qur'an: "We send down (stage by stage) in the Qur'an that which is a healing and a mercy to those who believe." Other hospitals have spaces, often initially created for Muslim physicians, medical residents, and other employees, where Muslims pray. While some other religious groups, such as Orthodox Jews, have beliefs and practices that make it impossible for them to share religious space with others, Muslims are the only group I learned about, apart from Christians and Jews in traditional chapels, that had space specifically designated for them in hospitals.[38]

In addition to renovating chapels and opening Muslim prayer rooms, a few hospitals also recently added additional quiet rooms, labyrinths, and gardens—all spaces that visitors might find restful and that chaplains believe are welcoming to everyone. When a new cardiovascular center was built at Meadows Hospital, a chaplain explained that "quiet/meditation rooms" were added that the chaplaincy department was "responsible for in terms of resources, literature, and such in there." "They're not chapels," the chaplain explained, implying that the name *chapel* is too Christian to describe them, "but they're . . . religious, spiritual places." Hospital gardens are nothing new, but some are being newly designed with notions of respite, comfort, and restoration in mind.[39] A few directors dreamed of "spiritual centers," what one described as a "place for people to come and be quiet in prayer, . . . with a labyrinth, prayer wall, space for Muslim prayer, [and a] way to access chaplains," rather than chapels or meditation rooms in hospitals of the future.

A Continuum

The chapel, prayer, and meditation spaces in these seventeen hospitals are best described along a continuum that represents the different choices that chaplains and hospital leaders make when faced with creating physical space for religiously diverse people in their hospitals. At one end are those with traditional chapels, built to serve people in one religious tradition (fig. 3.2). In the middle of the continuum are hospitals where traditional chapel spaces have been renovated or expanded into multifaith spaces that include symbols and objects from many religious and spiritual traditions. The majority of hospitals are at or moving toward the other end of the continuum, creating spaces, either through renovations or new designs, that are intended to be neutral and include few religious symbols or objects.[40] While some hospitals with two or more chapels have one that is more traditional and another that is more neutral, most hospitals with two or more spaces fall in consistent places on this continuum.

On the traditional end, one hospital has two dated chapels—one built by Protestants for Protestants and a second, much smaller, space for Catholics.[41] The Protestant chapel was built in the 1950s and appears today much as it did when it was built. Designed to seat more than one hundred, the chapel was constructed as a separate building connected to, rather than situated within, existing structures. Funded by a wealthy donor, the chapel includes numerous

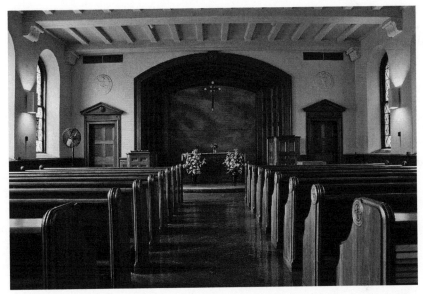

FIGURE 3.2 The Protestant chapel at Bellevue Hospital, New York, New York. The hospital also has a Catholic chapel, synagogue, and Muslim prayer room. Photo by Emily F. Olson. Published with the permission of Bellevue Hospital.

stained-glass windows, rows of fixed pews, and an arc of the covenant. Originally the chapel had a large oversized cross, which was removed in the 1970s. The chapel also has a choir loft and an organ, as do most large Protestant churches in the area, and an internal broadcasting system, with individual speakers for every bed so hospital in-patients can listen to chapel services and radio programs. The radio broadcasting system no longer works, and chapel services are today broadcast into patient rooms via television. When the chapel first opened, student vespers were held every Wednesday with the support of the affiliated nursing school and the hospital chaplain.

The chapel appears today—with its fixed pews, organ loft, and stained-glass windows—much as it did when it was built in the 1950s, although patients and staff are much more diverse religiously and spiritually. It is rarely used, and many are not comfortable in this clearly Protestant space. Several non-Christian groups have tried, informally, to create spaces for themselves outside the main sanctuary. Jewish services are held at the base of the stairwell leading to the organ loft rather than in the actual chapel. Led by the husband of a staff member, Muslims brought prayer rugs and other materials to a small room off the main sanctuary where they pray. These gatherings demonstrate the challenges that non-Christian staff and visitors face when trying to utilize a space constructed for Christians.[42]

In the middle of the continuum are a few hospitals with multifaith chapels (fig. 3.3). These were generally created as spaces specific to one tradition and were renovated over time. One such chapel, located near the main hospital lobby, was dedicated as a Christian space in the 1950s by the Board of Women Visitors. With the support of donors, hospital staff, and volunteers from a range of religious traditions, the chaplaincy department director renovated it in the early 1990s as an explicitly multifaith space. The crosses on the reredos, a decorative screen behind the altar common in Episcopal churches, were painted in during this renovation and are now flowers and solid-colored blocks. Other Christian symbols (e.g., words etched into the altar) were removed or covered—replaced by nooks around the edges of the round room that contain tapestries, symbols, and objects from Christian, Jewish, and Muslim traditions. Each tradition has its own nook with texts, symbols, and images.

"I suppose there must have been some people who weren't happy about the changes," the chaplaincy director commented, "but I never had a single

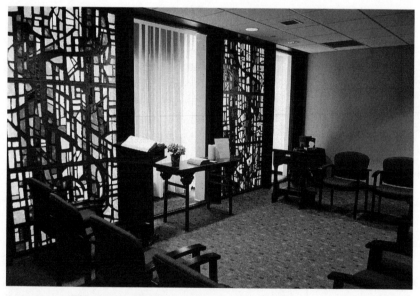

FIGURE 3.3 The chapel at Faulkner Hospital in Boston, Massachusetts, used to be primarily Christian but today includes symbols from a range of religious traditions, including praying hands made of olive wood from Israel and a sign pointing toward Mecca. Photo courtesy of Faulkner Hospital.

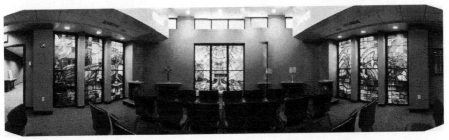

FIGURE 3.4 The chapel at Riverview Hospital in Noblesville, Indiana, includes symbols from several religious traditions donated by area religious organizations. Photo courtesy of Riverview Hospital.

complaint come directly to me about those changes that we made." A prayer book, lectern, and a few chairs sit at the front of the room, and there are a few plants below the decorative screen. Several pews sit in the middle of the room. In addition to the nooks representing different religious traditions, memorial boards made by family members whose loved ones died in the hospital are sometimes displayed in this space. This chapel seems to be well used by people praying, reading, writing in the prayer book, or just resting during the day. While other hospitals in this category do not have the same kind of tradition-specific nooks or areas of their chapel, they do tend to include a range of religious objects and symbols in the spaces. At another hospital, for example, one of the two chapels includes a movable altar as well as a menorah, Muslim prayer rugs, and a tabernacle in which to hold Catholic communion. "We have all kinds of literature in there," one of the chaplains remarked, as well as "prayer rugs, . . . rosary beads, . . . scapulas, . . . [and] yarmulkes."[43]

On the opposite end of the continuum are the increasingly numerous hospitals that have few to no religious symbols in their chapels—the spaces often appear more like art galleries or carefully designed waiting rooms (figs. 3.5 and 3.6). Overbrook sits between the multifaith middle and this end of the continuum as a space that includes no formal religious symbols on the walls but has some religious objects, such as the Muslim prayer rugs and tabernacle for Catholic communion, even though the director did not comment on them when she called the space "neutral." One of the chapels at another hospital at the extreme end of the continuum looked more like a conference room than a chapel, with its movable furniture, lighting, and wall designs incorporating leaf motifs. A metal sculpture with leaf designs divided the doorway from the room, and the same image was incorporated into the lighting and wall designs. Aside from a box labeled "Prayer Requests" and a sign outside the door that

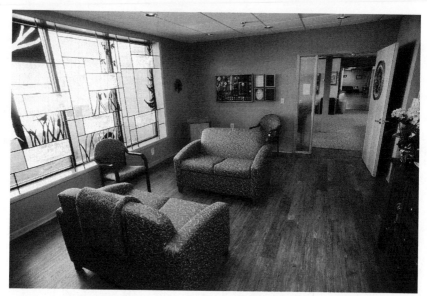

FIGURE 3.5 Samaritan Pacific Communities Hospital on the Oregon Coast opened this room, called the Pacific Sanctuary, in 2010 as a safe and protected place for all people. Photo by Karl Maasdam, Karl Maasdam Photography, for the hospital.

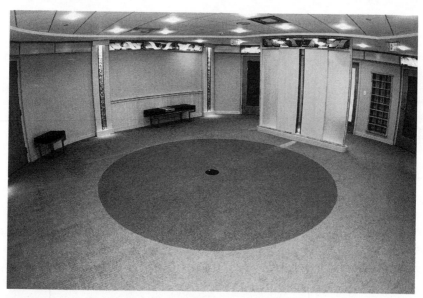

FIGURE 3.6 In November 2010, the Department of Pastoral Care at Virginia Commonwealth University Medical Center opened this newly renovated chapel. The space contains no religious images or symbols in an effort to welcome all. Photo courtesy of Virginia Commonwealth University Medical Center.

said "Chapel," visitors to the room might not be aware that the space was a chapel and taken care of by the chaplaincy department. A similar "meditation room" at another hospital—in which I never saw anyone meditating—had several pieces of abstract art on the walls, a large piece of art glass hanging at its front, and a constantly gurgling fountain in the corner. A press release issued when the space was opened described "six art pieces" that "express hope and healing through abstract imagery of nature and water." A wavy piece of glass separating the doorway from the room sits next to a small podium holding a book that reads "We invite you to write your thoughts, feelings, or a message." Signs indicate that "the room is dedicated to people of all faiths for meditation and quiet prayer." On this sign, as elsewhere, prayer is assumed to be a practice shared among people from a range of religious and spiritual backgrounds.[44]

Stepping Back

Given the range of hospital chapel spaces along this continuum, it was striking to hear chaplains describe these physical spaces as versatile, interfaith, and welcoming to all—regardless of how they actually appeared. The chaplaincy director at a hospital with a traditional Jewish chapel described it as having been "adapted to be more welcoming of many faiths . . . there isn't any blaring 'This is Jewish, if you're not Jewish don't come in,' which actually kind of upset the Orthodox Jewish community." The Torah scrolls inside the arc at the front of this chapel, which are regularly loaned out for bar and bat mitzvahs, in addition to other Jewish symbols (and the lack of symbols from other religious traditions) around the room marked the space to me as Jewish, though the director saw it otherwise. Similarly, chapels with stained-glass windows like those in Protestant and Catholic churches were described by directors as open to all people and had signs outside or over their doors that read "Interfaith Chapel for Meditation. All are Welcome" and "Whoever Will, May Enter Here." Pews remain in such chapels, directors explain, not because of what they symbolize but for functional reasons, "Families in grief have a tendency to pick up things and throw things, so we don't want folding chairs in the chapel," one director explained, even though pews mark spaces as connected to particular religious traditions and histories, and make it difficult or impossible for some other people—like Muslims—to use them for prayer.

The chaplain who said it "breaks my heart" to walk past the "Christian-like chapel with pews and an altar and all of that" and see Muslims trying to find a place to pray was not the norm. Few chaplains spoke directly about individuals or groups not welcomed, either explicitly or implicitly, in their chapel spaces. Almost no chapels, for example, included information in languages other than English, even when located in cities with large Spanish- or Chinese-speaking populations. While Muslims were sometimes granted separate spaces, chaplains rarely mentioned members of other religious traditions that do not use shared, seemingly neutral spaces. They also rarely mentioned traditional Catholics or members of religious traditions for whom a neutral chapel might be a pretty place to rest but not a religious or spiritual one in the absence of symbols, texts, or consecration by leaders of their traditions.

Hospitals like Overbrook that have tried to make their spaces more neutral but retain some religious symbols display the tension between the spaces that chaplains think they are creating and the spaces they actually create. These tensions are not new but are often present at the time the chapels originally open.[45] When the original chapel opened at Overbrook, the director drafted a policy about how the department would accept gifts. He saw the chapel as interfaith and "interdenominational," and aimed to accept gifts of items from a range of religious traditions so that the chapel could be used by people in different faiths. The items he listed as needed, however, were exclusively Christian, including "a chalice for the celebration of Holy Communion, kneelers for the Chapel chairs, . . . and custom-made hangings for seasons of the liturgical church year." Responding, in part, to the Christian-ness of this space, the current director tries to keep the chapel space what she considers neutral, though Catholic communion implements, Muslim prayer rugs, and several religious texts are inside. When a Catholic staff member asked for a kneeler in the chapel, the director said no, seeing it not as an addition to the symbols currently there but as a first symbol in moving the chapel away from being a neutral space. While movable Christian symbols marked the first chapel as versatile and interfaith to the first director, the absence of a kneeler—a symbol of the numerically dominant Catholic religious group in the hospital—indicated a neutral space for the current one.

CURRENT USE

Like their designs, the events that take place inside chapel spaces vary across hospitals, though there has been a shift over time away from more formal religious services and toward more individual, private use of chapel spaces.[46] Despite this shift, some formal religious services are still held, and memorial services for hospital staff take place in these spaces. In hospitals with small chapels, services also take place in auditoriums and conference rooms, depending on the size of the crowd.[47] "When there's a very large holy day," one chaplain explained, "we secure space in the various auditoriums and larger rooms." About 80% of the hospitals (14 of 17) have Catholic mass at least weekly. Sixty percent (10 of 17) have non-denominational Protestant services, and 47% (8 of 17) have Jewish services regularly. Four have meditation or Buddhist services at least weekly, and more than half have space for Muslim prayers, especially on Fridays. About 40% (7 of 17) have interfaith services, usually ten- or fifteen-minute midday interfaith prayers frequently focused on nature imagery and other seemingly neutral themes. Most of the services I attended were led by staff chaplains and were attended by fewer than fifteen people.

Although few people attend, chaplains continue holding services, perhaps out of habit or because chaplains see them as symbolically representing their value to the hospital. "You need to keep a modicum of these events," the director of chaplaincy at Grace Hospital told me, "but the expectation is they're not going to be attended as much and in the way they were years ago" due to declining hospital stays and the increasing severity of patients' illnesses. This increasing severity also means that patients and their families need more extraordinary than mundane religious and spiritual support services than they did in the past. Several chaplaincy departments regularly cancel services that people do not attend. "We have an ecumenical Christian service on Sundays," one remarked, "although often nobody comes—there's just not that much ability for people to get out of their rooms anymore." Sometimes it is only the chaplains who attend. "I play my harp for maybe fifteen minutes before each [interfaith] service," a chaplain at Southern Hospital explained. "Usually it's just the other chaplains that are there. . . . Even if nobody shows up, it gives us an opportunity to pray for all our patients" Several hospitals broadcast their services through closed-caption TV in an effort to make them more accessible to bedridden patients. Several departments also either offer or would like to offer music, meditation guidelines, nature photos, and other soothing sounds and images through these television stations.

Despite low attendance at regular services, most hospitals also offer services for certain religious holidays, though deciding which holidays to recognize and mark with formal services is not always straightforward. The chaplains at Overbrook, in addition to their daily interfaith service, organized services for several Catholic holy days, Christmas Eve, the eight days of Hanukkah, Yom Kippur, Rosh Hashanah, Passover, and Iftar (the breaking of the Muslim fast) during the time I spent with them. The Ash Wednesday service was the largest service, attended by more than one hundred people, and services for Holy Thursday, Good Friday, and Easter Sunday were also held. Chaplains and the chaplaincy director discussed whether to have a Good Friday service, concluding that it was important to do so because of the large number of people who usually attend. Chaplains at several other hospitals also remarked on the size of their own Ash Wednesday services, calling that day the busiest of their calendar year, perhaps because of its connection to repentance and to death. A few also mentioned offering Blessing of the Hands services in their chapels during Nurse Appreciation Week. Hospital chapels are also occasionally used for weddings, confessions, and meetings with large families. "A couple got married in it in May," one chaplain explained speaking of the chapel at her hospital, and a priest heard "confessions there that people need to do during Lent."

The few people who do attend religious services in hospitals, either regularly or on holidays, may be connected through them, either literally or metaphorically, in new ways to others in the hospital. The mix of physicians, clerical staff, and family members I observed at Catholic mass and Muslim prayer services, for instance, would probably not have otherwise been in the same room, and if they had been, medical hierarchies would have dominated. One Jewish chaplain commented on these connections, talking about how some of the Jewish services he leads challenge medical hierarchy and bring people together in new ways. "There's so much hierarchy in the hospital. I mean it's just the length of your coat," he explained, "and doctors and nurses, and the patient is always at the bottom of the hierarchy. They're always naked or half-naked and have no control over who comes into the room." During the high holidays, though, "we get doctors, we get young residents, we get nurses, we get the guy from the print shop, we have family members, we have patients with IV poles and gowns, ... everyone standing together, singing together . . . with noisemakers." These holidays lead people to be "bowing and singing together, . . . kind of bringing down a lot of those walls that divide people. . . . It is often very meaningful." More the exception than the norm, such experiences do happen for at least a few people occasionally.

More than for services, chapel spaces are used daily for private prayer and meditation, attracting people looking for a space to rest for a few minutes. In her study of the Millennium Dome in Greenwich, London, Sophie Gilliat-Ray described visitors as more tourists than pilgrims, much like the visitors to these chapels who enter and leave at will.[48] Sitting in the chapel at Overbrook one afternoon, I observed a staff member sitting in one chair with her eyes closed resting or praying. Someone else wrote a prayer in the hospital prayer book, while, in another part of the room, a woman kneeled, clearly in prayer, and a physician in scrubs prayed on a Muslim prayer rug. This combination

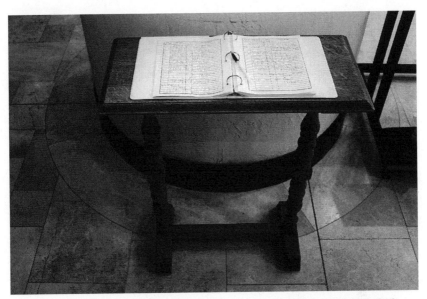

FIGURE 3.7 A book in which people write prayers in the Chapel and Multifaith Sanctuary at Cincinnati Children's Hospital. Photo courtesy of Cincinnati Children's Hospital.

of praying, resting, and sleeping was common in other chapels where it was physically possible, given the design and decor.

Prayer books, boxes, or boards were also focal points for visitors in almost every hospital chapel. These bound blank books and locked boxes are places where people can write, and leave behind, prayers and personal notes (fig. 3.7). Usually on tables or book stands, they have guidelines like, "Please feel free to write any concerns, worries, or joys." Some specify that only first names be used, to protect patient confidentiality. Prayers of thanks and petition fill these books in English, Spanish, Arabic, and other languages, alongside children's drawings and unintelligible scribbles. "Dear Lord," one prayer read at Overbrook, "Please watch over and protect my loving husband as he undergoes his surgery and recovery. Thank you for all the gifts you've given us." Chaplaincy directors describe these books as giving visitors something to do. "People feel so helpless usually when somebody is sick," Pat, the director at Overbrook, explained, "and it's so easy. I can write a name or a phrase. . . . I think it helps with people's helplessness." At some hospitals, chaplains read prayers out loud during services or pray them quietly; at others, prayers remain in prayer books in silent witness to people's experiences. When prayer books are filled, and when prayers written on bits of paper have been read by chaplains, they are stored or burned, similar to how sacred texts are disposed of in some religious traditions.

Researcher and hospital chaplain JoAnn O'Reilly writes about prayer books and the prayers they contain as comforting to people coping with their own illness or that of a loved one. She thinks people "meet the familiar" in hospital chapels, and prayer books help them converse with God. "When we converse with God," she writes, "the remembering of God's story in the light of our own is part of the dialogue. . . . When we write these stories in the context of prayer, the immediacy of the divine narrative as it intersects with our own story heals."[49] I analyzed the prayers in one such book, find- ing they are written like notes or e-mails to God. Authors primarily thanked God in their prayers, made requests of God, or both thanked and petitioned God. The majority of writers in the books I examined imagined a God who is accessible, listening, and a source of emotional and psychological support. Rather than focusing on specific discrete outcomes that might not occur (e.g., healing for a broken leg), writers tended to frame their prayers broadly, (e.g., asking for strength to get through the difficulty of having a broken leg) in ways that allowed them to make multiple interpretations of the results.[50] Chaplains remark on the gratitude evident in these prayers: "There's a certain amount of petition," one explained, "but the theme overall is gratitude."

CONCLUSIONS

Some hospital chapels are dark, dimly lit, "downsized waiting rooms" off of bleak corridors, in the words of architects Stephen Verderber and David Fine (2000), often almost empty and in need of renovation and repair. Most of the chapels described here are not. They have moved, been renovated, and in some cases been opened recently for the first time in the history of their hos- pitals. While many are close to empty when daily or weekly religious services take place, others—especially multifaith spaces—have people coming in and out otherwise, resting, praying, and reflecting in these spaces, more tourists than pilgrims and often happy for a space where they can simply sit quietly behind a closed door.

As spaces, chapels provide clues about how the hospital chaplains who cre- ate and maintain them think about religious and spiritual inclusivity in their hospitals. Like university, military, and airport chapels, these spaces range from those oriented around single religious traditions to multifaith spaces that include symbols from multiple religious traditions to seemingly neutral spaces that favor art and nature rather than religious symbolism.[51]

Directors of chaplaincy departments with multifaith spaces describe them as some of the few spaces in the United States where, as one director explained, people from various backgrounds might practice their religions at the same time. "We had a rabbi," this director explained, in the chapel "videotaping something about the High Holidays so that we could play it on the closed circuit system here. As she was taping this, . . . somebody came in and knelt at the kneeler on the other side of the chapel and started praying the rosary. . . . And while the two of them were doing that, somebody came in, took off his shoes, and began to prostrate himself and pray to the east. All three at the same time." The multifaith chapel space at this hospital made such simultaneous actions possible, though there was no interaction; each individual conducted his or her prayers and rituals privately. The director saw this as a metaphor for interfaith chaplaincy, explaining, "I keep saying that we do an interfaith model of chaplaincy here, partly because it was logistically impossible to do anything else. But even if we could do it another way, I wouldn't want to, because I think this is one of the few places where we can learn and encourage and experience what it is like to take each other at our best." The extent to which the individuals in the chapel or the chaplains whom this director describes really interact with and learn from one another, however, is an open question, as are the ways these practices fit within the broad spiritual frame of professional chaplaincy.

Simultaneous Jewish, Catholic, and Muslim prayer or practices by people from a range of other spiritual and religious traditions are less possible in the more neutral spaces that many hospitals are creating, which lack kneelers, Muslim prayer rugs, and other religious objects needed for such practices. As they replaced crosses with movable altars, furniture on wheels, chairs that can be stacked, and spaces that can—at least theoretically—accommodate people from a range of backgrounds, hospital chaplains and administrators remove some of the images, symbols, and rituals that have traditionally transmitted religion among and between people and illustrate the broader challenges implicit in trying to accommodate people from a range of religious backgrounds, including those with no such background or current practices.

Such challenges are reminiscent of broader questions about whether American religious pluralism includes space for everyone as they are or requires certain sanitized or least common-denominator approaches to religion for their use.[52] While multifaith chapels try to make room for many with their religious symbols, the movement toward neutral chapels shows hospitals and chaplains increasingly opting for new symbols of art and nature rather than those of religious traditions. Hospitals are thus creating an absence of obvious markers of religion or spirituality in the designated physical spaces where they might most likely be present. It is ironic that many hospitals are moving toward creating such spaces, even as they continue to hold Catholic masses and Protestant religious services in their buildings. These hospitals display a particular response to American religious pluralism that is less about recognizing diverse religious and spiritual beliefs and practices and more about efforts to remove such symbols and create generic spaces that seem to accommodate people and do not offend.

When I ask undergraduates how they would design hospital chapel spaces anew, almost none opt for multifaith spaces, instead preferring seemingly neutral spaces that they imagine will be welcoming to everyone. Like many Americans who view religion and spirituality as personal and private and who are comfortable drawing from a range of traditions and practices to construct their personal approaches, the students believe that chapel spaces should include cabinets or shelves of religious texts and symbols that individuals can select and use as needed.[53] While a person praying the rosary and one praying to Mecca could, theoretically, bring their prayer beads and rug into the same space, my students are uncomfortable with sharing space and also imagine cubicles in chapels where people would have privacy to sit, rest, or say their prayers. Their privatized supermarket or buffet approach to shared spiritual and religious spaces in hospitals illustrates the value we as Americans place on private religious expression, our hesitancy to share space with others who are spiritually or religiously different, and our concern—often based on our own lack of understanding—about offending people. They also reflect many people's doubts that truly neutral space that would be seen as such by all can be created. The decisions chaplains and hospital leaders are making to create neutral, generic spaces full of nature imagery reflect a similar hesitancy and discomfort about engaging with people from a range of religious and spiritual backgrounds and the belief that shared spaces are best empty, rather than full, of religious and spiritual symbols and objects.

As staff and visitors use these spaces in hospitals, the question that remains unasked is how they experience them. My observations suggest that more recently renovated chapels, those that are more central, and those with a bit more light are used more frequently than others. Chapels with comfortable places to sit—soft chairs rather than pews—seem to have more people in them. Overall, multifaith chapels seem to have more people in them than neutral chapels, though some of the chapels that chaplaincy directors see as neutral contain religious symbols, as at Overbrook, that are likely comforting to some people but not others. Prayer books play prominent roles as ways for people to connect with each other and the objects of their prayers; they are perhaps the most shared objects actually used in these spaces. Muslims increasingly have their own spaces, but I find light, nature, water, and art emerging as shared symbols in neutral chapels, not the symbols of messy, lived religious traditions in multifaith ones.

Similarly, it is silence that chaplains often see as accessible to all people, not ideas or symbols more specific to religious or spiritual traditions. Following 9/11, the hospital CEO called the director of the chaplaincy department at Oceanview to ask what the institution could do for staff. "I thought of what to do that everybody in the hospital could participate in," she reflected, "and it came to me about having a moment of silence for the whole hospital." She was given access to the hospital public address system, and at 9:00 a.m. she announced, "I'm going to ring the bell, and then we will all be in silence for a minute . . . to remember everybody we lost in the 9/11 tragedy." She told me, "For one moment this whole hospital, everything, stopped. And then a moment later I rang the bell. And there are people that tell me they've never had a moment of silence in the ICU except for that moment."

It is in this silence and the movement toward neutral or generic hospital chapels and prayer and meditation rooms that religion and spirituality are absent in hospitals—paradoxically—in the very spaces where we might most expect them to be present. Interestingly, chaplains were not eager to talk with me about these spaces. While I see them as physical indicators of religious and spiritual inclusivity in hospitals, chaplaincy directors preferred to emphasize other aspects of their work. "By focusing on the chapels and the services," one chaplaincy director asked me pointedly, "do you realize what a small percentage of what we do that reflects?"

Chaplains, like physician and religious ethicist Margaret Mohrmann, preferred to speak about their work in other areas of the hospital. In a recent *Hastings Center Report*, Mohrmann proposed a professional ethic for chaplaincy that encourages chaplains to "see themselves as professionals responsible for creating 'sacred space' within the hospital." Such spaces could be most visibly obvious in the hospital chapel, but they extend more invisibly to "Patients' bedrooms and family waiting rooms . . . operating rooms, nurses' stations, clinics. . . . The ultimate goal would be recognition by the institution as a whole that the entire health-care enterprise—now including board rooms, kitchens, record rooms, and communication centers as well—is sacred space, full of infinite meaning."[54]

I turn from chapels in the next two chapters to focus on the work of chaplains in these other areas of the hospital. While some begin their days in offices next to centrally located chapels, many more chaplains have offices in distant corners of buildings located in areas with less prime real estate. Few spend much time in their offices, however, as they move throughout the hospital, perhaps trying to quietly create in their daily work the sacred spaces Mohrmann describes.

CHAPTER 4

Wholeness, Presence, and Hope: The Perspectives of Hospital Chaplains

Ash Wednesday is one of the busiest days of the year for the Chaplaincy Department at Overbrook Hospital. Catholic patients, visitors, and staff "come out of the woodwork" according to chaplain-priest Father William.[1] While daily interfaith services in the chapel tend to be poorly attended, a sign on the chapel door directed me to the auditorium when I arrived at the hospital on Ash Wednesday. It was the only room large enough to accommodate everyone expected at noon mass.[2]

Before heading to the auditorium, I ducked inside the chapel, where I saw a staff member in blue scrubs and a woman in street clothes help an older man pulling an IV pole approach a table at the front. A do-it-yourself ashes station had been set up, with ashes in a condiment cup from the cafeteria and framed instructions about what to say as you placed them on your forehead or the head of another. Two more people in street clothes followed me into the chapel, and one turned to the staff member to ask where ashes were being given out. "I think it is self-service," he replied, pointing to the station. The second person seemed surprised and then laughed casually, "Self service? I guess food and everything else is these days."

I watched for a minute before heading to the auditorium for mass. I found a place to sit in the back with the close to one hundred others—mostly staff, judging from their scrubs, white coats, and hospital ID badges. A folding table covered in a white cloth was set up at the front of the room and held an electric candle, wine, hosts, and several more condiment cups filled with ashes on Styrofoam cafeteria trays.

Father William, a young-looking seventy, has worked as a chaplain-priest at Overbrook for more than ten years. He wore a white cassock over his usual black clerical collar and began the service of ashes and communion by welcoming his "sisters and brothers" over the sounds of pagers and the occasional cell phone ring. He followed the traditional order of Catholic mass, with two Catholic chaplaincy staff members doing the scripture readings. In his short homily he asked those gathered as a "community of faith" to look around and notice someone present they did not know was Catholic. His wish for the Lenten season, he explained, is that when "you do something for Lent you think of the person you just saw, pray for that person, and do what you do for them as well." By noticing and thinking of others, "we might become the very goodness of God," serve as "ambassadors of God in the world," and better take care of "one another as healers."

Father William prayed over the ashes, "as a mark of repentance, an indication that we are dust, and to help us keep our commitment to Lent," before he and three other Catholic chaplaincy staff placed them on the foreheads of attendees who formed lines at the front of the room. He concluded the distribution of ashes with a prayer for the Church throughout the world during Lent. Included in the prayer were "all those who are ill and those who attend them." A service of Communion followed before the mass ended, and people quietly filed out of the auditorium.

In addition to this mass and the ashes station in the chapel, the Catholic Eucharistic ministry volunteers, who distribute communion to Catholic patients daily, also offered ashes to Catholics throughout the hospital. As I was leaving the hospital, I watched an older visitor step out of the main elevator, notice a Eucharistic minister walking by carrying ashes, and request ashes. As the minister quietly placed the ashes on the man's forehead, five people lined up behind him to receive ashes in the lobby.

This strong Catholic presence was not so publicly evident at Overbrook the rest of the year. Catholic chaplaincy staff sometimes held Catholic services in the chapel, but regular Catholic masses were replaced by interfaith services in the 1990s in an effort to make services more welcoming to all. Of the hospital's nine full- and part-time staff chaplains, three were Catholic, three were Protestant, and one each was Unitarian, Muslim, and Jewish. The explicitly Catholic language present in the mass and the distribution of ashes on Ash Wednesday generally mixed with languages of other religious traditions, of spirituality, and of hope as staff in the Chaplaincy Department did their usual daily work.

To get a sense of this daily work, staff chaplain Meg agreed to let me shadow her soon after I arrived at Overbrook. By 9:00 a.m. on a Friday morning, we were sitting in a conference room filled with dirty plates and cups. "It looks like there was a party and no one invited us," Meg chuckled and began to clean off the table. Meg is assigned to the palliative care service, and as we waited for the weekly team meeting to begin, a nurse opened the door, stuck her head in, and asked Meg to see a patient who, in her words, "just won't die." He wants to die, the nurse explained, the family is ready for him to die, everyone who needs to be in has been in, but still he will not let go. Meg agreed, and after reviewing all of the current and recently discharged patients on the service with the health-care team, she began her rounds in the unit.

After visiting a few other patients, Meg met the wife of the patient the nurse had mentioned. They spoke about her husband's life, their family, his Catholic background, and how the time in the hospital had been for her. The woman then asked Meg to go into her husband's room and say a prayer with him. Although the man was unconscious, Meg entered his room, introduced herself, spoke with him briefly, and then said a prayer like one I heard her repeat many times in subsequent weeks. "I lay my hands on you in the name of God the Father and his son Jesus." Meg talked to God in the prayer, saying that "in God's mansion there are many rooms, and we know that you have a room, God, with those who have come before. God, we know you have things in store that are greater than our imagination, and we ask you to prepare us for them." She ended the prayer in the name of "God the Father, Son, and Holy Ghost" and crossed the gentleman on the forehead. She then sat with him in silence for a few minutes before leaving. Meg checked in again with his wife and was then approached by the family member of another patient I later learned she had never met. This woman was looking for advice about how to speak with her mother, who was dying in intensive care. They spoke for several minutes, and Meg said it was all right to tell her mother that she was dying, even through tears.

We made several more patient and family visits on Meg's other assigned units before she was paged by a social worker named Joanne, who asked for help in the viewing room. As we descended to the basement of the hospital in the service elevators, Meg told me that the chaplaincy and social work departments had been working together to find a space where family members who were not able to be at the hospital when a loved one passed away could see the person's body before it was picked up by a funeral home. A case had come up, and Joanne wanted Meg to help train two social workers. We went first to the morgue, where Meg, Joanne, and two young social workers discussed logistics about the key to the viewing room and how you sign out a body. They then retrieved the body of an older woman who had died that morning and took it to the viewing room to prepare it for family members to visit. When Joanne went back upstairs to meet the family, Meg showed the others how to move the gurney, take off the top sheet, and uncover the dead woman's face. She then sat down in one of the two chairs in the closet-sized room and tried to put the social workers at ease by asking about vacation plans. When family members arrived, the social workers and I left and Meg sat with the family and their relative's body behind closed doors. When the family was ready, Joanne escorted them back upstairs, and Meg and the others returned the body to the morgue.[3] Meg then took off the gloves worn to transport bodies, turned to me, and said it was time for lunch.

On our way to the cafeteria, I thought about how Meg first came to Overbrook Hospital. Unlike Father William, who had been a priest, high school teacher, and university chaplain for years before he was hired as a hospital chaplain, Meg first came as a volunteer to the Chaplaincy Department. She found the work compelling and decided to go back to school to train as a chaplain. She worked as a per diem chaplain as needed until a full-time staff chaplain position opened more than ten years ago. She is ordained as a deacon in a Protestant denomination, has a master's degree in pastoral counseling, and a doctorate of ministry from an area seminary. She is recognized as a board-certified chaplain by the Association of Professional Chaplains.

When I spoke with Meg later in a more formal interview, she told me that "people come literally from all over the world" to teaching hospitals like Overbrook. "We [chaplains] are the ones who make these people not be strangers here. . . . We invite them into the community . . . so that this becomes a safe haven in some regards and a place of hope." "I often say I have a theology of hope," she explained further. "I'll often say to families of patients that when you're five years old you want a red bicycle and when you're twenty-five you want a red convertible. . . . Our hopes do change . . . as we mature and grow, and through life's transitions, the same hopes have to change." In these large hospitals people can often lose hope, but "to lose *a* hope doesn't mean that you lose *all* hope. . . . Part of a chaplain's task is to help people find something to be hopeful about." Sometimes that hope is for a cure for a disease, but more often it is about healing, which Meg describes as "being made whole. Sometimes that wholeness includes a physical response but not always. . . . A lot of the work that we as chaplains do is about reconciliation that helps people to feel whole, to bring them back to what has been, to what is, to what can be, either in this life or the next life, depending on what their theological belief system is."

Although the terms they use are different, Meg's attention to community, to healing, and to hope has some similarities to the messages that Father William emphasized in his homily on Ash Wednesday. In an interview, Father William spoke with me about the "humanity" that chaplains bring to hospitals. While he did not use the word *hope*, he described how he encourages patients, especially those with terminal diseases, not to "die before you die," but to spend the time they have "living. . . . and trying to do whatever you're capable of doing." Father William thinks chaplains are the people in hospitals "who help mobilize the emotional and psychological strengths in people to heal themselves" by encouraging a positive attitude, which he believes "contributes to physical healing as well as spiritual healing." Like Meg, he conceives of healing more broadly than do medical staff members, who usually focus largely on physical cure. Father William believes healing is aided when chaplains talk with people, listen to their burdens of infirmity, and then try to "help mobilize their own resources—whether they be faith or family or friends or whatever" to recover some strength.

*

Father William, Meg, and the other staff chaplains I met at teaching hospitals across the country did not emphasize their specific tasks in conversations about their work. Instead they spoke of the distinct perspectives they bring to hospitals. They described their attention to wholeness and healing sometimes in language specific to their religious traditions, like Father William in the Ash Wednesday mass, but more often in broader, general languages of wholeness, presence, and hope.

These general languages have histories in individual hospitals and in the development of hospital chaplaincy as a profession. Much as Rev. Cook, the first chaplaincy director at Overbrook, described chaplains as those who try to "reflect the wholeness of the patient," the current department director, Pat, emphasized wholeness and healing as she situated the work of chaplains in the realm of spirituality. "I think sometimes chaplaincy is understood too narrowly in some places in the hospital," Pat told me. "It gets equated with religion rather than with spirituality and then can get undervalued." As people who attend to spirituality, or all of the ways people find and make meaning in the world, Pat sees chaplains as the hospital staff members who help patients and families make sense of the crises that bring them to hospitals. "Crisis evokes a spiritual crisis," or crisis of meaning, and chaplains are those who "help people to deal with that dimension of whatever is happening. . . . We're a nonjudgmental presence, and we're probably the only person that enters the patient's room that doesn't have a task. You know, I'm not there to get blood. I'm not there to ask you your psychosocial history. I'm not there to sweep the floor. I'm just there to say, 'How are you doing?'" Through empathetic listening and by being present and paying attention to individuals as whole people, Pat, like Father William and Meg, believes that chaplains contribute to healing, helping people "come to a sense of acceptance, serenity, peace, forgiveness."

This chapter describes how directors of chaplaincy departments and staff chaplains articulate the perspectives they bring and contributions they make to hospitals. After briefly describing who chaplains are and how they came to work as chaplains, I outline the moral, empirical, and policy arguments they make for their work. While some speak of the moral—rather than explicitly religious—basis for their work, others justify it using the secular standards of clinical effectiveness and of the Joint Commission. Much as we saw in increasingly neutral chapels, chaplains downplay images, symbols, and rituals that connect them to specific religious traditions in favor of broader frames. They see these broad frames as their unique contribution to hospitals and as what distinguishes them from other professionals, especially nurses and social workers, who are often their closest colleagues.

Like the neutral chapels, these broad frames are further evidence of what I call an absence of presence or absence of talk connected to particular religious traditions by the professionals trained in these traditions in hospitals. These frames demonstrate how chaplains have attempted to professionalize and extend their professional jurisdiction in religiously diverse hospital contexts. While speaking the language of specific religious traditions might restrict their professional jurisdiction, speaking of spirituality and of wholeness, presence, and hope as broad concepts are jurisdictional expansion strategies intended to make the work of chaplains accessible to as many patients, families, and staff members as possible.[4] While some chaplains sometimes speak within the frame of their own religious traditions—probably especially with patients in that tradition—it is broader languages and more seemingly inclusive frames that dominate when staff chaplains and department directors describe their work to others.

PATHS TO HOSPITAL CHAPLAINCY

Before considering how chaplains see and speak about their work in hospitals, it is helpful to consider who they are and how they came to the profession. As a group, they arrived along multiple paths, with many seeing this work as a vocation. Most of the chaplaincy department directors I met—who had directed their departments for ten years on average—came to chaplaincy work early in their careers. Most came through long-standing interest and experience in Clinical Pastoral Education (CPE), an experiential approach to theological education that takes place in hospitals and other settings. Three-quarters of the directors were ordained as ministers, priests, rabbis, or nuns, and three-quarters were men.

The director at Overbrook Hospital became a CPE supervisor before she became a department director. The director at another hospital took CPE after completing seminary and then began to train as a CPE supervisor before becoming a department director. Two-thirds of the department directors I interviewed were CPE supervisors, and other chaplains often see such training as informally required for such positions.[5] Department directors who were not CPE supervisors generally came to chaplaincy after long careers in congregational ministry. The director of the department at Southern Hospital, for example, was a rabbi for more than twenty-five years before gradually transitioning to chaplaincy after years of visiting congregants and recognizing how much he enjoyed the work. Two-thirds of the department directors I met were mainline Protestant, and the others were either Catholic or Jewish. Evangelical Christians tend to avoid chaplaincy work at the large academic hospitals I studied because of the increasingly interfaith and inclusive nature of the work.[6]

While most of the directors had intended to become chaplains, few of the staff chaplains I met had anticipated becoming chaplains or had come to the work early in their careers. They were older than the U.S. population, as a result. Most first worked as congregational clergy, teachers, campus ministers, or in fields as diverse as banking and entertainment. A few were motivated by personal or family health crises, while many more were trying to bring together personal interests in health and social justice. About half of the staff chaplains I interviewed came to chaplaincy after leading religious congregations. Some of them, like the oncology chaplain at Streamside Hospital, described their professional transitions in terms of substantive interest. "I was really enamored by the whole Elisabeth Kubler-Ross stuff about death and dying" this chaplain remembered, speaking of her experiences as a college student in the 1970s. Also deeply committed to social justice, she worked as a Protestant minister and then in pastoral counseling before finding her way to hospital chaplaincy. Others were less interested in health care than in finding work that was not in a congregation. A rabbi working as a chaplain at Grace Hospital came to the work because, in his words, "I was not finding that I was

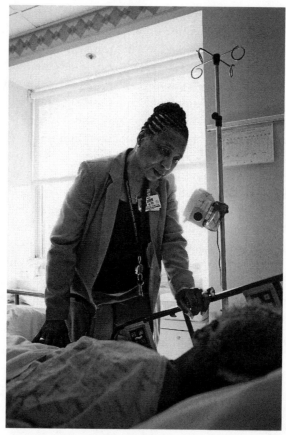

FIGURE 4.1   The Rev. Florine Thompson, BCC, on the clinical staff of HealthCare Chaplaincy and director of pastoral care at St. Luke's–Roosevelt Hospital Center in New York, with a patient. Photo courtesy of HealthCare Chaplaincy, New York, New York.

very happy in a lot of the other rabbinic kind of work I was doing. . . . I started the CPE program one summer really in large part because I hadn't come up with anything else to do." Some, like a chaplain at Southern Hospital, were "fed up with church politics and a lot of the stuff that goes on in churches" that has "nothing to do with ministry whatsoever" and were looking for a change. Some of these individuals settled on chaplaincy work, almost by default, while others had profound experiences in CPE training that drew them to chaplaincy. A chaplain at Forest Hills Hospital, for example, left the congregation she was leading after a "difficult personal situation" and decided to take a unit of CPE "to come to terms with some of my interpersonal issues." She explicitly told her CPE supervisor that she was "not there to become a chaplain" but realized in the process that she loved the work and thought it would suit her in the longer term.

In addition to chaplains who previously served as congregational rabbis or ministers, about half of the chaplains I met came to chaplaincy following unrelated careers.[7] Some raised children. Others worked in other fields. Sarah at Overbrook Hospital worked in finance before deciding in her fifties to do a master's degree in divinity. This led her to take a unit of CPE and then to work as a chaplain because, in her words, "the idea of talking with people about where God is in their lives at different times was very appealing to me." A chaplain at Streamside Hospital decided to become a rabbi on her fiftieth birthday as a second career and was then accepted into a year-long residency program to explore hospital chaplaincy, despite not having the prerequisites or being sure it was something she wanted to do. A chaplain at Sandy Point Hospital sought new work following a workplace injury that ended his first career. He was not aware of chaplaincy when he began his search, but the process of exploring gradually led him there. Only one of the chaplains I met who changed careers had intentionally came to chaplaincy as a second career. Trained as an actor, this chaplain was very involved in the early years of the AIDS crisis. He volunteered much of the time when he was not on stage to related groups, telling me, "The more I did that work, the more I realized that showbiz was becoming an interruption in the work that was filling my soul." He went back to school specifically to become a chaplain.

Staff chaplains trained to become chaplains and were certified as such in a range of ways. Most had master's degrees and were ordained as ministers, priests, rabbis, or nuns. The major professional chaplaincy organizations have attempted to standardize professional training for chaplains and regulate who can become a chaplain by creating the category of "board-certified" to designate those who have completed a related master's degree, have four units of CPE, have the endorsement of a religious organization, pass a committee review, and have paid professional dues to one of these organizations.[8] Despite these standards, few of the seventeen chaplaincy departments I studied required individuals to actually be board-certified to be hired. About half of the department directors told me that chaplains must be eligible for certification to be employed, with the exception of Catholic priests. In the words of the chaplaincy department director at Sandy Point Hospital, "We require that they [chaplains] have four units of Clinical Pastoral Education, that they have a seminary or a graduate degree in religion and an undergraduate degree, and that they're in good standing with their faith group. That's about it. We don't require that they be certified with the Association of Professional Chaplains, but they certainly could be if they wanted to. I leave it up to them."

While prospective chaplains have to be eligible for certification at about half of the hospitals, they do not need to be board-certified or eligible at the other half, illustrating the challenges that professional chaplaincy leaders and organizations have faced and continue to face in their attempts to regulate the profession. A few department directors told me that they are or should be moving in the direction of requiring certification, likely in response to related national developments in the profession. This includes Overbrook, where half the chaplains were board-certified and the other half were not.[9] At City Hospital, the director said chaplains have to be "committed to moving further on those steps to achieving board certification" but do not have to be certified to be hired or to maintain positions they currently have. Hospital administrators at City Hospital only recently learned that board certification was possible for chaplains, though many chaplains had known about the option for years.[10]

Becoming formally recognized as a "board-certified chaplain," often abbreviated as *BCC* after their names, is particularly challenging for individuals who have been chaplains for many years or do not have the master's degree required. As the director at Creekside Hospital explained, some of its chaplains "do not have some of the technical requirements they would have to have [to be board-certified], and they're at a place in their careers where it is not realistic to expect them to [become certified]." He supports the movement toward board certification within the profession and thinks it is what he calls a "luxury, to be in a position where . . . I know the people well enough that I can make exceptions and not believe I'm damaging the standards. . . . I'm not sure it is a luxury we can afford too much longer." Directors of other departments find the standards and process of board certification bureaucratic and unnecessary for chaplaincy as a profession. One such director requires full-time staff chaplains to have two units of CPE, to be ordained, and to have some experience as chaplains, but he does not think board certification is necessary. Absent professional licenses or requirements by regulatory agencies like the Joint Commission, individual department directors and hospitals can hire whomever they want as chaplains, regardless of their professional training and certification.

An important exception is for Catholic priests. Chaplaincy directors often do not require Catholic priests to be eligible for certification both because current national priest shortages make priests difficult to find and because some chaplaincy directors view the tasks that priests perform as largely sacramental and distinct from those of other staff chaplains. The director at Streamside Hospital explained, "Staff priests' functions don't call for the kind of knowledge and skill that APC [Association of Professional Chaplains] certification speaks to. In our design, to be a perfectly good staff priest, you just have to be a perfectly good priest." The majority of Catholic chaplains I interviewed, however, were nuns or lay women, as is the case nationally.[11] Hospitals with large numbers of Catholic patients need priests for sacramental reasons, so they often have them assigned by supervisors or hire them from abroad. In the words of the priest at Streamside Hospital, "I'm assigned here. I'm in effect a gift from the archdiocese to the hospital, and that is why I'm here." Other hospitals or archdioceses looked abroad, usually to Africa or Asia, for priests to meet the shortage. "I had about seven different hospitals that I visited for patient support, for sacramental purposes," in my home country of Nigeria the chaplain-priest at University Hospital explained. "When I came here six years ago, I was formally introduced to hospital chaplaincy as a full-time job." Chaplaincy was one of several things this priest was told he could do when he came to the United States, and he took six units of CPE to help him adjust to his new surroundings and learn about hospitals after he arrived and started to work.[12]

The chaplains and department directors I met came to the work of chaplaincy along multiple paths. Many were seeking a second career, and their training was diverse, like their motivations and professional certifications. Because working in hospitals requires chaplains to interact with people from a range of religious backgrounds, the majority are religiously or spiritually liberal. Those with strong or dogmatic religious positions that they believe to be the only truth (with a capital *T*), tended to be weeded out early in selection processes, either through their own decisions or those of CPE supervisors or department directors. The directors and chaplains I interviewed were much more likely than members of the general population to be mainline Protestant, Catholic, or Jewish. There are few non-Christian chaplains nationally. I met only one Buddhist and one Muslim chaplain during this research, along with a few others who considered themselves humanists and agnostics. Most of the chaplains I met had completed some CPE training, but most departments do not actually require them to be board-certified to be hired. From their positions in departments with different names, as I outline next, most spoke passionately about their work, framing their contributions in one of three ways.

FRAMING THEIR CONTRIBUTIONS

Mission Statements

Hospital chaplains have traditionally worked in departments with *chaplaincy* or *pastoral care*, in their titles. Emerging from the Christian tradition, the term *chaplain* is defined by the *Oxford English Dictionary* as a "clergyman who conducts religious service in the private chapel of a sovereign, lord, or high official, of a castle, garrison, embassy, college, school, workhouse, prison, cemetery, or other institution, or in the household of a person of rank or quality, in a legislative chamber, regiment, ship, etc."[13] *Pastoral care* describes the private support that Christian clergy, and leaders in other religious traditions more recently, provide to individuals, drawing on their theological and psychological traditions.[14] Trying to distance themselves from this Christian past and to become more religiously and spiritually inclusive, several of the hospitals I studied have dropped the words *chaplaincy* and *pastoral care* from their department names, replacing them with the word *spiritual*, a term they view as more inclusive and broadly welcoming.

Seven of the departments I studied include the word *spiritual* in their department names, most commonly using the names Spiritual Care Services or Department of Spiritual Care. Seven others continue to use the phrase *pastoral care*, as in Department of Pastoral Care, and three use the term *chaplain*, as in Chaplaincy Department.[15] The shift to including the term *spiritual* in the formal names of these departments is also marked by use of the term *services*, as in Spiritual Care Services, perhaps indicating the active role that chaplains play (or would like to play) in the hospital.[16] Whether such name changes have caused or are indicative of actual changes in what chaplains do in hospitals is an open question.

Regardless of their names, three-quarters of the departments that chaplains work in have formal mission statements, in which they frame their work in terms of spiritual needs, spiritual care, emotional support, and sometimes hope. Use of the word *religion* or reference to religious rituals is less common. A few departments frame their missions very broadly in terms of the "soul of the institution" or "helping [to] foster a caring presence throughout the Hospital." More departments say they are concerned specifically with the spiritual needs of patients as well as families and staff. Many refer to the holistic care they offer and include a clear statement of their respect for and appreciation of diversity. For example, "The Department of Chaplain Services cares for the spiritual needs of the Pines Hospital community, which includes patients, their loved ones, and Pines Hospital staff." Their services are "born of a respect for every person and for diversity of culture, belief, and religious practice." Members of departments that speak of hope see themselves, as does Meg, as people who can facilitate hope, describing themselves in the words of the department at Streamside Hospital as "a faithful and professional service counted on and supported for contributing hope."[17] Several also note their role as liaisons with local religious leaders who visit hospitalized congregants. Chaplains position themselves as secondary to patients' local religious leaders.

As a group, these departments are strategically vague about what they mean by *spiritual*, and what spiritual needs are in their written mission statements. They speak, for instance, of bearing "witness to the spiritual dimension of illness, suffering, and healing" at Pines Hospital and of "foster[ing] spiritual values for healing" at Lakeview Hospital, allowing patients and staff to come to their own conclusions about what that means. Only two departments refer to God or "the Holy" in their mission statements as related to or being a source of authority in what they do. The mission statement of the department at City Hospital says that its members help "people faced with illness and hospitalization [to] remember that they belong to God and their community," but the mission statement later seems to retract that idea, saying that they help people use their "language and framework of meaning,. . . . whether religious or secular," to "identify and draw on . . . spiritual strengths in facing present circumstances." The department at Streamside Hospital speaks of engaging people's spiritual needs as "intentional reminders of the Holy in our lives and in our care." Other departments tend to say a bit more about how they support people spiritually, explaining that they listen, provide support, and are a nonjudgmental presence in addition to offering tradition-specific and interfaith rituals and services.

Moral, Empirical, and Policy Motivations

In talking about how this spiritual work is important and what it contributes to their hospitals, department directors made three distinct arguments, none in terms specific to individual religious traditions. Moral arguments were most common and made most strongly. Some made these arguments easily, suggesting that they make them often in conversation with colleagues inside and outside of the hospital. Others, especially the four longest-serving directors of departments that have seen little change in staff or mission in the past ten to fifteen years, were surprised by questions about why their work is important and what they contribute to hospitals, and struggled to craft answers, perhaps suggesting that they rarely make the case for their work or talk about it with others in the hospital.

The majority of directors made moral arguments about the importance of chaplaincy, arguing that hospitals need chaplains because they represent an essential dimension of the hospital, because patients are struggling and attending to their spiritual lives is the right thing to do, and because the work chaplains do contributes to healing. The director of the department at Pines Hospital called hospitals not just "technological institutions" but "spiritual endeavor[s]" and "agents of God's care," making the question of why they need chaplains "almost a no-brainer." In his words, "If they [hospitals] propose to care for the needs of a patient, needs are also spiritual" and chaplains, obviously in his view, are the people who address these needs. The director at Oceanview Hospital agreed, arguing that "the higher tech the institution, the more they need spiritual care. . . . The more we need to have that healing touch, that human touch, that very intimate personal touch that the chaplains bring into the environment." Instead of emphasizing the human connection and relationships that chaplains bring, as his colleagues at Pines and Ocean-view Hospitals did, the long-term director of Center Hospital struggled to answer the question of why hospitals need chaplains. He finally answered by explicitly rejecting the dominant spiritual frames of his colleagues, which he finds too broad to be meaningful. Instead he said, "I think they [hospitals] need somebody to represent the religious dimension" but did not explain what that includes or why it is important to do so.

A large fraction of directors framed their moral arguments in terms of the needs of patients, saying that religion and spirituality are important to many patients and paying attention to them is the right thing to do, especially when people are ill. The director at Creekside Hospital said, "The first argument I think most folks will make is that whether the institution and its staff and leaders take religion seriously or not, the patients do." In particular, people who have come from out of town to be treated at these large medical centers, the director at Southern Hospital explained, "feel disconnected from their minister or their source of spiritual direction," and they "look in the hospital for a clergy person." Having these resources available becomes particularly important when people are ill: "Their world is often turned upside down, and if they have a strong faith, it is certainly tested," said the director at Brookfield Hospital. In the words of the director at Grace Hospital, "When people are ill is the time they most need—they're most likely to consider these issues. You need trained people to address that." Crises of health, as the director at

Overbrook explained, "evoke spiritual crises," and chaplains are needed to "help people to deal with that dimension of whatever is happening." These directors framed their constituents broadly and argued that patients, including those who consider themselves religious or spiritual and those who do not, both need and demand chaplains.

In addition to moral arguments, a smaller group of directors made empirical arguments for chaplaincy, pointing, in broad strokes, to social scientific and medical research that suggests a positive relationship between religious, spiritual, and emotional support and health or healing. The director at Forest Hills Hospital, for instance, said he was "convinced" by the "research of our colleague Harold Koenig at Duke showing that healing is fostered by attention to spiritual care. . . . I think there is growing empirical evidence that confirms from a scientific perspective what theologians, and pastors, and priests, and rabbis, and pundits, and imams knew all the way, . . . that if you're sick, . . . you suffer emotionally and spiritually" and attending to both kinds of suffering speeds the healing process. Another director made a similar argument, referencing research about spirituality and healing conducted by Larry Dossey but making clear that none of this research has focused specifically on chaplains. "I think that's what we don't know," this director explained, "how much what we do as chaplains contributes to the healing outcomes." Several chaplains that referenced empirical research did not see it as central to their conviction that chaplains are important in hospitals and make distinct contributions to healing. In the words of the director at Oceanview, "Whether that research proves that [that chaplains help people heal faster] or not, you just intuitively know [that they do] by the stories that the people will tell you. . . . I wouldn't be doing this if I didn't believe in it that much." Her belief comes not from the data or analyses in empirical studies but from her own perspectives and beliefs.

Some chaplains are motivated more empirically than the director at Oceanview and are actively doing their own research to help them understand their contributions. Called "outcomes-oriented chaplaincy," by national chaplaincy leaders, many such studies ask—and attempt to measure—how chaplains influence patient outcomes. This approach was explicitly evident at only one of the departments I studied.[18] This director's vision is to be, in his words, "more and more clear of what our contributing outcomes are," and he and colleagues have developed a model in the past ten years designed to facilitate spiritual care that helps patients and has a measurable impact on patients, their families, and the hospital.[19] The model focuses not on documenting what chaplains do but on documenting the effect their actions have. For example, the director explained, in heart surgery "a very common contributing outcome is [that] the person is able to identify a key value that he or she wants to maintain . . . on the other side of surgery. What we found is people who do that weather the surgery better as opposed to those who want everything to get back to normal." With his colleagues, this director has identified similar values and capacities for patients with a range of other health conditions and created a structured way for chaplains to provide care that contributes both to patients' healing and is documented empirically, published, and shared with others in the field. While some chaplains favor empirical approaches to chaplaincy, others are challenged by them and argue both that they require chaplains to come to patient interactions with too much of an agenda and that chaplaincy work is essentially not measurable.

In addition to moral and empirical arguments, a few directors motivated their work in policy terms, specifically in terms of the Joint Commission.[20] The Joint Commission has made statements about the religious or spiritual care of hospitalized patients since the late 1960s but has never required hospitals to have chaplains to provide that care. Professional chaplaincy organizations have tried to lobby the Joint Commission to require chaplains, and several directors used those arguments, at times slightly exaggerating the required role of chaplains. Two directors argued for chaplains by telling me that the Joint Commission "wants patients to receive spiritual care" and that "hospitals can get censured for not having spiritual care." Another said that the Joint Commission "began mandating some chaplaincy support" in the 1990s, and another affirmed that the Joint Commission "requires hospitals to have a method" for providing spiritual care and that chaplaincy departments are an efficient and cost-effective way to do so. All but the "mandating" of chaplaincy support is true, but only one department director interviewed explained that "you can meet the Joint Commission regulations without a very sophisticated or adequate program."

Unique Contributions

Underlying the moral, empirical, and policy motivations that they described for their work, department directors and staff chaplains emphasized the unique perspectives they bring to their work in hospitals that make them distinct from other staff and frame their professional jurisdiction or profession-specific work. This attention to unique perspectives rather than specific tasks or roles is shared among chaplains, although they do not always agree about what these broadly framed perspectives include. Their perspectives include attention to the whole person, the presence they offer, and the attention they pay to relationships.[21] While many chaplains acknowledged their work with hospital staff, they tended to focus on patients and families when talking about their unique contributions.

Whole Person

Attention to the whole person was one of the dominant themes as chaplains described what is unique to them and their work. "Whole people come into hospitals," the director at Streamside Hospital explained, "not just livers, and kidneys, and lungs, and part of what goes on in health care today takes absolutely every flat-out damn resource the person has if there's going to be healing and thriving as opposed to simple medical curing and recovery." Chaplains contrast themselves to medical staff who, in their view, focus only on the part of patients that brings them to the hospital. Chaplains describe themselves as people who pay attention to individuals as whole beings, caring for their emotional and spiritual needs rather than just their physical ones.[22]

Presence

Chaplains spoke of their unique contributions most frequently in terms of presence. Scott, the CPE supervisor at Overbrook, told me that what chaplains most offer in hospitals is their presence. "Just somebody who walks in, takes them [the patient or family] as they are, listens to their stories, shares their concerns. . . . I think the most we can offer them is just a listening ear, and a caring heart, and somebody who takes them the way they are, who has no expectations." Sarah, a staff chaplain at Overbrook, shared with Scott the importance of presence, saying, "There's a challenge to put words to what we do. . . . It is about presence, about being present for whatever happens."

Chaplains at other hospitals also spoke about presence. This emphasis on presence reflects the central role it plays in Clinical Pastoral Education across the country as supervisors try to teach CPE students to come to human interactions able to empathize with and to respond to whatever is happening.[23] "What I say to new employees" in their orientation, a chaplain at University Hospital explained, "is that pastoral care is about being in solidarity with someone. . . . We simply are present with people; . . . we are a spiritual presence." Providing two recent examples, she spoke first about sitting with a woman in the emergency room whose children were hit by a bus and then about sitting with the family of a man waiting for the clothes of a loved one who had just died and whose body was being sent to the morgue. She also described a chaplain colleague who was called to see a woman who was refusing to go home from the hospital because she felt she was not ready. "The chaplain was called because this woman was getting loud. What happened was the chaplain sat down with her and just listened to her for about an hour and a half and heard her out. And that's the great thing that we really have—the ability to take the time to visit with people that no one else has." The director at Center Hospital also emphasized the time chaplains have, in comparison to others in the hospital, to be really present with patients. "We're probably the only department in the hospital where we have time sitting around to listen to somebody for forty-five minutes. Doctors don't have time. . . . Social workers are into discharge planning. . . . So we're the best resource for patients who have concerns or are struggling over any life issue."

Chaplains can be present with people not just because they have the time but because they are trained through CPE to do so. Explaining a bit more about what it means to be present as taught in CPE, the director at Eastern Hospital explained, "We have a very unique philosophy here in terms of our educational method [CPE], which is don't ask questions; questions are evil. We stay away from an interrogative style because the other health-care disciplines are always about that. . . . There's a real challenge not to ask questions" but to allow the patient to bring up with the chaplain whatever is most relevant for him or her at that moment. Doing so, the Eastern director explained, "allows that person the freedom to make a choice about how to be in the relationship," which is unusual in our culture of questions. When asked what he most brings to patients, the Southern Hospital director reflected this perspective, answering, "My presence; . . . being able to sit down and to listen, to hear people's stories, to let them vent if they need [to]."

I hear chaplains doing much more than just sitting with people as they are present in these examples, though they speak of their contributions in a broad language of presence, rarely explaining how they learn to be present, how their presence differs from that of other health-care staff, and how they see their presence influencing the families and patients with whom they spend time. In contrast to the director at Streamside, who is focused on measuring and documenting what patients and families learn or gain through their experiences with chaplains, this emphasis on presence is much more general and much less concerned with any effort to validate that it has an effect. Many of the chaplains I spoke with were not clear about whether just sitting next to someone is being present or whether some kind of interaction is required and, if so, what sort. They were also not always clear about how their presence differs from that of nurses, social workers, or physicians. The Protestant history of this concept of presence—as developed by Russell Dicks, Carl Rogers, and others, and reflected in CPE and chaplaincy publications—was not an explicit part of conversations about presence, although it silently underlies them, as does a turn to the therapeutic as understood by Philip Rieff.[24] Like the silence arranged by the CEO at Oceanview after 9/11 to bring the hospital together, chaplains' general notion of presence may make them accessible to all, but the notion is so general that it is difficult to know exactly what it means or how patients and families from different backgrounds hear and make sense of it. It also exists in tension with the pressure that chaplaincy directors often feel from hospital administrators to document what they do and what effect it has—pressure and tension that motivate outcome-based chaplaincy efforts among national chaplaincy leaders.

Relationships

In addition to wholeness and to presence, chaplains emphasize the relationships they create with patients and the ones that they help patients create with others in their lives. The director of the department at City Hospital, for instance, spoke of the unique contributions that chaplains make through the example of a cancer patient who was refusing a follow-up course of radiation therapy after chemotherapy and surgery. The patient told her physicians that "God has healed me, and so I have no interest in that [follow-up radiation]." The physicians called the chaplain, expecting him to explain to the patient that treatment was needed. He agreed to meet with the patient, offering her the chance to build a relationship with him rather than to hear a speech about what decisions she should make about her care. He explained to me, "I will be happy to go in and meet this particular patient, but I am not going to go in with that kind of agenda [from the physicians]. . . . I am going to meet [patients]. I'm going to find out where they are today, where they are with their spiritual resources, and I am going to stay with them, and as they move, I am going to accompany them." His goal is to be present and to build a relationship of trust with this patient that will enable him to support her through her decision-making rather than to tell her what to do. A chaplain at Center Hospital described his perspective similarly, saying, "My job is to walk beside someone on their journey. . . . Doctors, and nurses, and staff here are very busy and don't have time to answer some very personal questions—to share

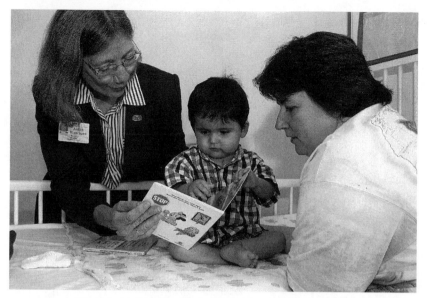

FIGURE 4.2 Chaplain Judith Blanchard visits with a family at the Maine Medical Center. Photo courtesy of the Maine Medical Center.

the experience with them. My job is to do that." This is made possible, in his experience, through the building of a relationship that "enables patients to know that they can share with you their darkest and deepest secrets, fears and wishes."

In addition to relationships that chaplains build with patients, they also speak of the ways they help patients build relationships or resolve issues in relationships with others. For example, the director of chaplaincy at Oceanview spoke of helping a patient with a terminal illness contact and reconnect with relatives. "We've actually watched that happen—watched that brother or sister who they haven't talked to for ten years fly across the country in a plane and walk into that room. That's a huge reconciling moment. It contributes to their peacefulness in death." Such examples are reminiscent of the attention other chaplains give to hope, though the Oceanview director makes clear that chaplains "don't take hope into that room. Hope is already there. We just help the patient discover it, articulate it, and see how they can embrace it."

Despite their formal location in Departments of Spiritual or Pastoral Care, many chaplains made no reference to religion or spirituality in talking about presence, or in describing the relationships they build with patients or the processes they go through to develop them. While chaplains do speak with patients and families about religion if that is where the patient and family are, the director of chaplaincy at Eastern Hospital went so far as to speak of religion/spirituality as a distraction. When he enters a relationship thinking about a patient's religion, "that means that right away I am unconsciously and consciously searching for a way to enter into religious or spiritual life with this person—which is a distraction to the kind of crisis the person is experiencing in the here and now," which is where he should be focused. "More often than not," he explained, "we have a person from a completely different [religious] tradition who is the chaplain. The care-seeker and the chaplain establish a relationship, and the traditions are then forgotten, which is, in my mind, the essence of great spiritual care." This approach, shared by other chaplains, is revealing in that it situates spiritual care outside the bounds of specific religious traditions and takes place when religious traditions are "forgotten" rather than being a source of engagement. This approach may be helpful for chaplains who interact with people from a range of religious backgrounds all day, but it is unique in setting the source of the relationship a chaplain has with them outside of these beliefs and practices. Chaplaincy from this perspective is less about religion than about building a supportive relationship with someone, whoever they are, as they are, that taps into what chaplains assume to be a sense of spirituality that is a universal part of human nature.

While many chaplains see religion or personal senses of spirituality as relatively unimportant in the relationships they build with patients, a few do describe their unique contributions to hospitals in spiritual or religious terms. A chaplain at Streamside distinguished her work from that of therapists by explaining to me that she incorporates a lot of information from the behavioral sciences but is ultimately an expert in the religious and spiritual aspects of people's search for meaning. She told me that, as a Christian and a chaplain, she "represents God," and her care for patients begins there. Staff chaplain Meg at Overbrook Hospital agreed. "I think, number one, we bring God with us. And that because we bring God with us, I think that there's an element of trust—not always—but I think more so than not, between families." She describes chaplains as a "reminder that God is there" and says she could have become a social worker rather than a chaplain but "it wouldn't have rounded me out in the same way because I wouldn't have had the theological touchstones that are important to me." She sees the reminder she brings of God not as a source of division or conflict with families but as a source of trust: "When a chaplain speaks, I think as a rule that people listen—the chaplain is seen as neutralizing, not coming in with an agenda."

Absent from These Perspectives

In emphasizing the attention they bring to the whole person, the value of presence, and their work on relationships, chaplains are silent about other topics that could be unique to their professional jurisdictions. First, although most chaplains are ordained, and those that are board-certified are endorsed by a religious organization, relatively few speak about their contributions to hospitals in the language of their personal faith tradition. Like the concept of spirituality, talk of wholeness and presence situates their work broadly and makes it accessible and relevant to more people than if it was framed in Christian or Jewish terms.

Second, none of the chaplains described efforts to proselytize through their work. Chaplains' professional codes of ethics have long forbidden this, and some chaplains spoke of their own shifts in perspective when transitioning from congregational ministry to chaplaincy. "As a local church pastor," a Protestant oncology chaplain at Forest Hills Hospital explained, "your call is to be evangelistic, to make converts, to know your brand. As a chaplain you're called to be inclusive and supportive of whatever tradition is there. . . . Theologically, I have moved myself from my very exclusivist 'only these people have it right, namely the Christians, since that's what I am' to a place where you're called to appreciate the diversity."

More notably, especially in light of public attention to conflicts over religion, spirituality, and medicine, there is little in what chaplains say to suggest that they regularly mediate in such conflicts. Unlike the physicians and nurses I spent time with who told stories about religion or spirituality as a source of conflict in their work before I asked, chaplains only spoke about conflict in response to my direct questions about it. One chaplain told me that dealing with conflicts is "not how most chaplains spend most of their time," and another said she had never been called to a situation of "conflict between staff and patients on religious grounds."

The few chaplains who did speak of working with conflict described end-of-life situations in which medical staff want to withdraw care, and families want to continue it. As in their other work, they perceived themselves as advocates for patients as whole people in these situations and as individuals who could bridge worlds, conversation styles, and approaches. A chaplain at Creekside Hospital spoke of an end-of-life conflict between a religious family and a medical team, saying that she came in "because I was the only person who they [the family] would accept as not being part of the medical team. So

I was able to build a relationship" not just with the family but with the medical team and the nurses who "felt like they were torturing this child." A chaplain at Streamside Hospital similarly described how chaplains provide space in such situations "for families to move through a process, where, for physicians, it seems very clear cut." She also described how she could help families receiving medical information from the renal team, the ICU team, and the infectious disease team, for example, translate it and "figure out the different pieces to the story" so that they would have "more insight into what's happening by hearing what else is going on."

As they spoke about conflicts around religion, spirituality, and health care, several chaplains mentioned reasons why dealing with them is not central to their professional jurisdictions. First, they told me that the nurses and physicians most commonly involved may not regularly think to call chaplains in these situations. A Jewish chaplain said he gets called by nurses "when there is someone on the unit who wants to celebrate Shabbat in a particular way that is disruptive" but not often for nonritual needs. Second, it may be that other staff members, such as those in Departments of Patient and Family Relations or those working around bioethics, are responsible for dealing with such conflicts in their hospitals. Third, even if they were called, chaplains do not usually have the status in the hospital to deal with such conflicts, especially if they include physicians. As a chaplain at Forest Hills Hospital explained, "In the hierarchy, quite honestly, the physician has way more power than a chaplain. And you don't tend to referee when you're in the lower power positions and it is not a definition of your job, after all. . . . Any chaplain who is going to go up against a doc is just not thinking straight because of the power difference."

While not called so often to deal with conflicts related to religion or spirituality, it is interesting to note that a few chaplains did speak of being the people called, almost as the last resort, to serve as a "calming presence" when there were other conflicts or problems in the hospital—usually involving patients or family members. One chaplain recounted, "There can be some pretty explosive situations . . . some doctors go off sometimes, nurses can go off with clerical people and vice versa." She tries to calm people down in such situations. This also happens with visitors. A chaplain told me about getting a call from a maintenance man who asked him to come to the front door of the hospital. "I thought, oh my gosh, what is this about? So I went down, and he [the maintenance man] said, 'You have to do something with those two women out there.' And it was two women who had their father in the hospital, they had been drinking, they were arguing, and so I went out and sat between them—it happened to be a warm day—and tried to do some kind of peacemaking, which I'm not sure worked at all."

Healing

Underlying the range of perspectives that chaplains see themselves uniquely bringing to patients and families are their commitments to helping people heal. Chaplains are quick to distinguish physical cure from broader notions of healing, which they define as helping people be made whole. While they do not see themselves curing, they do think they help people heal by, in the words of the director at Oceanview, "trying to bring some kind of meaning or some kind of wholeness, no matter what is going on." Explaining by example, this chaplain described working with a family whose infant had died to create a way they could bring their five-year-old daughter to the hospital to help her understand what happened and, with the chaplain's support, meet and say some words to her dead sibling in a way that could begin to bring her and her family some healing.

Chaplains, almost uniformly, believe healing happens when people feel

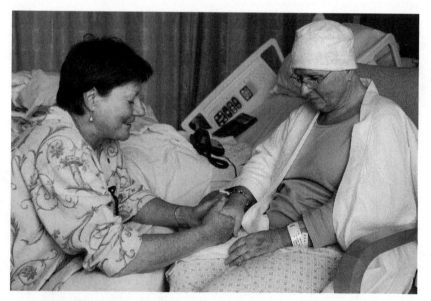

FIGURE 4.3 Chaplain Katrina Scott prays with a patient at the bedside. Photo by Steven H. Gardner, M.D.

cared for and can motivate their inner resources rather than when they themselves say certain prayers or call on an all-powerful God or higher power to magically intervene. As Scott, a chaplain at Overbrook, explains, "I think healing happens to people because they feel understood or cared for." Others say, "My work as a chaplain fosters healing for patients because it gives emotional support and assurance," and "I think it [healing] is 90% relational." Chaplains see themselves providing this support, in part, by entering into relationships with people as described above. "I think that we can be catalysts [for healing] if people invite us into their lives and are beginning to explore some of their own issues" explained a chaplain at Southern Hospital. And in the words of another, similar to Pat the director at Overbrook, "Spiritual care is not the work of the chaplain but the work of the patient. What the chaplain does is facilitate, lead, help."

CONCLUSIONS

Father William, Meg, and other staff chaplains at Overbrook and hospitals across the country see themselves contributing to people's healing as they are present with them, pay attention to them as whole people, and build relationships—even if a relationship lasts only until the patient is discharged. They conceive of the mechanisms by which people are healed as psychological and relational more than theological or God-centered. They talk of understanding people and offering emotional support rather than saying prayers or conducting rituals that they believe will call God or a higher power into the room in a way that may heal through supernatural presence. It is not that they or God or a higher power can heal, chaplains generally believe, but that people can heal themselves when they feel supported and loved.

While chaplains certainly pray and sometimes conduct religious rituals in hospitals, it is this particular relational perspective that they see as their unique contribution to their institutions, as they talk about wholeness, presence, and relationships.[25] These perspectives are informed both by the Christian, especially mainline Protestant, history of chaplaincy as a profession and by the fact that, in relation to national religious demographics, a disproportionate number of chaplains are themselves mainline Protestants. They are also informed by broad societal norms concerning individualism, pluralism, and the need in health care for seemingly nonreligious responses to moral problems, as described by sociologist Raymond DeVries to help explain the growth of bioethics.[26]

Chaplains offer different motivations—moral, empirical, and policy-related—for why their work is important, and they see themselves as among the few staff members in hospitals who can remind patients, families, and medical caregivers of the larger contexts in which they work and in which their patients live. In speaking of these contexts, however, chaplains are careful, even as they hold tradition-specific services (e.g., on Ash Wednesday at Overbrook) to articulate them in ways they believe are inclusive for all. Some clearly distinguish their work from that of social workers, nurses, and psychologists, saying, as does the director at Streamside, "There's a lot of overlap. The main thing is that the focus is different. The nurses' focus is the medical care of the patient. The social worker is psychological and placement as I understand it. And ours is primarily spiritual." Others are less certain of these distinctions among professions.

Like the language of spirituality, which has a history, means different things to different people, and is deployed by chaplains strategically as a jurisdictional expansion strategy in hospitals, the relational perspective of chaplains and their broader talk of wholeness, presence, and relationships is understood in various ways by patients, families, and staff. These understandings are complicated at Overbrook by the Catholic Eucharistic ministers, Protestant visitors, and CPE students, who also move through the hospital with "Chaplaincy" on their ID badges but do things quite differently than do staff chaplains. Many patients and families at Overbrook are unable to distinguish these students and chaplaincy volunteers from staff chaplains, nor do they understand what role each plays in the hospital. Even with staff chaplains there are disconnects—evident at Overbrook with some Muslim families and the Muslim chaplain. Explaining that chaplaincy and notions of presence are fundamentally Christian concepts, Aalam, the Muslim chaplain, told me that he brings Muslim patients practical information about Friday prayers, halal food, and local mosques while they are in the hospital. While Pat might describe Aalam's work in terms of her broad sense that chaplains "care for the soul of the institution," his own perspective points to the different needs of patients from different religious backgrounds that go beyond presence, a concept some Muslim patients would not understand.

Some chaplains, like the director of the department at Pines Hospital, are also skeptical that chaplains' perspectives on presence and relationships are clear and mutual enough to be the basis of their professional jurisdiction.[27] While the 2001 paper, "Professional Chaplaincy: Its Role and Importance in Healthcare," issued jointly by the major professional chaplaincy organizations, listed things that chaplains do, this director told me I would find that "chaplains do all kinds of stuff that other people do. . . . One could go through it [the list of chaplain's tasks in this paper] and say, 'Well, you don't have to be a chaplain to do that. A social worker can do that or a volunteer.' [You could] almost put yourself out of business that way."[28] Giving an example, he said, "Now if you say you're a non-anxious presence—well, lots of people can be a non-anxious presence. . . . We're not psychiatrists, psychologists, social workers, nurses, or physicians." Some of what takes place in his department, like religious rituals, require a chaplain, but much of the rest of it does not. He is, as a result, asking "our national [professional chaplaincy] certifying organizations as well as our chaplains" to think and say more about what chaplains do, apart from these religious rituals, that is uniquely their own. Professional chaplaincy organizations and chaplains rarely emphasize religious rituals as their unique contributions or professional jurisdictions because not all chaplains perform them; they can seem more exclusive than inclusive of all patients, and they frame the work of chaplains narrowly in terms of religion rather than broadly in terms of spirituality, which opens up their jurisdiction and constituents.

The flexibility and potential for jurisdictional expansion of wholeness and presence were evident among the chaplains with whom I spent time. Hope may be the frame of the future, as was evident when a Public Relations Department at an academic hospital related to one of those described here wanted to put together a new brochure to describe its chaplaincy department. The head chaplain had worked at this hospital for almost thirty years. At first, his services were mostly described as religious, a frame that has shifted to use of the term *spiritual* in the last ten to fifteen years. Describing recent transitions and efforts to create the brochure, this director said, "We had the perfect good storm." As the hospital was grappling with cultural diversity initiatives and privacy issues, "there was a subcommittee on spirituality" as part of this process that "started this journey of trying to define spirituality so we could put it in this brochure. . . . If you dilute the word too much, it loses everything. If you make it religious, then you're not being culturally sensitive, because there are those who do yoga, and that is their spirituality or transcendental meditation." In his view, all of these approaches are "different cars but you're driving the same, you know, the same purpose here." Eventually the committee decided on wording for this brochure that would be "sensitive to your spirituality" and that tried to "somehow define it without using religion." They sent the materials to Public Relations, and, in this chaplain's words, "they jumped on the word *hope*, which I never thought about because, if you look at it, hope personifies spirituality, regardless of religion, regardless of whatever. What I'm learning at my age," he reflected, "is that everything comes back," sometimes with a different name or title, but the same general idea. The resulting brochure says that the stress of seeing a loved one through a "frightening and traumatic time can cause both spiritual and emotional strain." At this hospital, "there is comfort; that comfort is hope," which is supported and nurtured by the chaplaincy department.

Whether they frame what they do in terms of hope, healing, presence, or wholeness, most of the chaplains I met believe—more intuitively than empirically—that they bring a human touch and connection that facilitates healing. The next chapter examines how the hospitals in which they work facilitate their ability to do so.

CHAPTER 5

Essential or Optional?
How Hospitals Shape the
Professional Tasks of Chaplains

Pat, the director of chaplaincy at Overbrook Hospital, stood in the doorway of the department office one afternoon wearing blue scrubs. She usually dressed in slacks and a blazer, so I was surprised to see her with a surgical mask around her neck until I remembered that she was attending an organ donation. Chaplains attend organ donations with the donor's family at Overbrook, and they recently also started to provide support to operating-room staff working on related cases. Chaplains bless the organ donors in the operating room, share details about the donor's life with the nurses and technicians, or pray as staff members prepare for the surgeries.

Working more closely with families and staff around organ donations is one of several ways that Pat has tried to increase the visibility of the Chaplaincy Department and the range of ways that chaplains are involved in daily life at Overbrook. When she became the director of the department several years ago, her boss, a vice president of Patient Care Services, asked her to develop a formal mission, vision, and values statement for the department. In her words, "to make ourselves more visible within the hospital. . . . It wasn't that we weren't doing good stuff, . . . but we weren't as known." Chaplains needed to get themselves out there, she told me, to be "more connected to the [other] departments."[1]

Staff chaplains have tried to do this as they visit the sickest patients in the hospital and sit on committees, including Ethics, Palliative Care, Organ Donation, Bereavement, Staff Support, Bioethics, and Domestic Violence. Chaplains lead or co-facilitate support groups for patients with specific health conditions and attend family meetings and professional education sessions with a wide range of staff. In addition to leading daily interfaith services, the Chaplaincy Department celebrates Nurses Week, during which chaplains push a cart around the hospital offering tea to nurses and blessings for their hands. A chaplain is physically present on call in the hospital, twenty-four hours a day, seven days a week. To help staff chaplains with increasing amounts of work and prepare more people to be professional chaplains, the department started a program for several chaplain residents who work full-time as chaplains for one year while completing three units of CPE and preparing for future work as chaplains.[2]

Staff chaplains see themselves as more involved in day-to-day work at the hospital than they used to be, but not all staff members know who chaplains are or understand or respect what they do. There are still nurses, a chaplain resident told me, who are surprised to learn that the hospital has chaplains, even though they are introduced to them at new employee orientation. "It [chaplaincy] is becoming more accepted," another chaplain resident explained, "but I think sometimes the [medical] professionals don't recognize that we're professionals and that we have something to bring forth." Catholic Eucharistic ministers say nurses do not always take their efforts to bring communion to patients seriously, and in a recent internal survey, the department found that about one-third of the time nurses do not ask patients whether they would like to see a chaplain, as they are supposed to do. When the question is asked, and the patient says yes, nurses do not pass that information along to chaplains in more than half of cases. About 90% of people referred to the Chaplaincy Department are eventually seen, but finding that nurses do not always pass along requests makes the task of connecting patients and families with chaplains that much more complicated.[3]

Such problems are not limited to nurses, who often work more closely with chaplains than other staff members. According to Scott, a staff chaplain and the CPE supervisor at Overbrook, chaplains get more respect than they used to, but there are still physicians who interrupt and "take over" the conversations that chaplains have with patients. In a large hospital like this one, space is also an issue. Just back from a meeting about the design of a newly planned building, Pat was frustrated one afternoon that the Nutrition Department was automatically given space in the new building, but when she asked for one office that two chaplains could share, the project manager replied, "Do you really need it?" and "Couldn't they [chaplains] just work from the offices over there [in another building]?" These questions, Pat told me, show that the project manager did not grasp "the significance of the work that we do and how it would be helpful, particularly for the families, if we were closer.

They're not going to come across the street looking for us." Such interactions reflect Pat's continued efforts to educate colleagues about the work of chaplains and to increase their professional profiles and legitimacy in the institution. Pat is closely in touch with evolving national standards, and changes in the Chaplaincy Department at Overbrook under her leadership reflect the department's transitional status and continued efforts to meet emerging professional norms.

*

Professional statements, standards of practice, best practices, and quality-improvement efforts in the last ten years have aimed to improve the professional standing of chaplains nationally. This chapter focuses on how the unique perspectives that chaplains see themselves bringing to hospitals are shaped by hospitals as institutions and translate into specific tasks. I focus less on the broad range of tasks that chaplains describe themselves doing than on what, if anything, all chaplains do that defines their professional jurisdiction or unique work in action.

I find that chaplains across hospitals do not agree on what their essential tasks are, though most listen to people's stories and work with ethics. They also manage death for hospitals. In addition to the commonalities, there are many differences. Differences in what chaplains do and when they are physically present demonstrate that chaplaincy directors, individual departments, and broader hospital contexts, rather than nationally shared professional practices or policies, strongly influence how chaplains spend time.[4]

I delineate differences in the work chaplains do at these hospitals and when they are present by first identifying three ideal types of departments that emerged inductively on the basis of what chaplains do at their hospitals *in addition* to the common tasks of hearing stories, working with ethics, and managing death. These types reflect the work of chaplains as well as where they are administratively situated in hospitals, whether they are paid by hospitals, whether they must be trained as board-certified chaplains to be hired, whether they are part of hospital protocols, and how volunteers and Clinical Pastoral Education (CPE) students are included in departments. I name these ideal types professional, transitional (like Overbrook), and traditional and then explain variations among them in terms of how departments developed, how directors built the professional jurisdiction of chaplains over time, and how broadly or narrowly directors conceived of chaplains' work.

Underlying discussion of these ideal departmental types are questions about legitimacy, or the authority on which chaplains do their work in hospitals. While board certification, standards of practice, and professional statements are recent strategies that chaplains have utilized nationally to try to establish themselves professionally, the stories that emerge in this chapter show many chaplains—like Pat as she explained to the project manager who chaplains are and why their work is important— struggling locally, which contributes to their seeming absence even when they are physically present. I conclude this chapter by describing how department directors and staff chaplains are trying to establish their legitimacy and improve their low status through staff education, writing in the charts of patients, and continued efforts to make the case for their profession.

ESSENTIAL AND CONSISTENT WORK

Arriving at Overbrook on a Sunday afternoon, I met staff-chaplain Tricia and spent three hours shadowing her through the hospital and learning about her daily work. She visited patients on her assigned units, those preparing for surgery the next day, and anyone else who seemed in need. We checked waiting rooms for family members who could use an ear or some supportive words and talked to staff members, patients, and families as we moved through the hospital. Tricia's longest visit, for which she had to put on gloves and a paper gown, was with an immune-compromised patient secluded behind curtains and glass doors. With some patients, Tricia talked; with others she prayed, and with others she recited psalms, or Hail Mary's, or simply reminded them that chaplains are available at any point.[5] In some cases, Tricia told me, she aims to connect with the patient, while in others—especially when the patient is not conscious or seems likely to die—she spends extra time with family members to build a relationship that might be supportive for them down the line when, in her words, "the bottom falls out." While there were no administrative meetings on a Sunday, Tricia tidied the chapel before she left for the day and made sure to check in with the CPE students also working in the hospital to see if they needed any support.

Chaplains like Tricia have many tasks in hospitals, usually more on weekdays than weekends.[6] The 2001 paper "Professional Chaplaincy: Its Role and Importance in Healthcare" listed no fewer than forty-eight different services and tasks that chaplains perform, grouped into ten main categories. These tasks and actions include serving as "a powerful reminder of the healing, sustaining, guiding, and reconciling power of religious faith"; extending care to those of different religious groups without proselytizing; providing spiritual care through empathetic listening; working as part of interdisciplinary patient-care teams; conducting religious rituals and worship; serving as leaders or participants in hospital ethics programs; educating hospital staff and students about the "relationship of religious and spiritual issues to institutional services"; providing mediation and advocacy for patients, families, and staff; making assessments for referrals; and being involved in research regarding pastoral care assessment and efficacy.[7] Chaplains at all of the hospitals I studied do some of these tasks, but almost none of the chaplains I met do all of them.

Chaplaincy researchers, including the authors of the 2001 paper, have spent considerable time documenting what chaplains do to improve understanding about the profession and increase its status in health care. Several studies suggest that chaplains spend about half their time with patients/families and the other half doing educational/administrative tasks.[8] Chaplains spend the most time with patients in traumatic situations, including at the end of life.[9] In addition to the 2001 paper, chaplaincy researchers have developed other frameworks to describe the most common roles of chaplains. A 2005 study divides the tasks into seven categories, including grief and death, emotional support, community liaison, directives and donations, religious services and worship, consultation and advocacy, and prayer.[10] Despite these studies, chaplaincy researchers tend to conclude that there is little consistency in what chaplains do.[11] Despite the energy that national chaplaincy leaders are putting into outcomes-based approaches, few studies focus on outcomes or attempt to demonstrate what effect chaplains have on patients and families—a question often of more interest to physicians, nurses, and hospital administrators than long lists of the tasks chaplains perform.

Essential Work

Rather than adding to typologies that delineate the tasks of chaplains, I ask when hospitals see the work of chaplains as essential and on what occasions they are always present. In what kinds of situations in these seventeen hospitals, in other words, are chaplains always called? I find that there is no single situation at all of these hospitals in which chaplains are always called.

At about three-quarters of the hospitals, there are situations in which chaplains are always called, but the nature of these situations varies among hospitals. At one, chaplains have become a part of multiple protocols, so they are called automatically, so that, in the words of one director, "another member of the team [does not have] to make an independent judgment that a chaplain is needed [and make] a phone call [to get] us there." They are called at Stream-side Hospital "for all deaths, partly because we're the grief folks, and we're also the designated requesters for tissue and organ donation [i.e., the people trained to ask family members about donating a loved one's tissues or organs]. We're called for all level-one traumas, . . . all cardio-pulmonary resuscitations, . . . all stoke patients, all victims of violence, all transplant patients." At most hospitals, chaplains are automatically called in only one or two situations, usually code blues when a patient's heart stops, deaths, deaths if family members are present, or traumas. At Creekside Hospital a chaplain gets the same page the surgeons do when there is a trauma. "We are the people who place the calls to the family" in these situations, a Creekside staff chaplain explained, "and then we meet and greet the family" when they arrive and stay with them when they talk with the physicians. While some chaplains grumble about getting such calls, especially in the middle of the night, many recognize being automatically called as a mark of professional recognition and status—an indication that they are needed in the hospital. Recalling the time and energy that has gone into becoming a part of protocols and seen as essential to hospitals over the years, the director at Eastern Hospital said that these calls are "part of the professional recognition that we have worked hard to achieve."

At the other quarter of hospitals, there are no situations in which a chaplain is always called or present. Particularly when someone dies, the directors at two of these hospitals said they thought a chaplain should be called but were uncertain about how to balance doing so against their limited staffing resources. In the words of one, "We don't get called for all the deaths, . . . which is all right because we're not always needed, and we just don't have enough resources to get to all of them." He went on to say that he thought chaplains should be there, especially when infants die, because "families are often there and traumatized, and need the support; teams are often traumatized; . . . roommates are often traumatized." In these situations and other code blues, he saw a need for someone "who is not caught up in the tasks of trying to resuscitate, who might be identified as a supportive presence." Another director, relatively new in that position, was surprised to learn that chaplains do not go to all deaths at his hospital. He thought this "ought to be a minimum requirement" for their work but had not yet tried to make the change. Other department directors thought the burden of always being called to deaths or code blues outweighed the benefits. "You end up focusing all your energy on calls, on codes," the director at City Hospital explained. "I've been just as pleased not to put us in that position." Others said it was just not possible, given their staffing limitations, or that it was "not the best use of our time," given that "the code team knows that we exist and certainly, if need be, we are called."

Consistent Work

Since there is no work that these chaplaincy departments and hospitals agree is essential for chaplains or times when chaplains are always present, I next consider what chaplains at these hospitals consistently describe as aspects of their work. Apart from when they are paged to emergencies, chaplains spend roughly half of their work time devoted to patient and family visits on hospital units.[12] They tend to focus on the sickest patients—in intensive care—and their families, as well as on trauma patients, often in the emergency room. They see their roles as secondary to those of patients' own religious or spiritual leaders, but they describe meeting many patients who are not involved in conventional religious or spiritual organizations and have no such leaders to call, especially when facing end-of-life situations.

A primary way in which Tricia at Overbrook and chaplains across the country consistently put their perspectives on wholeness, presence, and relationships into practice is through stories and the facilitation of storytelling by patients and families. Many of their interactions are short—a single ten- or twenty-minute visit—but chaplains speak of stories even in these contexts.[13] Only one hospital trains chaplains to follow a specific approach when working with patients and families to determine how they can best spend time. It has little to do with stories; instead, it is outcome-based, focused, in the director's words, "on literature in the field" that moves beyond being present with another to "take it to the next level." This next level is oriented toward making chaplains "accountable," in the words of the director, for offering interventions that lead patients to have certain kinds of experiences and outcomes during their time in the hospital. At all the other hospitals, chaplains make their own decisions about which patients to see and how to interact with them, and they consistently emphasize the opportunities they create—in the process—for patients to tell their stories. Chaplains describe their authority in so doing not in terms of God or other religious or spiritual sources, nor in terms of particular therapeutic, psychological, or pedagogical models. Rather, they speak in terms of their intuition and the healing value of stories.

Scott, the CPE supervisor who trains the chaplain residents at Overbrook, told me that "our intuitions are our biggest servants." He tries to teach the residents to "pay attention to their intuitions, . . . to give people openings and tell them that you're interested in hearing their story." Ninety percent of the time, he says, people respond to that and share their stories, which he and the chaplains at Overbrook believe is inherently healing and a central part of their work.

The value of intuition and of storytelling in chaplain-patient relations was particularly evident in the graduation ceremony for chaplain residents at Overbrook that marked the end of their year of residency. Scott opened the thirty-minute ceremony, held in the hospital chapel, by quoting *The Little Prince* and describing how wonderfully the residents cared for patients in the hospital and for each other. He went on to say that "as chaplains, we are inviting people to share their soul prints with us as they tell stories about what it is like to be who they are." I understood "soul prints" to be like fingerprints—unique to each of us but held in common He then spoke about each resident, not mentioning their personal religious backgrounds, or rituals they conducted with patients, or even speaking of spirituality in a general way. Instead he focused on how each resident facilitated storytelling with particular patients by following his or her intuition. He described residents hugging patients, bringing photos of Winnie the Pooh printed from the web to help them connect with patients, singing to patients, and communicating with non-English-speaking patients in gestures. He spoke of one resident sitting with a patient who was waiting for her stem cells to arrive; together, they placed their hands on the cells to say a prayer before they went into her body. Interactions between chaplain residents and patients that were celebrated at the ceremony were impromptu, improvised, and centered on helping patients tell their own stories. While social scientists and individuals working in the field of narrative medicine think carefully about narrative and sometimes analyze stories to determine what effects they have on the listener and the storyteller, these questions of cause and effect are far from the ways that chaplains speak of stories as facilitating relationships between themselves and patients.

At hospitals other than Overbrook, the value of stories was also emphasized among other things that chaplains described themselves doing in their interactions with patients and families. A chaplain at Oceanview Hospital described his interactions with patients as a dance. "I kind of introduce myself and usually let them do the leading to see where they want to go. . . . I definitely want them to know that they're in control because there is very little in their experience that gives them any control." Chaplains emphasize sitting with people, touching them, and leading meditations or visualizations as standard parts of their visits. Some leave patients with business cards or objects like small rocks to symbolize their conversation and time together. In only a few hospitals are chaplains explicitly not allowed to engage in certain practices with patients. One staff chaplain told me she is not allowed to do Reiki—a hands-on healing technique—with patients, to massage patients, or to perform exorcisms intended to remove bad spirits. She interpreted these guidelines broadly, though, saying, with reference to the exorcisms, that there was a patient "who was convinced that the visitor who had come to see her" had done "something really evil to the room and had left a mysterious butt indention in the chair." The chaplain said she "did what could be loosely called a blessing in the space" to "cleanse" it.

In addition to visiting with patients and families and facilitating the telling of personal stories, staff chaplains spend about half their time on educational and administrative work—mostly sitting on committees and supervising students and volunteers. In the words of one chaplain, "I think that's what the public would be most amazed by. . . . They probably picture chaplains, and it is this way in some hospitals, you hit the ground running and you're seeing patients nonstop all day. But I think the reality is, in a lot of hospitals, chaplains who have been around for awhile are on hospital committees, they're doing administrative things, they're teaching. . . . I think it is kind of a juggling act. It probably is for most." Through this administrative work, chaplains

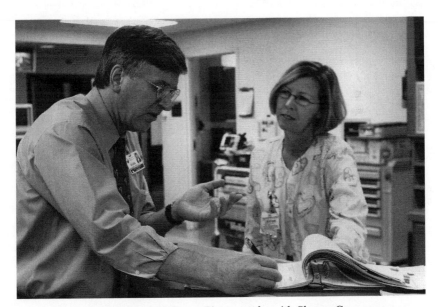

FIGURE 5.1 Chaplain Mark LaRocca-Pitts consults with Sharon Crampton, a nurse. Photo by Terry Allen.

consistently describe paying attention to ethics and specifically sitting on ethics committees, where some describe themselves having a "pretty strong presence." In a few cases, a chaplain is actually the co-chair of a hospital ethics committee. Particularly at the teaching hospitals described here, chaplains also spend time mentoring chaplaincy residents in year-long programs or interns participating in ten-week or longer CPE programs. "I'm one of the mentors for the CPE students," one chaplain explained, "so the first thing that I do when I come in [in the morning] is I'll make up these lists, . . . the lists of the patients I want them to visit." Another explained, "Part of the job of a senior staff chaplain is the oversight of care, . . . helping students get on board."

THREE IDEAL TYPES

Tricia, Meg, Father William, and the other staff chaplains I met at Overbrook enact their commitments to wholeness, presence, and relationships as they encourage patients and families to tell their stories, sit on hospital committees, mentor CPE students, and manage death for the hospital. They also attend organ donations, co-facilitate support groups, host Nurses Week, and engage in a range of other tasks as Pat tries to raise their visibility and improve their collective status in the hospital. Looking at *what else* chaplains do—in addition to facilitating storytelling and working with ethics and death—at these seventeen hospitals suggests that chaplaincy directors and the historical context of a hospital rather than broad norms or standards of professional chaplaincy organizations strongly influence chaplains' work, which helps to explain decisions about when they are called to be physically present and the variation in their tasks across hospitals.

Three ideal types emerge from descriptions of these additional actions by directors and staff chaplains, reflecting three distinct approaches to chaplaincy at large academic hospitals.[14] These types reflect not the size of departments, but the extent to which chaplains are seen and treated as professionals—individuals with distinct contributions to make to medical teams—who are integrated and involved in daily hospital life. These types reflect the tasks that chaplains perform and emerge from the positions in which chaplains are situated administratively in hospitals, whether they are paid by hospitals, whether they must be board-certified to be hired, whether they are part of hospital protocols, and how volunteers and CPE students are included in their departments.[15] I describe each ideal type in turn before discussing the factors that explain some of the variation among hospitals. While leaders in professional chaplaincy have focused a significant amount of attention on preparing individuals to be professional chaplains, these three ideal types point to the central and significant roles that hospitals as institutions play in facilitating or impeding the ability of chaplains to do that professional work.

Professional Departments

Four of the seventeen departments I studied are what I consider professional departments in which chaplains are treated as professionals with distinct contributions to make to medical teams. These are the hospitals that most allow chaplains to do what they are trained to do through the process of becoming board-certified. Chaplains in professional departments tend to be well integrated into hospitals and are automatically called or regularly integrated into hospital protocols; they are seen as essential by the hospital and are always present in some situations. They tend to sit on many committees, participate regularly in interdisciplinary teams, and to be clearly oriented to patient and family care as a first priority. The directors of such departments generally report to high levels in the administration of the hospital—to a vice president or above. Staff chaplains are paid directly by the hospital rather than by outside organizations, which makes them more accountable to the institution, and they normally must have the equivalent of board certification in order to be hired. While these departments may include CPE students or volunteers, these individuals are mentored by staff chaplains and clearly understand what they can and cannot do and how they can and cannot represent themselves in the hospital.

The director of one such department stated that its members "intend everything about" the department "to start with our patients, their loved ones, and the hospital staff." He and similarly oriented directors recognize that staff chaplains, students, and volunteers bring different training, skills, and expertise to departments, and they divide work among them accordingly. Many prefer not to have many volunteers, both because volunteers need to be supervised and because they are not well trained or as accountable to the institution as are staff chaplains. They also do not rely on CPE students for the bulk of patient and family care. As one director explains, "Our [chaplain] residents do a good share of pastoral care as well as [being] on call, but we don't hire them to do that as some programs do because they have a small staff. They [other programs] almost have to exclusively rely on their CPE students to do that work." Directors of professional departments tend to share a vision of high-quality care for patients and families provided by staff chaplains who are as visible and integrated into the hospital as possible.

Departments in Transition

Three of the seventeen departments are not fully professional departments as described above but are oriented to the same goals and are in processes of transition. They tend to have directors, like Pat at Overbrook, who are relatively new to the job and are trying to orient the department toward patient and family care and the broader needs of the institution. As at Overbrook, these directors are often trying to make chaplains more visible by placing staff chaplains on interdisciplinary teams and committees and trying to convince their hospitals to hire and pay all staff chaplains directly rather than relying on financial support from dioceses, synagogue councils, and other religious organizations outside the hospital.

These departments also tend to have two tiers of staff—an older group of staff chaplains who were hired with less training and certification, and a newer group of staff chaplains more oriented to the developing professional standards and norms of the profession. Some of these departments continue to rely on volunteers or CPE students, in lieu of or in addition to staff chaplains, either because they feel it is necessary or because they are slowly trying to decrease the size of their volunteer pools. As one such director explained, "When I got here [one year ago], we had a plethora of volunteers. I immediately started to establish some protocol and criteria, and we had a lot leave once that became established. My reasoning behind that . . . is that we are establishing a professional discipline, and traditionally volunteers in a hospital system are not prepared to become professionals. . . . My interest is again becoming on parity with the health-care team to establish a very rigorous set of criteria in terms of compliance, in terms of CPE training, and so forth." It is not that volunteers do not add to hospitals, in this director's view, but that retaining volunteers to provide some care while aiming to establish chaplaincy as a professional field undercuts the idea that chaplains are professionals with distinct training and skills. While transitional departments may not automatically become professional departments, their directors are oriented to the same standards and are trying to facilitate the transition.

Traditional Departments

The remaining ten departments are more traditionally oriented, and the work that chaplains can do in these hospitals is more limited by their institutional contexts. While some chaplains who work in these departments are board-certified, the standards of their training and the responsibilities they have in their institutions do not always match. Simply put, they are less physically present as a group in these hospitals. Many chaplains in traditional departments tend to "fly below the radar" or to work as "lone rangers" or "cowboys," in their own words, rather than on interdisciplinary teams with other health-care professionals. There are few to no situations in which chaplains are always called, and chaplains are less likely to sit on committees or collaborate with nonchaplain colleagues. The directors of these departments tend to report to lower levels in the administration, and more staff chaplains are financially supported by organizations outside the hospital. Such departments also tend to rely more heavily on CPE students and volunteers to provide services to patients and families. These departments tend not to require chaplains to be eligible for board certification when they are hired and to employ chaplains with a much broader range of educational backgrounds.

Several of these departments consist of a director, a CPE supervisor, volunteer chaplains paid by outside organizations, and CPE students who rotate through the hospital in ten-week or year-long intervals. Rather than focusing on patients and families as the primary recipients of chaplaincy services and orienting their mission statements and goals to them, several department directors spoke largely in terms of the CPE they are providing, orienting their goals and main contributions to the hospital in terms of the education they provide for CPE students. One director explained, "The [CPE] program has been so well received by patients, families and, staff that sustaining the CPE program has become an essential priority." One of these departments hired its first senior staff chaplain only recently, previously relying on CPE students to do all of the work with patients and families.

Unlike the transitional department described above that was trying to limit the number of volunteers and distinguish them from staff chaplains, several of the directors of traditional departments wanted to build their volunteer programs as a way to serve more hospitalized patients. Building a stronger volunteer program, one director explained, "would enable us to do a lot more visiting of patients who haven't requested a visit—which, I think, is in keeping with my understanding of a good theological thing, to be able to reach out to folks and make them aware of our presence." Another described volunteers less kindly, saying, they "kind of fumble around. . . . They're harmless; . . . they visit people, they go to patient rooms, they're just sort of well intentioned; . . . they're useful." Rather than setting clear limits on what CPE students or volunteers can do based on their training and seeing these individuals as educationally and professional distinct from staff chaplains who are board certified, traditional departments tend to use students and volunteers as the equivalent of staff chaplains, or at least as the people in the department who spend the most time with patients and families.

In addition to CPE-oriented departments, other traditional departments have been built around a single, long-term chaplain, who is either still at the hospital, or who recently retired and is much missed. Some long-term chaplains are well known and loved by staff throughout the hospital. They have built their departments, however, on the strength of their personalities rather than by collaborating with other chaplains, CPE students, or health-care staff. As a result, many in the hospital do not understand who chaplains are, what they do, or even how to contact them, except for the single, well-loved chaplain. Such departments tend to have few vibrant programs or other chaplains who are involved in the hospital apart from the long-term chaplain. When this chaplain retires, departments falter, as there are few to no other chaplains with any institutional memory and no well-established initiatives or protocols that include other or newer chaplains in hospital routines. It is not uncommon for hospital staff to have the long-term chaplain's pager or cell phone number, and, when that individual retires, to not even know how to contact another chaplain. Newer chaplains in these departments are, not surprisingly, frustrated that medical staff do not refer patients to them more or better understand what they do.

UNDERSTANDING PROFESSIONAL, TRANSITIONAL, AND TRADITIONAL DEPARTMENTS

I view differences in the work chaplains do in these three types of departments and the ways they are oriented in their hospitals in terms of individual department and hospital histories rather than in terms of the demographic or geographic contexts in which they are located. The religious history of these hospitals also seems less relevant, since hospitals originally founded by religious groups fall into all three of the ideal types described above. Many of the differences are related to how departments were founded, the strategies that department directors used to build the professional jurisdiction of chaplains over time, and the broadness of the department's vision.[16]

First, departments that were started by people within hospitals or with financial or other direct support from hospitals tend to fall into the professional or transitional type. One hospital, for example, had a volunteer chaplain for several years before a physician started a foundation to raise money to pay the chaplain. The hospital then formed an administrative team to investigate the possibility of hiring and expanding the chaplaincy service, which included consulting with relevant professional chaplaincy organizations and conducting a survey of hospital staff to assess the need. These surveys identified a clear need, and the department was started with financial and administrative support from the hospital.

Directors of several other departments described the support of the administration as central to their successful development. This was not automatic; some departments were started with chaplains being paid for by organizations outside the hospital. The chaplains were permitted to work in the hospital but were not actively welcomed or integrated physically or financially. In some cases institutional support came from directors, connecting the work of chaplains to the spirit and values of the institution. The director of chaplaincy at one such hospital said that their support comes from, "the spirit of what this institution is about."

In other cases, institutional support was not complete but developed from a positive relationship the director had with one or more hospital administrators. When the director of one professional department was hired more than ten years ago, the department was in a period of transition. A well-positioned administrator outside the department told him that growth and development of the department had to happen "through the back door." "You need to let me quietly get you on [as the director]," the administrator told him, "and then see what you can do." The new director even came in over the weekend to paint the chapel rather than asking for funds from the hospital to do so. He explains, "She [the administrator] was right to a significant degree. I'm not sure that the CEO who was here at the time ever was particularly supportive of pastoral care, but there were enough other people around that we actually managed to expand the department and its facilities . . . quite a bit, even before the CEO left." Reflecting now on his experience as a director and his observation of other departments, he explains, "I think that health-care institutions that have strong chaplaincy departments almost always have or had some administrator who really believed in pastoral care. We were a fairly small expenditure in a big institution, and if an administrator wants to have a strong pastoral care department, it is not a make-or-break financial matter. They can do it if they want to. On the other hand, if they're not really committed to it, they can just sort of tolerate it as window dressing . . . always keep it just sort of on the verge of survival." Several other directors agreed that at least somewhat supportive administrators who could help department directors access various resources in institutions were essential for the development of professional or transitional departments.

Professional and transitional departments have also grown and become integrated into their hospitals through the efforts of directors who became familiar with the language and priorities of the health-care system. By using that language and understanding those priorities, directors systematically worked to include chaplains in the institution, as Pat is trying to do at Overbrook. These directors recognize that hospitals are primarily concerned with the health outcomes of patients, the satisfaction of patients and families, and the financial cost, and—as a result—they think about the ways chaplains might influence each of these outcomes. Such directors then worked to demonstrate the value chaplains have for the institution, either by gathering systematic, empirical data, in line with the evidence-based orientation of modern medicine, or by proactively communicating with staff about who they are, what they do, and how they might influence outcomes of concern.

The director of one such hospital, for example, was hired in the 1990s and built the department by doing outcomes-based research and having staff chaplains work closely with medical teams in ways that demonstrated their value and encouraging health-care teams rather than the chaplaincy department to ask the administration for more resources for chaplaincy. This director describes his orientation in terms of the contributions chaplains make to patient care, saying, "We have kept the focus away from activity and on contributions. A risky conversation I've had more than once with a new administrator is—you know, I can tell you how many visits we make. It will take me awhile, because we don't capture that right now. But I can tell you now, if that's what you really care about—a lot of visits—you can do it a lot cheaper and you don't need me. But if you want to talk about what difference it [chaplains' visits] makes for the reasons people come to this hospital—let's talk. And they've always wanted to talk." Such attention to the contributions chaplains make is evident in softer ways at other hospitals, such as Overbrook, where directors place chaplains on committees and work to integrate them into hospitals. At a very few hospitals, the value of chaplains' contributions has been recognized as physicians who have appreciated their work write salary support for chaplains into grants so that chaplains will be able to work directly with the seriously ill patients in their care.

The directors who learned the language and priorities of health-care institutions—who are not the majority of those interviewed—and then developed strategies to build their departments did so individually and through informal networks rather than as a result of particular courses they took in their training. Some had other relevant experience. Current and former directors of professional and transitional departments are more likely than directors of traditional departments to have had prior administrative experience outside of chaplaincy departments. Through these experiences, they learned to see patterns and communicate with other hospital staff, including administrators. Such experiences also broadened their perspectives, as they did for Pat at Overbrook, and led them to take risks or to try new things with people and departments of the hospital with whom they had not previously worked. In the words of one such director, who came to direct her department after other administrative experience, too many department directors at other institutions approach their positions by trying to "stay below the radar." This is absolutely the wrong approach, in her view, to making the department as visible and integral to the culture of the hospital as possible.

Finally, as part of operating within the norms and priorities of hospitals, professional and transitional departments have continued to broaden their visions over time. This has happened particularly as they transitioned from focusing primarily on teaching CPE students to working with patients and families, since that is where hospitals focus, even in teaching hospitals that are also training medical staff. It has also happened as departments transitioned from relying largely on volunteers to relying primarily on staff chaplains. Professional and transitional departments founded with strong emphases on CPE have come to situate their training of students within the context of providing high-quality care to patients and families rather than making CPE training their primary goal and marker of identity. In the words of one such director, "My vision is much broader than CPE." While some departments are professional or are transitioning in that direction, it is important to remember that the majority of departments I studied were traditional departments whose directors reported to low levels in the administrative hierarchy and whose staff chaplains were not well integrated into their hospitals.

STRIVING FOR LEGITIMACY

Since chaplaincy began to emerge as a profession in the early twentieth century, chaplains have struggled to articulate and demonstrate their value to the health-care organizations in which they work. Nationally these efforts have taken multiple forms, including joint statements from professional chaplaincy associations and efforts to articulate standards of practice and best practices and improve quality. As a group of multifaith professionals working with religious and spiritually diverse patients in secular health-care organizations, the staff chaplains and department directors I interviewed carefully negotiated their views on their profession, broadening them to focus on spirituality in recent years.

Whether it is because of the ways chaplaincy has developed as a profession, the church-state issues in the background, broader historic tensions between religion and medicine, the issues of religious and spiritual diversity central to chaplains' work, or the simple fact that chaplains work in medical institutions but are not medically trained, chaplains have often experienced their work as having low status and being poorly understood by others in health care.[17] Those who work in what I call professional chaplaincy departments may struggle with questions of status and professional legitimacy less than those in traditional departments—perhaps because they are more integrated in their institutions—but even in transitional departments like Overbrook's that have long institutional histories of chaplaincy, department directors like Pat find themselves regularly explaining to project managers, nurses, and other hospital staff who chaplains are and what they do.

Almost all the chaplains and chaplaincy directors I met spoke of efforts to explain their work and improve their status in their specific hospitals in terms of staff education, efforts in recent years to write in patient charts, and continued efforts to advocate for themselves and their colleagues. At Overbrook, Father William described "a lot of skepticism" among staff about aspects of his work, even though he is well known (and liked) throughout the hospital. He tries to get to know medical residents, fellows, and other physicians in training "as they are coming up the ladder," hoping they can "see the expertise as well as the humanity of chaplains" in ways that will lead them to respect and work with chaplains in their future professional work. Such concerns were echoed by chaplains across the country who are frustrated and want to be called more often and known better in their hospitals. At Forest Hills Hospital, the director said there were "still many parts of the health system who do not know about pastoral care" and are "surprised" to learn that chaplains are there and available. Chaplains there and across the country spoke over and over of trying to educate staff to call them. In the words of the director at Southern Hospital, "Our biggest challenge is to educate, . . . [to foster] the ongoing education of the staff" with the message that "all you need to do," if you need a chaplain, is "call, and we'll come, . . . if it is an emergency, right away." Such education mostly takes place in individual interactions as well as in new employee orientations and through Pastoral Care Week, which many chaplains organize in their hospitals once a year.[18]

In addition to trying to educate health-care staff, chaplains since the mid-1990s—earlier at some hospitals—increasingly document their interactions with patients in their medical records to show they have been there (fig. 5.2). In the mid-1990s, a national chaplaincy leader explained to me, "the Joint

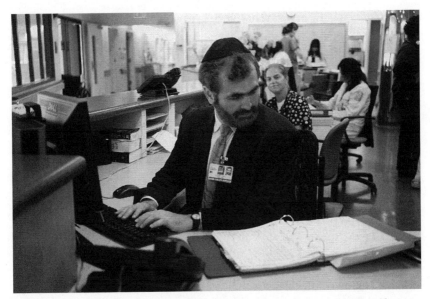

FIGURE 5.2 Rabbi Ralph Kreger, BCC, on the clinical staff of HealthCare Chaplaincy and chaplain at the Hospital for Special Surgery in New York, works on patient records at the nurses' station. Photo courtesy of HealthCare Chaplaincy, New York, New York.

Commission said that if you're a professional group in the hospital and doing anything with patients, you have to document it." This led more chaplains to do so. This shift was challenging for some chaplains who, like religious leaders, considered their conversations with patients to be private, confidential, and not appropriate to summarize in medical records accessible to everyone on health-care teams. To provide such summaries, chaplains also needed to be able to describe what they do to others on the medical team in a way they would understand and hopefully respect—a process of translation that was often a challenge.

Chaplains today document their visits in medical records in many ways, ranging from stickers that chaplains fill out and put in charts to multiple forms of documentation for the hospital and for chaplaincy departments.[19] At one hospital, the department created a charting sticker with boxes to check for what kind of visit it was (initial, follow-up, etc.), where the referral came from, the person's religious tradition, and what the chaplain did with the patient (read scripture, said a prayer, etc.). In some departments, chaplains simply write in the medical chart that they have seen the patient, while in others they are encouraged to note anything they learn about the person that might be relevant to their care.

Chaplains in even the most professional departments I studied, however, are hesitant about what they write in charts, reflecting their low status as non-medical professionals and the continued challenges they face in communicating with medical staff.[20] One chaplain explained how he charts, saying, "I don't go into a lot of detail" because "it might come back to haunt you. Like if you dare write 'Patient was depressed,' as a chaplain, you can't give a diagnosis, so you have to be really careful. I pretty much only write 'I was here.'" Most chart notes that chaplains write are a version of "I was here." At only one hospital do they follow the more standard medical model of diagnosis (obtained through a spiritual assessment), a care plan, and a plan for follow-up. Many chaplains began to chart in order to demonstrate the care they were providing and potentially to improve their status with other medical professionals, but this may have backfired at some institutions where, as described in the next chapter, medical staff told me they were confused by "I was here" notes in different patient charts that all look the same. Without more details of how the chaplain interacted with different patients, medical staff members are uncertain about the care chaplains provide. The ways chaplains write in charts are inconsistent across hospitals—"loosely goosey" according to some directors—and reflect the ambivalence some feel about writing in them.

In addition to charting, chaplains continue to make the case for themselves as professionals in multiple ways. In the words of a national chaplaincy leader who regularly advocates for the profession, "Our biggest challenge is always going to be advocating for our place within the professional team. . . . And part of it is, we simply need to show our worth." She describes that worth in terms of chaplains' abilities to meet Joint Commission standards. Other directors I interviewed focused more on research and training. "We need to be doing real research," one director explained, that reflects current standards in evidence-based medicine and directly informs how chaplains do their work. "I don't care if it is quantitative or qualitative or a blend, we need to be doing some research so it isn't just 'I'm John Smith, I'm going to do chaplaincy the way I want.' There's literature." Such literature would help chaplains to focus not just on the patient they are working with and his or her story but to understand broader patterns in patients' experiences that would enable them to provide more systematic, targeted care, according to this director.[21]

Other directors spoke about training, pointing to the fact that chaplains have not become an integral part of the spirituality in health care movement. In the words of one, "Those grounding issues, about spirituality as part of healing and patient care being written about in *Time* magazine, have never really taken hold within chaplaincy in the hospital setting, . . . so the issues being discussed out in the culture and [by] chaplains are running on a separate track." It is not just that chaplains have missed raising their professional profiles by contributing to this broader conversation, this director argued; he sees no strong academic base for people preparing to teach CPE, which, in his view, has not been as patient-focused as it should be. "I think we have some raising of the bar to do in terms of what it really takes to be a professional chaplain and be certified as such."

CONCLUSION

Hospital chaplains put in a lot of miles walking from one end of rapidly expanding academic hospitals to the other as they meet with patients and families, support staff, attend committee meetings, and lead services in hospital chapels. Where in hospitals they walk and how they work with other staff in the process is influenced by their personal background and training, and perhaps more by their departments and how their hospitals shape and define their daily work. While chaplains are increasingly members of departments with the word *spiritual* in the title and articulate their contributions broadly, their actual tasks vary significantly according to their institutional contexts.

Chaplain Martha Jacobs describes chaplains as "the health-care professional expert in providing spiritual care" in an issue of the *Hastings Center Report* focused on quality improvement.[22] Speaking of their tasks, she writes, "Chaplains do what needs to be done, in the setting in which we find ourselves, to ensure that care is focused on the emotional and spiritual needs of the patient and the patient's family, particularly in times of suffering, stress or grief."[23] While this may be the case, the departments I studied show that the actual tasks of chaplains vary in different hospitals depending on how individual departments were started, the extent to which directors learned to speak the language and articulate the priorities of the hospital, and whether they continued to broaden their department's vision over time.

The liminality that many chaplains experience in this work was particularly evident in the language and metaphors they used to discuss it. As they tried to "make space," "provide space," or create openings for people's stories, chaplains saw themselves acting as bridges between patients and medical teams and between the world of the hospital and broader religious and moral worlds. When they brought physical objects like communion supplies, prayer books, and candles, they also saw themselves as bringing the intangibles of presence, peace, and silence in ways clearly shaped by the medical institutions in which they worked.

Chaplains are different in this respect from nurses and physicians, whose work is shaped not just by the hospitals in which they work but by long-established, if changing, national standards of care in their fields and the requirements of professional licenses and continued education. National chaplaincy leaders strive to standardize their work as they grow into their own profession and develop similar national standards of practice and best practices. As Martha Jacobs writes, "We need to standardize our practices, both in the interest of quality and so we can negotiate with institutions over funding and deployment."[24] Chaplains need to be clear as a professional group about when they should always be present in health-care organizations and then be so present.

Standardizing the work and physical presence of chaplains, however, requires dealing with the religious and spiritual diversity of the chaplains, patients, families, and hospital staff. To date it appears that this is happening more through broad talk of spirituality than in the standardization or regulation of tasks that are explicitly part of all chaplains' professional work. While some chaplains have picked up additional tasks—like working with organ donation at Overbrook or serving as the contacts for funeral homes at another hospital, chaplains at the hospitals described here do not agree on when their services are always needed and how they can best provide them in hospitals. Beyond intuition, they are also not clear about the authority on which their work is based, which undermines their efforts to make a case for their profession to colleagues in their hospitals.

Chaplains also do not agree, in some departments, about who can provide chaplaincy services. At Overbrook, a patient who calls for a chaplain could be greeted by a Meg, a staff chaplain with ten years' experience and a doctorate in ministry, or a local divinity-school student doing a summer unit of CPE who has been working in the hospital for just a few weeks. Such variation, not just among individuals but among chaplaincy departments, illustrates what sociologists Rue Bucher and Anselm Strauss call a "profession in process," or a professional group with many segments in transition.[25] Chaplains are historically in the midst of a transition from the "subjective" to the "official" labor force and are still developing a clear and consistent sense of who they are, when they need to be present, and what tasks are unique and specific to them as professionals.

The extent to which chaplaincy remains a profession in process, at Overbrook and nationally, was particularly evident to me one morning in a conversation with George, a chaplaincy department volunteer. George told me that he introduces himself to patients by saying, "I'm a chaplain from the hospital chaplaincy department and I'm making the rounds." Sarah, the staff chaplain who supervises the volunteer visitors, reinforced his identifying himself as a chaplain when she told me that the volunteer visitors "function exactly the way chaplains do, . . . but they can't get into the [patient] chart" as they used to before changes in health-care privacy laws. "The only difference [between a volunteer and a staff chaplain] would be that they wouldn't go to an inter-disciplinary meeting or something like that." George has no formal training in chaplaincy or permission from Pat, the department director, to call himself a chaplain. The fact that he works in the chaplaincy department at Overbrook, which Pat is trying to professionalize and orient to developing national pro-fessional standards, reminds me of how diverse the people are who claim to be chaplains as well as how wide-ranging their tasks are.

Some of the looseness and variation in the identity and tasks of chaplains may indicate that hospitals see religion and spirituality as an extra, not some-thing that must be addressed with patients by health-care professionals, de-spite Joint Commission guidelines. Although patients are sicker, and the ethi-cal decisions that families are asked to make more complex than in the past, there does not seem to be stiff competition between groups of professionals trying to talk about religion, spirituality, or other broad issues of meaning in hospitals. Nurses, social workers, and physicians often spend more time with patients than chaplains, however, and may be more likely to be around when issues related to religion and spirituality are present. I shift my focus from chaplains to ICU staff in the next two chapters, listening first to how staff members in two ICUs see and respond to religion and spirituality in their daily work.

Spirituality and Religion in Intensive Care: Staff's Perspectives and Professional Responses

Nurses described the mid-sized, mostly windowless neonatal intensive care unit (NICU) at City Hospital–close to Overbrook–as a cave that had the same lighting, temperature, and smell regardless of the weather outside. Up to eighteen premature and critically ill infants were cared for in the space, some in beds called giraffes that cost more than most new cars. Between the beds were additional pieces of medical equipment, wooden rocking chairs, colorful infant jump seats, and handmade blankets and beanie babies. Medical protocols, photos of growing children, and thank you notes covered the walls.

While waiting for the nurse I was there to interview, I listened to the whishing and whirring of ventilators helping some of the infants breathe and chatted with Lisa, a staff nurse who has worked in this NICU for more than twenty years. Wearing a scrub jacket covered in small blue handprints, Lisa stood next to baby Rose's bed, telling me she weighed less than three pounds. I noticed drawings made by Rose's siblings and cards from other family members hanging around her bed. One of the cards, signed by her parents, included words by a Hallmark author about how God only gives you what you can handle and must think you are very strong right now because of all you are being asked to bear. In addition to the beanie babies and medical equipment actually in bed with Rose, her parents had placed a small green book—a New Testament. On other visits to the NICU, I saw Qur'ans and Catholic medallions in beds with babies, often carefully sealed in plastic bags with identifying hospital labels.[1] I saw wooden saints strategically situated to protect babies and overheard parents, nurses, and the pediatric chaplain talking about prayers, miracles, and angels.

I noticed fewer religious and spiritual symbols and less related talk several months later as I waited to interview a respiratory therapist who worked in an adult medical intensive care unit (MICU) at this same hospital, which was three to four times the size of the NICU. Eighteen adults were cared for in the MICU in individual, glass-walled rooms arranged in a U shape around banks of computers. Awards, recently published articles, and announcements about medications hung on the walls, and young staff members clad in blue scrubs moved quickly through the space. With the exception of a note-card-sized image of the previous pope that one of the nurses kept, I saw few explicitly religious or spiritual symbols during my visits to this unit. As in the NICU, I saw members of the chaplaincy department though, both one of the hospital's Catholic chaplain-priests who was assigned as the unit chaplain and Eucharistic Ministers offering communion to hospitalized Catholic patients and their families.

As I waited to interview the respiratory therapist, I thought again about what two attending physicians in this unit had told me in recent interviews. The first, Dr. Ackerman, explained that religion and spirituality do not "interfere" much on the unit. "Most people in the hospital go about their business—the doctors, the professional side go about their business doing whatever is required for medicine," he explained. "Every now and then, ... you might deal with a Jehovah's Witness, and then it really does make a huge difference ... and interferes with ordinary, everyday treatment." Despite the inconvenience such cases present, he said "there is a lot of respect from the staff for ... people who want to believe that way." The second physician, Dr. Brown, sounded more like physicians and nurses in the NICU when she explained that "some people would think you should leave religion out of this [ICU care] because it gets in the way." She disagrees and teaches young doctors to "take time to understand other people's faith perspectives."

*

This chapter shifts from discussion of hospital chapels and chaplains to staff in ICUs. I also move from Overbrook to nearby City Hospital, a similar, secular, academic medical center with a traditional chaplaincy department. While the director of chaplaincy at City Hospital, like Pat at Overbrook, frames the work of chaplains broadly in terms of spirituality, medical staff in these two ICUs mostly spoke of religion in terms of specific religious traditions, practices, and rituals, especially related to Catholicism. In a paradoxical way, religion and spirituality seem to be more present among ICU staff than among chaplains, as staff saw and named religious symbols, practices, and rituals—up to a point.

This awareness of religion may reflect the fact that more Americans die in hospitals than elsewhere and that ICU staff often care for them before they die.[2] Intensive care units are therefore places where many American families spend time, often making difficult treatment and end-of-life decisions in the process. Religion and spirituality—however understood and framed—may be important parts of those decisions. A 2005 survey showed that more than 65% of the public and 60% of trauma professionals say their religious beliefs would be very or somewhat important in making decisions about their own medical care if they were critically injured.[3] Close to 75% of people in a national survey said physicians should open up discussion of spirituality, refer patients to chaplains, or suggest prayer as part of treatments. That number rises to 90% when survey questions ask about patients who are approaching death. Many of these discussions and referrals would likely take place in ICUs.[4]

Despite this survey data, little is known about how hospital staff members understand and talk about religion and spirituality, generally or in ICUs.[5] I ask such questions here, focusing on how religion and spirituality come up, when staff members think the topics are particularly relevant for patients, and how they respond as professionals. I pay attention to how staff members conceive of religion and spirituality and how their hospital and unit cultures shape their talk and actions, especially with regard to unit chaplains, physicians, and nursing leaders.

I find that most staff view nurses in collaboration with chaplains as the professionals most responsible for engaging with families around spirituality and religion. With the exception of the chaplain in the NICU at City Hospital, who consistently spoke a broad language of spirituality, staff members talked about spirituality and religion almost exclusively in terms of religious traditions, beliefs, and rituals. As at Overbrook, the majority of patients and nurses at City Hospital were Catholic, which helped to explain some of their focus on rituals, especially baptism and last rites or the Sacrament of the Sick. Staff members saw spirituality and religion as most relevant in crisis situations, while making difficult decisions, and especially when a patient was dying, though they were not always sure how to offer spiritual or religious support to families. Overall, they described spirituality and religion as more of a help than a hindrance for patients as long as it fit within the biomedical orientation of the units. Once they spilled outside this frame, however, religion and spirituality were sources of conflict—often as families made faith-based arguments for continued medical care against the advice of medical teams.[6]

Few staff members—nurses, physicians, or respiratory therapists—reported learning about spirituality and religion as part of their formal training. As a group, those in the NICU were more attuned to religion and spirituality and more comfortable talking with families in those terms than those in the MICU. These differences likely result from the greater involvement and accessibility of the unit chaplain in the NICU and more related leadership over a longer time period from physicians and nurses in that unit.

THE NEONATAL AND MEDICAL ICUS AT CITY HOSPITAL

It is in ICUs, sociologist Everett C. Hughes (1971) reminds us, that lay people's emergencies are turned into the routines of medical professionals.[7] These professionals include physicians, nurses, respiratory therapists, social workers, chaplains, and administrators. At City Hospital, physicians—including medical residents, interns, and medical students—worked in teams led by an attending physician who rotated into and out of the unit every two weeks. Nurses, overseen by a nurse manager, were typically assigned two patients per shift of eight to twelve hours and worked for a total of forty hours per week. Nurses at City Hospital practiced primary nursing, working with the same patient throughout that individual's hospital stay. Of all of the staff, they had the most sustained contact with patients and were empowered by nurse managers and the hospital nursing leaders to work directly with physicians.[8] The ICUs also had case managers, who helped to coordinate care, as well as respiratory therapists, social workers, and chaplains assigned to provide support to patients as needed.[9]

The NICU at City Hospital was a level-three medical-surgical unit prepared to deal with the most severely ill newborns. It was staffed by six neonatologists, two neonatology nurse practitioners, and sixty nurses when this research was conducted. The unit cared for babies born at the hospital and those transferred by ground and air ambulance from a radius of several hundred miles. Infants were placed in the NICU because they had respiratory problems, were born prematurely, had congenital abnormalities, or suffered from a genetic syndrome. Babies born as early as twenty-three or twenty-four weeks (usual human gestation is forty weeks) were treated in this NICU. Many premature babies suffered from respiratory distress syndrome because their lungs were not fully developed, and they relied on mechanical ventilators to help them breathe.

The MICU at City Hospital was staffed by twelve attending pulmonary critical care physicians and sixty-five nurses at the time this research was

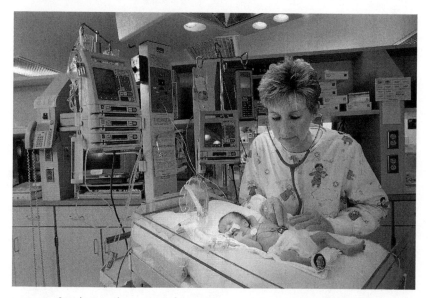

FIGURE 6.1 A nurse in a neonatal intensive care unit cares for an infant. Photograph by David Joel/Photodisc. Reproduced by permission of Getty Images.

conducted. While the physicians interviewed in each unit had similar levels of experience, the nurses in the NICU had almost twice as many years of experience in intensive care (13.8 years) as did those in the MICU (7.5 years). Patients treated in the MICU generally had severe pulmonary issues and other medical problems, such as kidney failure. Adults waiting for liver transplants were also cared for in this unit. This medical ICU is the place, one nurse told me, where "you can literally see a bit of absolutely everything. If you work here long enough, . . . you'll see patients that would normally be in every other ICU environment." Many patients were sedated or on ventilators due to respiratory ailments, which left them only minimally able to communicate verbally with staff and their families.

Karen and Julia, the nurse managers of the NICU and MICU, respectively, described them as "family centered," or oriented to the care of the patient and his or her family. They welcomed visits from family members at any time and found places on the unit where loved ones could spend the night, if needed. Speaking strongly, Karen, the nurse manager of the NICU, said, "I feel like we shape the lives of American families here." Focusing more on the specifics, Julia, the manager of the MICU, described changes in the last five years toward open visiting hours that made the unit more family oriented. An empty wait-

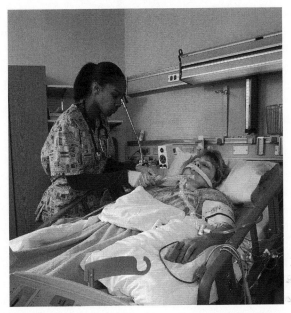

FIGURE 6.2 A patient in a medical intensive care unit is checked by a nurse. Photograph by David Joel / Photographer's Choice RF. Reproduced by permission of Getty Images.

ing room is now the sign of good care, she explained, because family members are with their loved ones inside the ICU.

Daily Work

Work in these units is fast-paced, intense, and sometimes unpredictable. Staff members saw medically and ethically complex cases daily, often requiring them to work with families to make difficult decisions. Both units host regular ethics rounds or lunchtime meetings for staff, often mostly nurses, to debrief them and discuss challenging cases. Rounds in the NICU were led by an attending physician trained in ethics and included discussion of ethical decision making, end-of-life issues, and chromosomal and other medical abnormalities. Ethics rounds in the medical ICU, also led by a physician trained in ethics, focused on recent difficult cases. If there were none, the physician read the names of patients who had recently died in the unit, inviting reflection and comment. These rounds in the MICU grew out of weekly meetings that a psychiatrist held for medical residents as a way for them to "get things off their chest . . . and learn how to deal with [the] sometimes horrendous things" that they observe and must do to patients, an attending physician remembered. Julia described ethics rounds in the MICU as "group therapy for nurses."

As discussed in ethics rounds, patients die in both of these units—less often in the neonatal than medical ICU. About 20%, or three to four of the eighteen patients on the unit when the beds are full, died in the MICU, and about one baby died per month in the NICU.[10] Each unit took steps to support grieving family members. In the NICU, nurses put together memory boxes, including photos of the child, footprints in clay, and a lock of hair that they gave to parents. The MICU had been working to develop a stronger relationship with palliative-care professionals at the hospital when this research was conducted so that they could better support dying patients and their families. As in the NICU, dying patients were moved to the most private part of the unit, and a single nurse was often assigned to support them. After a patient died, the nurse who took care of the patient "sent out a sympathy card, just a "thinking of you" type of written sentiment to the family members of the loved one that [had] passed on our MICU within days or a week of their passing," as Becky, the nurse who started this effort, told me. She began what she calls the "sympathy card project" after getting close to families and, in her words, "experiencing a really important part of the life cycle; when their loved one passes, you feel that bond." She wanted to reach out to families following their time in the hospital.

The Religious and Spiritual Context

City Hospital is officially secular but, like Overbrook, it has a strong Catholic ethos. Fifty to sixty percent of the patients in the hospital were Catholic, according to the question about religion asked at admission.[11] Nurses in these two ICUs confirmed these demographics, noting that they have seen increasing numbers of non-Christians, including Hasidic Jews, Muslims, and people from Arab countries in recent years.

Catholicism was also the dominant religious affiliation of the staff, particularly the nurses, although they rarely discussed their personal religious or spiritual backgrounds with one another. The majority of attending physicians described themselves as agnostic or atheist (41%) or as Jewish (18%).[12] The majority of the nurses, almost three-quarters, were Catholic. All the staff saw their religious and spiritual backgrounds as private, as in the "back seat" at work, according to one physician. Religious or spiritual topics only came up with other staff when the conversation concerned social engagements, such as baptisms or weddings, or in discussion of current events, such as the Catholic priest scandal. "It is so infrequent that it comes up," a respiratory therapist told me. "I don't even know the religions of half of the people I work with." Another nurse said, "There's a girl here that I work with who is Jewish." "I was here two and a half years before I knew she was Jewish."[13]

The Chaplains

Traditionally oriented, the Chaplaincy Department at City Hospital sought to support patients, families, and staff regardless of their personal beliefs or experiences. Joseph, the director of the department, divided the population they work with into three groups. The first included those with "traditional religious beliefs"; the second, those who might be considered spiritual, who "do not have a particular religious tradition but instead have some belief in something beyond them, which people give different names to or sometimes simply the name *higher power*"; and a growing third group, those "who don't fall into either of those first groups, but who are looking to find meaning and purpose in their lives." The "fundamental principle" of the chaplaincy at City Hospital, he told me, "is in as broad and inclusive a way as possible to determine what group or groups [an individual belongs to] . . . and then to be able to provide that listening and understanding, that support, because what we find here in this hospital is that . . . people [often] forget where they're gaining their spiritual support from." When chaplains remind them, he explained, "it is almost like you can see people being reenergized, or refreshed, or renewed because they're back in touch with whatever is giving them that support on one of the deepest levels."

The Chaplaincy Department does this reminding in multiple ways. Chaplains lead daily Catholic mass, daily interfaith prayers, and weekly Jewish and Buddhist services in the hospital chapel that are broadcast through the hospital's in-house television network. Items like prayer shawls, meditation cushions (*zafus*), and texts required for practices in many religious traditions were available. The department also staffed full and part-time chaplains financially supported by groups inside and outside of the hospital from a range of religious and spiritual backgrounds. Chaplains are available in the hospital and on call twenty-four hours a day, seven days a week. Most chaplains were assigned to particular units in the hospital and were responsible for the patients in that unit. They also carried pagers specific to their personal religious traditions and could page colleagues from other religious backgrounds when needed.

Unit Chaplains: Elizabeth, the Pediatric Chaplain

The neonatal and medical intensive care units each had an assigned chaplain who was responsible for all of the patients in the unit. Elizabeth, the pediatric chaplain assigned to the NICU (and several other units) had a broad approach to all patients that mirrored the transition to spiritual care in chaplaincy as a profession. An ordained Protestant minister, Elizabeth was trained in a year-long, full-time chaplaincy residency program before being board-certified by the Association of Professional Chaplains and coming to work at City Hospital four years ago. In the past, chaplains were only involved in the NICU when a baby died. During her first few years on the unit, Elizabeth found that physicians worried when they saw her, asking which baby was dying. Gradually she taught staff to see her as a support person and counselor for them, as well as for families. One of the physicians spoke about appreciating her presences because "support is there for the families if need be. Not just your social work." Karen, the nurse manager, described Elizabeth's presence as strengthening "people's [both staff's and families'] consideration of spirituality and also their freedom to talk about the spiritual aspect of care work."

Elizabeth circulated through the NICU at different times of day, aiming to meet all of the families. Rather than asking specific questions about religious beliefs or spiritual practices, she spoke with families generally about how they were doing. "Often," she explained to me, "I walk through [the NICU], and I just stop near each bed space, and . . . I usually think to myself, 'Blessing to you little one.' And I just take a moment to look at the baby and appreciate [him or her] as a wonderful life." Even if the baby cannot hear her, Elizabeth trusts that somehow the infant "senses my presence and my goodwill." To the parents, she says, "'I think your child is beautiful and wonderful.' . . . I mean, often the children are really sick but to say, 'You have a beautiful child,' and really mean it I think is a gift." It is this kind of framing of the child's life in a context beyond the NICU that Elizabeth offers.

She further illustrated the broader context that she provides in a story about a nurse who jokingly asked her one day if she could pray for a baby to pee. "I didn't actually pray it," Elizabeth told me. Instead she whispered to the baby, "Please pee!" and then spoke with the nurse about how "there isn't a separation between body, mind, and spirit, especially in the hospital." Reflecting back, Elizabeth told me, "I have to sometimes say that distinction because it helps people understand my role," a role she describes as moving beyond the biomedical frame to tap broadly into humanistic themes of goodness connected to wholeness and presence.

Elizabeth additionally illustrated her broad perspective in describing a ritual, the blessing of a baby's bed space, that she sometimes leads for staff when an infant dies. Karen, the nurse manager, explained, "She'll bring the staff together, and she has the most moving prayer and way about her, blessing people's hands, and the space, and the care providers. . . . I think that's been very meaningful." Elizabeth describes this blessing as a "prayerful recap" intended "to create a moment that's different from the other moments in the day." She often conducts the ritual after she has finished working with the baby's parents, and she sometimes accompanies the nurses who take a baby's body to the morgue. The blessing is rarely planned ahead of time and usually takes place in just a few minutes. Whoever is around participates—people "from different beliefs and also people that don't necessarily believe in God," Elizabeth explains. Recalling the intense experiences they have shared in caring for a baby, Elizabeth begins by saying, "Let us take a moment to reflect on all that has happened in this place, and we will take a moment of silence.'" After that moment, she says something like, "May all of the work that we have done be acceptable as we celebrate the life of [name of the child] and all that this family has meant to us." Staff members might add their comments before she concludes, "May we be prepared for the next baby that comes to this place. May this be a place of healing and wholeness, and may our hands be blessed . . . with skill and compassion for all of the children that we will work with today." While some nurses interpreted this ritual as a prayer for God's blessing, others viewed it as a broadly secular ritual that could, in the words of one nurse, "still our thoughts and [help us] realize that we're all feeling the same way and that, you know, we're all in this together." No staff members spoke critically with me about the blessing. The lack of language about God or symbols specific to individual religious or spiritual traditions is notable in the blessing and reflects Elizabeth's efforts to find acceptable ways to express what is meaningful to all the patients and families she works with and to provide support around that. She also writes short notes in patient's charts after visiting with them and communicates regularly with staff, especially nurses, about the patients and families in their care.[14]

Unit Chaplain: Father Fu, the MICU Chaplain

Blessings of bed spaces and other broadly framed rituals did not take place in the MICU where Father Fu, the Catholic priest assigned as the unit's chaplain, mostly focused on providing traditional Catholic sacraments to Catholic patients. While Elizabeth dressed in street clothes and was only identified as a chaplain by the ID badge around her neck, Father Fu wore a clerical collar, marking him as a priest. He was born and ordained abroad and worked in a seminary for several years before deciding to pursue chaplaincy work in the United States. He was not board-certified as a chaplain, though he had completed some CPE training. He was hired by City Hospital primarily to provide Catholic sacraments. Rather than making rounds through the MICU, Father Fu met patients and families when they were referred to him, mostly by nurses. He explained, "In general, we are called for the sacraments. . . . I go there usually for the sacrament, connect with the person, what their needs are, or their concerns." Not surprisingly, in a hospital with many Catholic patients, he was called regularly to the bedsides of people who were dying or to consult with family members seeking guidance from a priest about end-of-life decisions. He tried to help in these situations by, in his words, letting people "express what is on their minds, what their concerns are" and letting them know what the Catholic Church teaches at the end of life. In addition to Father Fu, lay Catholic volunteers regularly circulated through the unit, offering communion to Catholic patients and families through the Chaplaincy Department's Eucharistic Ministry Program.[15] Because Father Fu did not usually meet with them, non-Catholic patients did not have their spiritual or religious needs met by hospital chaplains.

As a group, staff members in the MICU were puzzled and somewhat dissatisfied with Father Fu's role. He was rarely on the unit, and few physicians or nurses knew his name. Reflecting the low profile of the Chaplaincy Department at City Hospital and the lack of easily accessible information about the chaplains who were available to staff, few staff were aware that they could page chaplains other than Father Fu. Julia, the nurse manager, did not know if chaplains were always on call, and the phone number of the Chaplaincy Department was not included in the bedside reference manuals available for nurses in each patient room. Attending physicians in the MICU told me that the unit lacked "adequate spiritual care" and, in the words of one, that the "chaplains don't fit in with the [medical] team." Dr. Coyle said that chaplains could "really help you," but that they did not fit in with the medical teams because they were continually coming and going, and there was "very little communication back and forth" with the medical staff. He thought that a "spiritual social worker" might better meet their needs as "someone savvy" who could also "do family supports, transportation, . . . the whole package." While Elizabeth might have fit this role for him, Father Fu did not, as he was rarely on the unit, almost never saw non-Catholic patients, and communicated only minimally with staff either in chart notes or in person.

Other physicians on the unit echoed these concerns, stating that the chaplains did not help them in their work. Several mentioned that the chaplain always left the same note in charts, which basically just said that he had visited, leaving them unclear about what chaplains actually did and how the visit might have helped the patient. A number of (Catholic) nurses were hesitant to criticize a priest, but also felt that Father Fu did not fit in on the unit. Several were also uncertain about what the Chaplaincy Department volunteers do who offer communion. Some viewed them as what one nurse described as "volunteers that go in and say prayers with the patients almost every day," while others more accurately saw them as only visiting Catholic patients and offering communion or just prayers if the patient was not able to receive food by mouth.

IDENTIFYING RELIGION AND SPIRITUALITY ON THE UNITS

ICU staff mostly spoke about religion and spirituality in terms of objects, rituals, and prayers. They spoke of each primarily in relation to specific religious traditions, mostly Catholicism, reflecting their personal backgrounds and those of the majority of their patients.[16] The hospital formally gathers information about religious affiliation when patients are admitted and in nursing assessments on specific units. In the NICU the nursing assessment included a question about the family's "religious" preferences as well as questions about whether they had any beliefs that would affect their child's treatment and whether they would like to be visited by a hospital chaplain. The chaplains were the primary resource that nurses offered. As one nurse explained, "We ask these questions to identify what their needs are, and then we call the chaplaincy." In the MICU, the questions on the nursing assessment were more general. Nurses asked whether there were "any practices we can assist you with while you are here" and whether the patient or family would "like a chaplaincy consult call." Whether nurses called Father Fu when the answer to the chaplaincy question was yes is an open question.

Objects

Staff spoke about spirituality and religion in intensive care primarily in their descriptions of objects that families brought into the unit and ceremonies, such as baptisms and last rites, that they observed and sometimes participated in. Researcher Joseph Barr and colleagues describe holy books, notes written by rabbis, pictures of rabbis, and other items that parents placed on their children's beds in a pediatric intensive care unit in Israel.[17] Similarly, City Hospital doctors and nurses spoke of crosses, rosary beads, sacred books, images of Mary, and holy water that families placed in bed or close to their loved ones in these units. One nurse, caring for a Muslim baby for the first time, made a sign for the infant's bed outlining her parents' wishes that the Qur'an remain at her head at all times. Another nurse explained, "This baby I have now, she has a book of Psalms in her bed. . . . I always try to make sure that it's in there and don't drop it on the floor. . . . I wonder what that means." Nurses described these items as, in the words of one, "important to the family because [they give] that baby an identity—the role in the family that the baby would take if it was at home." Staff in the MICU also encouraged families to make "get to know me posters" about their loved ones to help staff get to know them, which sometimes included spiritual or religious symbols or messages.

Rituals

Staff also described and sometimes participated in rituals in these units. In the NICU, baptism was the most frequently discussed, if not conducted, ritual.[18] "The sacrament of baptism is really big," Elizabeth, the pediatric chaplain, reflected. "Some people [staff] that maybe aren't even Christian have a real sense that baptism is important for a child to go to heaven. That's something I'm always doing education about." The strong feelings nurses have about baptism were evident over and over again in interviews. As one nurse explained, "Any baby that is going to code [have his or her heart stop], or it looks like is going to pass away—all nurses in the NICU will baptize it, whether they're Catholic or not." "If the baby's dying and there's a question in the mind of whether the family would want them baptized," a respiratory therapist explained, "we do it by sprinkling water on the child's head and saying a short prayer. If they didn't want it, we don't have to mention it."

Nurses learned how to conduct, or improvise, these rituals shortly after they started to work on the unit. Lisa, a Jewish NICU nurse, described learning early in her time in the unit that, in her words, if a "baby is dying, . . . you have to baptize the baby." "Ok," she told me but, "I have no idea how to do that. Just give me a clue and I'll do that." She learned from other nurses, but after performing a few baptisms, she felt uncomfortable, as if they would not count because she is not Christian. She consulted with a Catholic priest at the hospital, who waved her concerns aside, saying, "It doesn't make a difference.

Don't worry. It's just a lovely thing," which made her feel a bit better but still "somewhat uncomfortable because it is not my religion."

In addition to performing emergency baptisms, nurses attended planned, bedside baptisms conducted by chaplains and sometimes served as godparents if they were Catholic. "If they [families] ask me to participate," Alexis, a nurse practitioner, explained, "I'll do that." Other nurses are listed on the baptismal certificates that the chaplains prepare as godparents. "I am actually a godmother to several babies," said Sarah, a nurse. As in the blessing of the bed space, Elizabeth sometimes performed baptisms creatively in the NICU, improvising in ways that brought staff together. In one situation, for example, she baptized a baby who had been in the unit for a long time and was going to die. She signed the baptismal certificate and then invited anyone who wished to join her to also sign it. "It was so interesting," she told me, "because surgeons signed it, nurses signed it, secretaries, . . . I mean almost everybody signed it." Struggling with the sadness of this child's impending death, Elizabeth interpreted hospital staff as "just want[ing] to do something" for this family, and she saw in this ritual a way for them to come together.

In addition to baptisms, nurses also described observing and participating in a number of other rituals, especially in end-of-life situations. "A lot of the Pentecostal people will bring a group of people in and pray over the baby," Nancy, a nurse, explained. "I love to join in any of those things that I can." A respiratory therapist similarly described the mother of a Muslim patient who was dying and wanted a blessing from a chaplain, which she helped to arrange. Kimberly, a neonatal nurse who worked nights, cared for another Muslim baby and wrote a detailed protocol, in collaboration with the baby's father, about how the child's body should be cared for if she died before he and the baby's mother could get to the hospital.

While a child's parents were normally involved in end-of-life rituals, in some instances they did not want to stay as a child died, and the nurses and chaplains performed the rituals on their own. Sarah, a nurse, described one such case in which a Buddhist family had decided to withdraw care from their infant but did not want to hold the child or be with him when he died. After a visiting Buddhist leader said a prayer and sang a song, she remembered, the parents left, and the medical staff disconnected the infant's mechanical support. "We pulled the tube," Sarah remembered, and I held the baby, and the Buddhist leader asked if she could stay. "At this point, I was like sobbing. . . . It just kind of hit me . . . that they didn't hold the baby." Sarah and the chaplain spoke about reincarnation, which led Sarah to feel comforted, "That that baby . . . the life goes on."[19]

End-of-life rituals were similarly common in the MICU, especially as Father Fu did the Sacrament of the Sick or last rites for patients who were dying.[20] Judy, a nurse, described offering the chaplain to families to "come and give last rites if they want that," and liking being a part of it. "I find that it is a big deal for me to be part of that. . . . You can be in there and just be with the family, pray with them, or encourage them." Another nurse described trying to respect the "many different cultures" she sees in the unit and "really try[ing] to do what you can to accommodate" them at the end of life. She felt comfortable standing with families, "even if I'm not saying the prayers, . . . just to even stand in there with them and hold their hands, or hug them, or whatnot." Linda, the social worker in the MICU explained, "I've seen nurses . . . sing at the bedside. We pray at the bedside, you know, whatever seems to be important and not invasive to families is what we will accommodate here."

As in the NICU, end-of-life rituals in the MICU generally included families, but sometimes the staff conducted them alone. A nurse named Jean, who sometimes prayed for her patients, explained, "If I'm the only person in the room, and somebody's dying, . . . I'll often sing . . . to kind of help them with the passing." Reflecting her own personal background, she sings "Amazing Grace," "An Irish Prayer," and "Ave Maria." Jean described a particular case in which a patient was dying, and his sister, in her words, "took one look at him and was like, 'I can't do this . . . I'm going to go home and say my goodbyes now. Call me when he passes.'" Jean assured her that she would not "let him die alone," and as the patient's heart rate went down over the next few hours, she went into his room and started to sing "Ave Maria." "I was singing it over and over again while he was dying. . . . I sang it the full time he was passing." When Jean called the patient's sister after he had died, she told her, "'He's passed and I want you to know that I was with him, and I was singing to him 'Ave Maria' as he was passing." His sister gasped when she heard this, saying this was their mother's favorite song. Their mother, herself dead, the patient's sister interpreted, must have had something to do with it. Revealing her own belief in God and an afterlife, Jean told me the whole experience gave her the chills, saying, "Weird connection with the other side I guess."[21]

While most of the rituals in both ICUs took place within mainstream religious or spiritual traditions, there were a few exceptions that the nurses mostly laughed at, reflecting their lack of comfort and familiarity. One patient, a nurse in the MICU remembered, had made a decision to stop treatment and pass away but had a friend come to the ICU to conduct what she called a Klingon death rite first. The staff made space for the ritual but were surprised, barely accommodating the different religious and spiritual assumptions potentially embedded in a ritual so different from mainstream norms. "You know," the nurse remembered, "3,000 years of Catholic and Jewish tradition. . . . It [the ritual] was just too much. . . . I understand he was a fairly strange guy."[22]

Prayers

In addition to rituals, staff in both units—mostly the nurses—also described prayers for patients that they observe and sometimes join. Prayers were most often initiated by family members, the staff reported.[23] A respiratory therapist in the neonatal ICU explained that if a family is saying a prayer, and she knows it, like an Our Father, "I've joined in. . . . If they're religious, or if they're Roman Catholic, I let them know I prayed for them. I think it usually gives them a nice, a good feeling; . . . definitely I think it helps them out." Another nurse explained, "I have joined in prayer as [part of] a group. . . . I don't feel uncomfortable about that. I feel kind of, you know, it's a privilege that they include me in that moment in their life." Christina, a nurse who described herself as "100% Catholic," said that she joined with families when the chaplain did a blessing. "I pray right with them, and I think that does bring a sense of comfort to my thoughts as well . . . you have to kind of turn it over to a higher Being because there's nothing else we can do." Nurses who participated in prayers waited to be invited. "I tend to want to give them their privacy, because I think it's a personal thing," Karen explained. "If they invite me to join in, I definitely will. . . . If they're holding hands around the bed, and I'm doing my work around the bed, and they reach for my hand—I'll put my materials down and medicines or whatever and join them." All are clear that they participated only if they were invited by the family or were working at the bedside, knew the prayer, and felt it would not be intrusive or disruptive to their work. While some framed the prayer as supportive to the families, Christina also saw it as a source of personal support. Dottie, an older nurse in the MICU, agreed, explaining, "If the priest comes, and he's going to say a prayer when the family's there, I'll stay with them. I'm taking care of their mother for twelve hours. I'm going to stay there and pray with them."

Other staff, often not Catholic, observed prayers but were more ambivalent about participating. Marie, a nurse, for instance, told me that "a lot of nurses have prayed with parents," but she has not, because "there's a little bit of a wall" she likes to keep between her personal life, which includes her religious or spiritual life, and her patients. A neonatologist described a much larger wall, feeling that religion generally and prayer more specifically were "very personal. . . . I really don't want to share that part of me here at work." While he was respectful the few times families asked him to pray with them, he was actually offended by the request, explaining, "I'm an employee here. . . . I have rights as well." Other nurses spoke about standing to support families at bedside prayer services but not participating unless they shared the families' religious or spiritual background.[24]

WHEN STAFF SEE SPIRITUALITY AND RELIGION AS RELEVANT

Staff spoke about spirituality and religion being especially relevant to patients and families in times of crisis, of difficult decisions, and at the end of life. At these times, nurses said, they were especially likely to check in with patients, and more often families, about spiritual and religious issues. Wanting to offer support around spirituality and religion in crisis situations did not always translate, however, into knowing how to do so. Julia, the nurse manager in the MICU illustrated her attempt to do so in a story about a man who was rushed from the MICU into surgery. "I stood with the wife and her daughter," as the man was whisked into surgery, Julia told me, "and it occurred to me that maybe we should offer a chaplain to come in to say a prayer with this family or to provide support." She was nervous to do so, however. "I was aware that they might think I was alluding to the fact that the man should get last rites before he goes," she explained. She did not know if the family was Catholic, Protestant, or something else and was stuck not knowing how to offer spiritual or religious support without scaring the family into thinking the man was dying. They picked up on her discomfort, she told me, and after some misunderstanding, she said to them, "I don't know what faith you are, . . . but it would be something that I would want someone to offer me." In telling me this story, Julia reflected, "I think that we want to look at all the resources that are available to people and not leave anything out. . . . If this man didn't make it, I wouldn't want them later to say, 'Wow, why didn't anybody offer us some spiritual guidance because we're in the middle of this crisis?'"

Julia used the word *spiritual* in telling me this story and may have wanted to offer this family the kind of broad support that Elizabeth, the pediatric chaplain, offers in the NICU around meaning-making. She was stuck in trying to articulate what she wanted to offer, however, in her own assumptions about chaplains being connected to death and to last rites, as well as by the fact that it is last rites that Father Fu, as a traditional Catholic chaplain, so often provided in the MICU. Julia was clear that spiritual and religious issues "come into play when we're having these crisis experiences with families," but she did not know how to offer families such resources gracefully or to teach the nurses she supervises to do so.

In addition to crisis situations, staff spoke about the important roles that religion and spirituality play when families are faced with difficult decisions, often concerning death. A nurse in the NICU spoke about how important spirituality and religion are in these situations by describing herself as standing at a door. "Open the door . . . this is your life. And sometimes it is close the door, that was your life. . . . I think when you're the person standing there opening and closing the door, you may think about that [religion and spirituality] more often." A neonatologist said she does not normally get into conversations about religion "unless the baby's in extremis, and I feel like we should get them to have the clergy come in or something like that." Similarly, a respiratory therapist said that if a patient is not doing well, "I'll say to the nurse or doctors or both . . . maybe we should call whatever their religion is down— have somebody to support them in that way." This connection between religion, spirituality, and death was especially strong in the MICU, where many nurses said the only time they called the chaplain was when a patient was going to die. "Honestly, I always ask [about the chaplain] at end of life," a nurse explained. "Any other time, it's kind of like a dropped priority." Some nurses always called when a patient was dying, while others said they "try to remember," but "it doesn't always happen." When a chaplain or religious leader was present at the end of life, staff generally welcomed him or her, feeling like they helped families and staff cope, perhaps by taking some of the burden of care away from others on the medical team. In the words of one physician, "I know that's a traditional role for chaplains, but people—staff included—really appreciate having somebody around in those times. It's hard."

The assumptions that many nurses have about religion or spirituality and death were further evident when some explained why they did not feel comfortable asking patients about religion or spirituality. For some, it was because they equated religion or spirituality with the chaplain and thought a chaplain might not help in a specific situation. More often it was because, like Julia, they did not want to scare families into thinking death was near—even when it was. One mother told a nurse that when the nurse asked about a chaplain, it really "freaked her out" because she thought it meant her child "was going to die." Sometimes staff were not sure how to phrase the question. A respiratory therapist bumbled through her approach, saying, "There's been many times when I've said, 'I don't think I need to ask you because I feel like you need to be asked, but I want you to know I'm not asking this because I think something's terribly wrong—I wanted to know if you wanted to, if it would it be helpful to you to have a chaplain come by and say a prayer for your baby—just because it's here, not because I think something terrible is going to happen. You know I feel myself sometimes rambling on." Because talk of religion and spirituality was so closely connected to death in the minds of many staff in these units, some nurses hesitated to bring up the subject and were not sure how to do so without upsetting family members.

In listening to ICU staff talk about religion and spirituality, I was struck by how their language differed from that of the chaplains. Unlike Elizabeth and other chaplains, who conceived of spirituality and religion broadly in terms of all the ways people make meaning, ICU staff members understood the topic more narrowly. They focused less on broad, existential types of meaning than on people and rituals—even improvised—that are connected to specific religious traditions, especially Catholicism. Some participated in prayers and rituals themselves—not seeing the mention of miracles, prayer, or end-of-life rituals by patients and families as reasons to automatically call a chaplain. When they did reach out to chaplains, especially MICU staff, they tended to equate their presence with impending death and were not always sure how to offer the services of chaplain without scaring patients and families into thinking death was near. While staff in the NICU also felt this way, Elizabeth's conscious efforts to enlarge her professional jurisdiction in the last few years beyond providing support for grieving parents seems to have been successful, as evident in the referrals staff now made to her for a range of other reasons.

STAFF RESPONSES

As a group, staff members described trying to respect what they understood of patients' religious and spiritual values, from varying distances. Attending physicians tended to take a bit more distance, speaking of the need "to respect a patient's religious beliefs" or to "respect it [religion] and always offer the option for them to have a clergyman present." Nurses were a bit more willing to engage with patients about spirituality and religion, perhaps because they were more likely to share such concerns, as they improvised rituals and spoke about life being "precious" and fragile: "If life is hitting you over the head with terrifying things such as your loved one being in the ICU—if you want to pray you pray. . . . You respect that," one explained bluntly. Family members have faith in these ideas, many staff members recognized, which is why they should, in the words of another nurse, "respect their religion [and] . . . make sure the rosary beads don't get lost in the laundry."

As long as the religious beliefs and practices of families fit within the biomedical orientation of the intensive care, staff generally viewed them as important sources of emotional support. A neonatologist stated, "I don't frown upon people's religious belief. I totally think that it's a great thing that they have something to be there that they can believe, . . . to provide support and comfort in times of need." Religion is "very often a solace to them," explained another physician and "almost universally a help," said another. Nurses concurred, calling religion a "help," meaning a source of emotional support that, in the words of one nurse, "family members call on" in "the very difficult times."

A number of nurses noted that religion and spirituality help family members to cope more easily with the impending death of loved ones. "This is what religion helps you do," a neonatal nurse explained, to "give you up to whatever afterlife [you] believe in." A nurse in the MICU agreed. Not only can religion and spirituality be a source of comfort when people are ill, helping them to maintain a few of their usual routines in a foreign ICU environment, but it can help them to die. "I find that . . . patients who are more comfortable and have some sort of faith, whatever it is," do a "little bit better" as death approaches, a nurse told me. Whether this is actually the case or just appeared that way to nurses is an open question.

The spiritual or religious beliefs and practices of patients became a barrier or hindrance in the eyes of ICU staff when they did not fit within the biomedical orientation of the units. For example, families frequently make religiously based arguments for continued medical care against the advice of medical teams. In these cases, as anthropologist Sharon Kaufman explains, God is a part of medical decision making, and for those families, God trumps the advice of physicians.[25] The extent to which religion and spirituality help rather than hinder in the ICU, Dr. Davis explained, "all hinges on really whether there's conflict about what we think as . . . caregivers and what the families think." When there is conflict based on religious beliefs, Dr. Davis says they try as physicians to be "rational," and religion "can be in a way irrational." Conflict between families and medical teams often result.[26]

Such conflicts took place in both units and were described by attending physicians and nurses alike, often before I asked. A neonatologist, for example, spoke of a family who listened to the team recommend withdrawing support and letting their child die, but refused to do so on the basis of Catholic beliefs about the sanctity of life. In these situations, there can be "quite a conflict," a nurse practitioner explained, because the "parents don't want anything done because of their religious background. They feel like God will take care of everything." Staff described trying to convince families by saying that "God is helping, but he has given us the tools to help," generally without their desired result. Such cases were frequently referred to the hospital's Ethics Committee, not the chaplain, which could make a recommendation but could not force parents to make specific decisions. In most of the neonatal cases that staff described, they said care was not withdrawn, and the child was eventually discharged to a hospital for children with special needs. The child then returned frequently to the neonatal or pediatric ICU as what staff described as a "frequent flyer."

Similarly, in the MICU, it was not uncommon for families to believe that "God [would] decide" when a loved one would die. Some were convinced that a miracle would come. Maura, a nurse, remembered a case in which a woman was dying, "and we were just coding her [trying to start her heart] over and over because her husband stood there with a cross in his hand, saying, 'God's going to save her.'" This was traumatic for the staff and family, as this patient "died with her children screaming at the doctors outside," according to a nurse. "And they came back the next day. They wanted to see her in the morgue." Another nurse described a similar situation in which a woman was waiting for a miracle to save her husband. Judy remembered, "It's hard because you want to be accepting of their belief that God is so powerful that he could perform a miracle right now," but when the man died, the woman was devastated. Such cases were not uncommon and reflect national survey data, which indicate that just over three-quarters of Americans believe God or the saints can cure people who are given no chance of survival by medical science.[27]

Religion and spirituality were welcomed by staff in these two ICUs as long as they did not get in the way of biomedical care or were called on at the end of life, when staff, patients, and families agreed there was no more that biomedicine could offer. When spirituality and religion got in the way of biomedicine or were used by families to contradict it, however, they were not tolerated. Attending physicians and nurses tried to deal with the conflicts that resulted by engaging with families in terms of their different beliefs, often in family meetings. One physician described trying to "engage people and say, well, God also instructed us in medicine. . . . We're not working against God," but this approach usually did not work. Another physician also described trying to negotiate with families. "I always think our duty is to the patient, so I think the family members are asking for something that is actually somehow harming the patient; then . . . I wouldn't necessarily acquiesce to their wishes." Most staff said these attempts at negotiation rarely worked. Reflecting their low status in the hospital and on these units, chaplains were not usually involved in these cases and could not help to bridge these different languages, faith positions, and broader perspectives that were central to them. Linda, the social worker in the MICU, sometimes did this bridging, and the hospital's Ethics Committee, the group with the status to potentially bring the conflict to an end, regularly investigated and made recommendations in such cases.

CONCLUSIONS

Staff in the neonatal and medical intensive care units at City Hospital saw and responded to spirituality and religion in a number of ways, making it visibly present where an observer might expect it to be absent. As groups, staff members in the NICU were more aware of and attuned to spirituality and religion among patients and families than were those in the MICU. They were more aware of the range of religious and spiritual traditions that families brought to the unit, more aware of how to inquire about them, and more sensitive to how their own personal beliefs might influence the care they provided. Many nurses spoke in interviews about looking on the Internet for information about unfamiliar religious traditions and asking colleagues for resources. Several nurses also said they wished they had "more awareness" of religion and spirituality and were excited when they learned of colleagues planning to attend related seminars and share information with them. In this awareness, staff members in the NICU were more oriented to religious traditions, rituals, and practices—especially Catholicism—than to broader notions and languages of spirituality, such as those espoused by Elizabeth, the pediatric chaplain, or leaders of the national spirituality in health care movement. Reflecting national trends that show women to be more religious than men, it was largely women—the nurses—who provided spiritual and religious care in the units.[28]

In the MICU staff members were less aware of spirituality and religion and less certain about whether and how to inquire about it. Nurses mostly asked related questions on the nursing assessments, but they were often uncertain about what to do with the information they gathered, especially from patients not seeking the Catholic rituals that Father Fu provided. Linda, the unit's social worker, was the staff member most versed in the ways that spirituality and religion inform people's experiences and decision making, but she often spoke with families about such issues only after a conflict developed, and she said that was usually too late. While physicians and nurses respected and made space for families' spiritual and religious beliefs and practices on the unit, they did so in a narrower range of circumstances than in the NICU—mostly related to death. Although they used the words *religion* and *spirituality*, they mostly spoke of these issues in terms of religious traditions, especially Catholicism, like their colleagues in the NICU.

Differences in the extent to which staff in these two units felt comfortable with religion and spirituality related primarily to the influence on unit cultures of unit chaplains, nursing staff, and physician leaders. Several senior physicians and nurses in the NICU had long been interested in ethics and consistently sought out additional training that included attention to spirituality and religion. They brought what they learned back to the unit and shared it informally with colleagues and in ethics rounds. They also mentored younger staff, who regularly applied to participate in special courses on related topics. What some staff described as the "touchy-feely" nature of talk about spirituality and religion was welcomed rather than pushed away in the NICU, especially by the nurse manager and current and former unit chiefs, who did much to set a context in which such issues could be discussed.

This sensitivity to spiritual and religious issues led leaders in medicine and nursing in the NICU to advocate several years ago for a pediatric chaplain who would be well trained and board-certified, able to work across religious and spiritual traditions, and assigned to the unit. While Elizabeth's broad spiritual frame was markedly different from the specific religious categories that most staff used to think about these issues, her presence gave staff permission to raise such topics and an easily accessible contact person when they had questions. Her attention not just to families but to creating inclusive rituals that included and supported staff also shifted her profile from someone present only in end-of-life situations to someone who might be helpful if consulted on a wider range of topics.

Almost no staff in the MICU completed additional courses related to spirituality or religion or advocated for more comprehensive care from a chaplain. A few nurses described wanting to feel more comfortable talking about spirituality and religion, more in terms of their personal experiences than of work on the unit. One nurse, for instance, described how Reiki was helpful to her mother when she died, leading her to want "a little bit more education about various cultures and religions because . . . for instance, [in] the Muslim religion, . . . all sorts of things . . . need to be done at the end of life, and it would be nice if we had some sort of book to refer to when, you know, you want to try and . . . again, make the experience [good] for them as best as you can." While medical staff members were directed to ask a question about spirituality when talking with families about withdrawing care from patients, the topic was otherwise little discussed. Absent strong leadership, these individual desires did not cohere into a strong culture of talk and knowledge about spirituality and religion on the unit.

Beyond the features of these specific units, it is possible that staff members who care for ill infants have different sensitivities to religion and spirituality than do staff who care for ill adults, though more systematic research is needed about a greater number of units and hospitals.[29] Different sets of people, especially nurses, choose each of these specialties. Pediatric nurses and neonatal nurses, in particular, tend to be more oriented to holistic care and care of the whole family than are nurses in the MICU, many of whom are there to gain experience for other specialties. Many neonatal nurses spoke in interviews about wanting to do this kind of work to support and educate new families, potentially making them more aware of nonmedical family factors like religion and spirituality that might influence this care.

Many staff also perceived the infants cared for in the NICU as young, new, blameless, and certainly without the complicated interpersonal histories of the adults in the MICU. Words like *angel* and *miracle* were regularly used in public relations materials for the unit, just as small handprints and footprints adorned the sweatshirts, fuzzy coats, and other staff attire. These symbols and NICU staff members' sense of working with innocent children point to broader cultural ideas that link innocence and traditional religious and spiritual themes in ways that lead them to come up more on the unit. Regardless of the causes, it is notable that few staff—even those recently hired—learned about religion and spirituality as part of their formal nursing and medical educations; instead, they usually learn about related issues on the unit from other staff and occasionally from chaplains. For staff in both ICUs, the important professional questions about religions are not about whether they are true but about whether they help patients or interfere with medical care.

Beyond the visible presence of religion and spirituality in these units—as brought up by patients and families in the objects, rituals, and prayers described here—some staff personally drew on spirituality and religion as they moved through their shifts in other ways that were largely invisible both to me as a researcher and to their colleagues. I turn to these invisible experiences in the next chapter.

CHAPTER 7

Why Sickness and Death?
Religion and Spirituality in
the Ways Intensive Care Unit
Staff Make Meaning

At City Hospital, respiratory therapists are members of the medical team who "take the tube out" or "redirect care" after a family decides to withdraw care from a loved one. They do this by turning off and removing the ventilator that has helped the patient breathe. Sitting in a small conference room in the medical intensive care unit (MICU), I asked Shawna, a young respiratory therapist, what the process is for turning off a ventilator. "We have a procedure," she explained. Several members of the medical team are there, and one asks loved ones if they would like to be present in the room. They then "take the tube out," and try to "make the patient as comfortable as possible." Loved ones usually stay until the patient dies. "I've had family there," said Shawna, "and you can feel the sadness . . . you can touch it . . . you just want to get it done and just step out of the way and let them have their time."

"It's almost like you're not there," she continued. "You separate your job, . . . how you are feeling, from what you're actually doing so you can deal with it. If I actually had to be in that moment with them, . . . I'd probably end up crying." To make this a bit easier, Shawna, a self-described Baptist who regularly attends church, has personal procedures that she conducts along with the hospital's procedures. "I'll say a silent prayer before I do it [remove the tube]—bless them, bless the family, hope they're doing well after the fact." She says these silent prayers not only when withdrawing care but "all the time" on the job. "You know, just like, real simple like 'God bless this person,' or whomever I'm taking care of. And, you know, . . . hope we have a good day . . . and bless their family members who are suffering with them."

Joy, a young Asian American woman who works as a respiratory therapist in the NICU, described similar experiences. Wearing green City Hospital scrubs, Joy briskly entered the conference room where we spoke, a pager attached to her hip. Thirty minutes into our conversation, her tone was somber and her eyes filling with tears as she described having to withdraw support from an infant. "Sometimes you'll come on your shift, and you'll find out that's what you're doing, and you take a big breath, and you do what you have to do, and you walk out." Sometimes, she says, the pain "hits me right on," and other times "it'll hit me later on in the day. . . . It still breaks your heart every time. Never gets easier. . . . I mean, I can remove myself to be quick and fast and get it out of the way, . . . but it usually hits me at some point in the day, and I mourn every one of our patients that we lose, because it is always really a heartbreak."

Joy went on to describe a recent "horrible week" in which she had three deaths. "I felt like the angel of death. . . . Some people are lucky enough to be there sporadically, but if you're doing a stretch, and you happen to be there for all of this, it can be painful." In such situations she lets herself cry, more at home than at work. "I give myself a good bawl. And then I just pick myself up. I mean that's always how I am, and how I've been in life." She seeks the comfort of other staff, her family, and her dog. Occasionally she goes to a patient's memorial service. Like Shawna, Joy also says silent prayers during her shifts. "I always say a prayer when I turn [adjust] the machines. I think that's just force of habit. I was raised Roman Catholic. I'm not devout—but I believe in God, and I pray to Him, and always for the babies, always for the babies." She says these prayers "not just when I'm turning off the machines," but a lot of times when working. "I believe it helps me. . . . I mean, I know they're all little angels. At least that's my comfort." As for the content of her prayers, she says, "I talk to God. That's pretty much what I do. You know, bless and protect, keep them safe, do what you must—kind of thing. I usually go home, and I'll do a rosary when a baby dies."

Joy and Shawna have developed ways of coping with the suffering and death they witness in ICUs that combine aspects of their personal religious and spiritual backgrounds with other parts of their lives. They developed these strategies on the job; Shawna said that such responses "are probably more talked about rather than taught" in school. "You figure it out as you go, because nothing really trains you how to handle this." Comparing aspects of her job to her cousin's work in the military, Shawna tells new respiratory therapists, "You are going to have some good days, and you're going to have some bad days," while encouraging them to have "healthy ways to deal with stress" and to remember "you're not alone." Joy attributes her own coping abilities to her "big and loving family that's so faith-driven." Catholicism, she says, gave her a "strong heart" and "compassion." In her work in the NICU, it is that compassion, she says, that helps her "to feel for other people and to reach out to them and do the right thing." When a tragedy is happening in a person's life, as it is so often in intensive care, "you just can't turn away" she says, you have to engage.

*

This chapter shifts from considering how ICU staff respond to religion and spirituality on their units to focusing on how they personally make sense of and cope with the sickness and death they witness in their work. While such processes are not always visible in hospitals, they are there—an important way in which religion and spirituality are present even when they are not visible. Some staff, like Shawna and Joy, draw on personal religious or spiritual beliefs and practices. Others respond using languages of science, randomness, and personal responsibility. Most staff members combine these languages and practices in hybrid ways not clearly connected to how they personally identify religiously or spiritually.

I explore the often invisible—seemingly absent—presence of religion and spirituality in the personal experiences of staff members on these units in three ways. I begin by describing, in their own words, what they view as the most difficult aspects of their work. While a few described the administrative and bureaucratic headaches that come with working in a large medical institution, most spoke of the suffering of patients, the constancy of death, and the grief they so often face in their work. I then describe how staff members personally conceive of and understand this suffering, asking them why they think patients and families in their units become sick and die. Framing it less as a biomedical question than an existential one, I follow sociologist Renée Fox's attention to the human condition and experiences of health-care professionals in asking it.[1] I delineate a range of scientific, behavioral, higher-power, and randomness-focused languages that staff use, in hybrid forms, to respond to these questions.

Second, I consider what staff members describe themselves doing—their practices—to cope with the difficulties they witness in their work. As they talk with colleagues, spend time with family, exercise, cry, and engage in a wide range of hobbies, they also engage in personal religious and spiritual practices to varying degrees, most commonly through personal prayer. To illustrate how different people combine various practices, I briefly describe the experiences of three staff members. Their examples illustrate points along an analytic continuum ranging from those who explicitly draw on religious and spiritual beliefs and practices to those who do so more implicitly to those who do not do so at all. No one draws only on religion and spirituality, and the ways they combine these beliefs and practices with others is part of the story I tell.

While my attention to language and to practice gets at religion and spirituality indirectly via the ways staff members talk about them in discussion of difficult aspects of their work, I conclude by considering the issue more directly. Specifically, I asked staff members how religion and spirituality influence their work, and I outline their responses. Their answers to such direct questions raise different themes, especially related to vocation and moral guidance, that further enrich our understanding of the multiple ways that religion and spirituality invisibly inform the personal experiences of some staff in ICUs.

Medical sociologists and others who view ICU staff as emotionally detached or unfeeling may be surprised to hear them, especially the nurses and respiratory therapists, speaking about sickness, death, spirituality, and religion in emotionally rich language. There is rarely space for such emotions or reflection in the public, technical, biomedical culture of intensive care.[2] Such talk is evident here because most of the experiences that staff spoke with me about took place privately, out of public view. Glimpses of these languages are occasionally evident in studies of ICUs, though usually only in passing, as most studies focus on their public dimensions. Sociologist Robert Zussman, for example, in his classic study of ICUs, describes a rare exception to public ICU norms in what he calls one of the "strangest moments" he witnessed. Realizing that a young patient was going to die, medical staff briefly lost their awareness of the public norms, he writes, and "the discussion somehow drifted to voodoo cults, the use of drugs to stimulate brain death, and, finally, to zombies and the 'undead'—as," Zussman interprets, "the ICU doctors, apparently unaware of what they were saying, dropped the guise of science to search desperately for any way of defying death."[3] Glimpses of such conversations suggest that ICU staff members think about and try to make sense of sickness and death, even if they rarely share their thoughts publicly. They have been trained, as sociologist Renée Fox and others argue, to embody "detached concern," keeping sensitivity to patients at an emotional distance.[4] This detachment is part of the hidden curriculum in medical education, and staff members generally maintain it publicly.[5] But as Shawna and Joy silently adjust mechanical ventilators, physicians commute home, and nurses prepare for their shifts, there is another layer of awareness and meaning-making—

seemingly absent and initially invisible to me as a researcher and to staff colleagues—connected with the sickness and death that are central to their work.[6]

In exploring this invisible awareness, it is primarily differences in sense-making between physicians, nurses, and respiratory therapists as professional groups, rather than differences between staff in the NICUs and MICUs or among people with different religious histories or affiliations, that are most striking. I briefly explore reasons for these professional differences in the conclusion. Staff members' experiences are private and do not easily fit within the broad spiritual frame that chaplains use to describe their work or the narrower religious—mostly Catholic at City Hospital—frames that staff use to identify professionally and respond to religion and spirituality in their units. Nevertheless, they add an important layer to this story about religion and spirituality in secular academic hospitals by showing again how they are present even when they seem to be absent. They suggest that for staff, perhaps much as for patients, many of the ways religion and spirituality are present in hospitals are invisible on the surface, rarely the subject of public discussion, and difficult to trace historically. They also suggest that religion and spirituality take different forms for staff that are not obviously connected to their own religious or spiritual backgrounds and that depend on whether the topics come up in conversations about suffering or are inquired about directly as staff members go about their daily work.

DIFFICULT ASPECTS OF WORK

Staff members in the neonatal and medical ICUs at City Hospital find many aspects of their work difficult. Challenges from the hospital's administration, issues in the medical hierarchy, personality conflicts with coworkers, diagnostic dilemmas, and conflicts with families all make for challenging days. Most frequently, however, staff described the suffering and death they witness and experience as *the* hardest part of their work. "Dealing with people dying," a nurse in the MICU said simply, is the hardest part of her job. In addition to death, grief is a constant companion in both units. In the NICU, Karen, the nurse manager, said that all patient admissions involve grief, because parents are grieving the loss of their perfect baby. "We experience grief for every single admission." It is cumulative and wears on the staff even as they try to cope with it. Patients admitted to the MICU and their families are also grieving a loss of functioning as some face the next (or final) round of illnesses. Even when patients do not die, the grief and suffering their illnesses create in families are constantly present on the units.

In both units, staff described the death of patients as the hardest part of their jobs. A neonatologist who has worked in the NICU for more than ten years said, "The most difficult part has remained the same, . . . those incredibly difficult times around loss and death." "If you lose a patient," another physician agreed, "that's just a horrible thing." Nurses agreed, and one, Sarah, called "dealing with a baby dying" the "absolute most difficult" part of their work. In addition to describing the actual death of a child, nurses described how hard it is to support parents when their child is dying. A young nurse named Penny explained, "It's one thing to see a baby that's sick. . . . You feel very badly for them, but when the parents come in, and you have to tell them that their son or daughter is pretty sick, or that . . . we had to change something because it wasn't working, or when they look at you and say, 'I just don't want her to die,' it's—that's sort of the hardest. I mean the science is the science, and you can always get help from people about the science of it, but having to deal with those . . . difficult family moments . . . " "You get attached to these people," Sarah told me. When a child dies, there is nothing to do, a nurse named Joanne stated, but to "be in the moment and be with the parents."

Physicians and nurses in the MICU agreed. In addition to speaking about their personal reactions to death, several of these physicians also spoke of institutional problems with how death is managed in the hospital.[7] "It is always difficult when there's a young person that you know is not going to make it despite your best efforts," Dr. Ari explained, "but I think actually you kind of come to terms with the fact that you're not always going to win, and it's just the way life is." Sometimes, however, physicians say the hospital's medical bureaucracy does not manage these patients well. Families are estranged from one another, families and medical staff are not in agreement, and people have unrealistic expectations that cause everyone pain as they try to negotiate making difficult decisions. In Dr. Jackson's words, "I think the most difficult part is the end-of-life issues. . . . They're frequently difficult because things have not been handled well before a patient gets transferred to us," and families arrive with unrealistic expectations.

Nurses in the MICU compared their work to that of individuals in combat and were especially affected by deaths that took them by surprise. "I'm not sure that there's another profession that sees people die with so much regularity over a long period of time," Martha, a nurse, stated. "I mean, people in combat, they go out and see very intense death and destruction for maybe a year, . . . but we see people bleed to death. We see people code and die, and we see this with frequency. It's very hard." Another nurse explained, "There are patients that you start taking care of when you know they're going to die, and you're like, 'It would be best for them to die.' But then there are patients that you . . . you just pray they get a chance. Those are the ones that, when they don't make it, it really hurts you." It is the deaths that take nurses by surprise that they describe as the most difficult; times when, in the words of another nurse, "someone's young, and just codes, and we don't bring them back." Linda, the social worker in the MICU, explained that "with deaths that we know are going to occur," I can "help the patients sit with that, and the families. But also I have to help myself sit with that as well." The unexpected deaths are the most difficult because they do not allow her to prepare herself or the patient's family.[8]

Respiratory therapists in both units, like Shawna and Joy, monitor patients connected to ventilators or heart/lung bypass machines. Not surprisingly, given their proximity to the very sick, they also spoke frequently about how hard it is for them when patients die. "Seeing them [patients] being wheeled out on stretchers going down to the morgue," Shawna explained, "I mean, there is obviously nothing to do about it, because this unit has the sickest patients in the hospital. . . . It's just their time, but, you know, it hurts when they come in fine, talking to you. . . . You get to know them a little bit for a couple of hours during the day, and then they can turn around just like that [snap]." "The death and dying are tough," Melinda, another respiratory therapist, explained, "especially with kids." While she has gotten more used to adults dying during her ten years as a respiratory therapist, she still gets upset when children die. Other respiratory therapists agreed. "Watching the kids that we are unable to save is so difficult," said one, "and their families—watching some of the families go through what they go through only to lose a baby is just horrendous. I think that's clearly the biggest negative of my job." When an infant dies, another said, "you take it hard, . . . because more often times than not you've been involved with the parents and developed relationships with them."

In addition to talking of patients dying, staff vividly described the pain and suffering they witness, experience, and sometimes cause on both units. "The hardest things," said Dr. Karker in the NICU, "are seeing the fellows in pain, the nursing staff in pain, the respiratory therapists, people on the phone; . . . there's pain all around." Karen, the nurse manager, made clear that she would be "out of touch with the nursing staff" and not able to do her job well "if I didn't understand the suffering that goes on" as the nurses "walk side by side with families that are suffering." She encourages staff to rely on each other and hospital resources as sources of support as they respond to "the anguish people experience in the work that they do."

Nurses described different dimensions of the suffering they see and experience. This work is "physically demanding and draining," said Dottie, a nurse in the MICU. "Sometimes you go home, and you just think there are so many people that are young, much younger than yourself, and are suffering and dying. . . . It is a very, very difficult place to work, . . . but I always go back, I just love taking care of the patients." Some describe the physical pain that patients are in or that they inflict through procedures. "It's just hard when you see a baby suffering," Judy, a nurse, commented. Others describe the pain they experience in their relationships with patients and families. "You're not dealing with just the baby," explained Hannah, a nurse in the NICU. "You're dealing with the whole family. . . . It can be difficult, because you've got to put yourself right there. And you have to open up all your emotions." This is a bit easier when relationships are short, but sometimes patients are in the hospital for long periods of time. Christina cared for her last primary patient throughout his seven-month stay in the NICU. In her words, "The hardest part is when you develop that relationship, and you want the baby to do well, and they don't." Learning to "listen and hold pain, the pain of children and families, . . . disappointments, heartbreaks" without being overtaken by it is a daily challenge for Elizabeth, the pediatric chaplain, and for many of the nurses.

Many nurses also spoke of ethical dilemmas they face and are a part of in the intensive care. Nurses in the NICU spoke of the challenges of treating infants who are, in the words of one nurse, "severely brain-damaged, and you know the baby's never going to have any good quality of life." In the MICU, nurses described difficult end-of-life situations when they felt like medical teams were "torturing" people by continuing aggressive treatments, while families did not see how much a patient was suffering. "We all know what the outcome is going to be, and yet the family wants to press on, the team wants to press on," Jean, a nurse, explained.[9] As in the NICU, nurses found these situations more difficult if they were sudden or if the patient reminded them of someone they knew. "It's a lot tougher for me when it's the younger patients or the patients close to my age, and [you have to deal] with family members," a nurse told me, who "could be your mother or father." Erica, a nurse in her twenties, told me how she used to encounter ethical dilemmas in taking care of patients with liver failure, because she felt they were suffering from a disease of their own making. It was not until her best friend's mother died of liver disease that she remembered that every woman she takes care of is somebody's mother, wife, or daughter. That realization and others made her more aware of the sadness she described as "always inside" of her, coming out in tears that she shares with patients and families.

The struggles that ICU staff at City Hospital face in their work, especially those involving death and suffering, are not new.[10] Their words illustrate the findings of other studies that document both the effects that ICU work has on individuals and the failure of nursing and medical schools to prepare people for them.[11] Staff members at City Hospital cope with these challenges in multiple ways. They rely on their colleagues—"the team"—for support and seek solace in families, pets, exercise, food, entertainment, and hobbies. Some join like-minded groups at the hospital to network with others who share their approach to end-of-life situations, while others focus on the "successful" patients who recover, or, in the NICU, grow up and send photos and cards as motivation for continuing this work. Before focusing on the actions of staff members and the role of religious and spiritual practices among those actions, I step back and listen to the languages they use in trying to make sense of the sickness and death central to their work.

SENSE-MAKING LANGUAGES

I asked ICU staff directly why they think people get sick, why they suffer, and whether illness is random.[12] Many of them think about such questions regularly, both privately and in discussion with patients and families. When I asked Lisa, a nurse in the NICU, if families ask her "why" questions—"Why me?" or "Why my baby?"—she replied, "Oh God. They always ask me that, and they always say, 'Did I do something wrong?' and 'Why did I get chosen?'" Three-quarters of the physicians and nurses in the N ICU described similar conversations. "Every woman feels guilty . . . that her body let go of her baby," a nurse explained, "There's a lot of guilt that people carry around. It's like a driving force." Nurses and doctors alike spoke of trying to reassure mothers and alleviate that guilt. "One of the most general ways I try to respond," Dr. Cohen explained, "which I think is applicable in about nine out of ten cases—I very much make sure that the mother doesn't feel like she is to blame. That is the key, key, repeated theme in my clinical practice." Family members also raise such questions in the MICU, though less frequently. A nurse in the MICU explained, "It all depends on the family. It depends on people's backgrounds; it depends on other experiences they've had."

Beyond conversations with families, staff members think about these questions privately as they drive home, review their shifts in their heads, and move through their lives outside the hospital. They draw on overlapping languages I identified inductively as focused on science, individual behavior, higher purpose, and randomness in trying to make sense of why people become ill, as well as saying there is no reason or they do not know what the reason is. Almost all of the staff draw on more than one of these languages, constructing their own hybrid ways of thinking about such questions—which include religion and spirituality in varying degrees—in the process. The ways staff think and talk about these questions do not map clearly onto their personal religious or spiritual backgrounds, current affiliations, or practices, as I describe later. Before describing the hybrid languages most common within each staff group, I describe each individual language in turn.

First, not surprisingly, many staff responded to questions about why people become ill by using languages of science, with particular attention to genetics, evolution, and environmental exposure.[13] Neonatologist Dr. Alley, for instance, replied, "It's evolution, I think. It is mutations in the gene pool that lead to these weird neuromuscular diseases." Dr. Martin in the MICU agreed, adding environmental exposure to genetics as a factor in illness. Using cancer as an example, he explained, "There's been a lot of cancer in my family, and why, you know, is there some gene that we inherited, or was it from living in [a certain state] and being exposed to toxic chemicals, and so forth?" He answered his own question by saying he was "very comfortable" with scientific explanations of cancer "as sort of [a] random mutation, or some of it environmental exposure but not really determined by more than that." A neonatal nurse agreed, explaining that some infants do not do well in the NICU because of their genes: "It's genetic or biological. I think some people just don't have good protoplasm." And nurses in the MICU agreed, describing "bad genes," "medical histories of patients" that have been "inherited through genetics," and "genetics, hereditary things" as factors in why people become sick.

Second, some staff looked to the behaviors of patients or of infants' parents for explanations. Mothers who took drugs, the neonatologists explained, could harm their babies in utero. Similarly, Dr. Shapiro argued that much of the illness he sees in the MICU is self-inflicted: "A lot of it is self-imposed in the sense of people abusing themselves. Alcohol, tobacco, drugs. If we took away that, I think we would cut our population in the ICU probably by at least thirty or forty percent or more." Nurses and respiratory therapists pointed to similar behavioral explanations. Jean, a nurse in the MICU, said, "For the most part, I would say probably 75% of our patients, . . . a lot of it is lifestyle. It is people who . . . don't take care of themselves, wind up with an ulcer that makes them septic. You know a lot of coronary artery diseases, a lot of alcohol

withdrawals, a lot of drug overdoses, suicide attempts, . . . stuff like that."
Maura, a nurse, agreed, saying, "A lot of our patients have self-inflicted illness," as did Nancy, a nurse: "A lot of it is the way people live, . . . lifestyle."

In addition to these two approaches, a significant number of staff referred
to a higher power, a broader purpose, or a reason that exists for patients' illnesses but that they could not identify, at least not in this lifetime. People used
such ideas regardless of whether they considered themselves to be spiritual
or religious. Few staff explicitly mentioned religious or spiritual traditions or
beliefs by name; they more often referred generally to God and what they
called "spiritual ideas," alluding to purpose and reason in a general sense. "I
think everybody comes into this world with their own purpose," Dr. Chang,
a neonatologist and self-identified atheist, explained, "and the babies who are
born at full term, they have their purpose. And the babies who are born at
twenty-four weeks, they have their purpose in life." She did not know what
these purposes were, however. Similarly, drawing on the language of reason,
Lisa, a mostly nonpracticing Jew and neonatal nurse, said, "I think that there
is a reason for a lot of things that happen, but I don't know what that reason
is. I'm hoping that one day, . . . which I don't think will be down here, I'll
find out what the reason is, and I'll find out . . . why children have to suffer."
Speaking more directly of God, another nurse said, "There is a theory that
God gives you what you can handle. . . . I do believe that." Another nurse said,
"Everything is happening for a reason, and God does have a plan." Mark, a
respiratory therapist who identifies as a nonpracticing Catholic, similarly explained that "there's only one guy that is making the decisions, and we always
say it is the guy upstairs [i.e., God]. . . . We have the ability to lengthen the
decision that's made and override the decision sometimes, but not always."
For some, this God or higher power is all-knowing and all-powerful, while
for others, it is simply present and part of the explanation for why illness and
suffering happen.

Some staff also believed illness is random. "Life is extremely unpredictable," a critical-care physician in the MICU explained, "so I think it is just
luck of the draw." "Why moms go into preterm labor, or why the babies are
full-term and get so sick," a neonatal nurse told me, "it's random." Phrases
like "bad luck" and people being "dealt bad hands" were common, as were
statements like this one from a nurse: "Some illnesses I feel like do happen
randomly."

Finally, many staff members stated that there is no reason why people suffer
or become ill. A neonatologist replied thoughtfully, "It's a great question; I do
ask it. I don't ever get answers." And a critical-care physician in the MICU im-

plied the limits of scientific knowledge and thinking, saying, "We often don't know the cause," of particular diseases. "That's true in a lot of medicine." Referring to the broader existential questions, he said, "I don't think there is an answer for those kinds of questions" either. Nurses responded simply by saying, "I don't know" or, more broadly, "Who could answer that question?" implying no one. A nurse in the MICU responded to a question about why people get sick, saying, "I don't think there's a reason for it. I think there are a lot of good people that have really bad things happen. I don't have those answers for myself either."

Rather than drawing on one of these five themes alone, most staff drew from two or more as we talked about why people get sick and why there is so much suffering and death in their units. Individual staff members constructed hybrid languages as we talked, with particular explanations being more common in the hybrids of certain professional groups. The physicians in both units, for example, generally privileged scientific explanations combined with "no reason" explanations for suffering when the limits of scientific knowledge were reached, even as they drew on other themes. "Most of the time you can't explain" why infants in the NICU have certain diseases, Dr. Cohen said. "If there is a true genetic reason, we give it to them [the parents], . . . but otherwise the answers aren't clear, at least initially." Sometimes additional medical tests make clear the cause, but "the majority of times we don't know what caused" the illness or the infant's suffering. Genetics and medical testing are sometimes helpful in explaining illnesses, he said, but beyond that, he did not know why these things happened. Similarly, combining languages of genetics, randomness, and the possibility of a higher power, critical-care physician Dr. Waver explained, "We all have different genetic predispositions to different diseases, and to a large degree I think it is the genetics and actually the environment." He continued, "I believe that there's some sort of higher sort of power that exists and some days I guess I believe . . . it may have some sort of interaction with the world, and some days maybe I believe it does not." Privileging genetic and random explanations, Dr. Waver is uncertain about the higher power: "Maybe there's something that helps that is behind it all, but I don't even pretend to understand what that is anymore."

Nurses and respiratory therapists also drew from multiple themes in interviews, tending to draw less from scientific explanations and more from higher-power or purpose-oriented explanations, especially the neonatal nurses. While some neonatal nurses referred to genetics or randomness alone to explain why their patients were ill, the majority also spoke of God, purposes, and higher reasons (even if unknown). Penny, a nurse, said she thinks that randomness determines who goes into preterm labor and ends up with a child in the ICU, but that a higher power may also be involved. "If it's really bad," she explained, "you try to think . . . God obviously gave us this baby to learn something, learn from the family. . . . You kind of know in your heart that God wouldn't give somebody more than they can handle." Also referring to God, Tamara, another nurse, said that "we don't know what God's plan is," but "things happen for a reason. . . . There may be a reason why he [an infant] is going to suffer." Making clear that she does not know how God's plan will work out, Tamara said that "God made us smart enough to be able to make those machines [in the ICU] and to use them in the best ways possible while trying to understand God's plan.

Other nurses and respiratory therapists in the NICU referred to plans and reasons without specific reference to God. "I believe that things happen for a reason," Abby explained. "I don't have to know what the reason is. I can accept that. . . . Maybe some day I'll know." Absent this knowledge, she aimed to turn negative or difficult things in her life and work into positives, saying, "Well, this happened. What can I learn from it? And how can I move on in a positive direction?" Neonatal nurses struggling to answer questions about why people become ill and suffer, as evident in these examples, struggled not primarily within strictly scientific frameworks but within frameworks in which questions about the presence or absence of a higher power were very much in play.

Nurses and respiratory therapists in the MICU also referenced God, a higher power, or broader reasons in the hybrid languages they developed but not to the same degree as the neonatal nurses. "In some cases," Jean, a nurse, explained, things are random, but in many more "it is lifestyle." Laura spoke of genetics and individual behaviors as influencing the course of people's illnesses. Dottie pointed to randomness, individual behaviors, and a higher power in explaining why people get sick. "There's a little bit of randomness," and some things result from people "smoking, . . . drinking, or eating too much," she said. In addition, a higher power plays a role. "I usually say to them [patients] that I won't know the answers until we meet again, and then we'll be able to ask why. . . . I believe in an afterlife, and I believe in seeing God and understanding. . . . That's what gets me though." As Lisa explained, these things are parts of plans yet to be revealed.

The different emphases in the hybrid explanations for illness and suffering offered by physicians and by nurses and respiratory therapists likely relate to their training and their orientation to patients. Physicians have more years of training, and most are actively involved in ongoing scientific research in labs, which may influence their inclination for scientifically based explanations.[14] The nurses and respiratory therapists in this study (and likely nationally, though systematic data has not been gathered), are also personally more spiritual and religious than the physicians, which may influence their orientations to broader, nonscientific explanations. Nurses and respiratory therapists in their daily work also spend more time with individual patients and are more oriented to the whole patient, which may lead them to more holistic approaches to life and death that include spiritual or religious dimensions.[15]

SENSE-MAKING PRACTICES

Thinking about why a person is ill or dying does not change the fact that the person is in the ICU needing care. As they provide that care, Shawna and Joy silently pray. On difficult days and with hard cases, other staff members get support from coworkers, supervisors, and the hospital's Employment Assistance Program. They spend time with family, exercise, and have hobbies. Some cry and occasionally go to funerals. All have developed ways of setting boundaries with patients and families to manage the emotional components of this work.[16]

Personal religious and spiritual practices are present to varying degrees in the practices that staff members use to cope and take care of themselves in this work. I illustrate three points along an analytic continuum to describe the presence or absence of religious and spiritual practices that staff use to take care of themselves. I first describe Barbara, a nurse in the MICU, who explicitly draws on her personal religious beliefs, memberships, and practices. I then describe Jamie, a nurse in the NICU, who is more distant from organized religion but draws on religious practices implicitly when she talks about praying as one of several things that help her cope with her work. Finally, I describe Martha, a nurse in the MICU, who makes no mention of religious or spiritual practices when explaining how she copes with the difficult parts of her job. Staff who personally identify as religious or spiritual are spread among these three groups. Personally identifying as Catholic or as spiritual, in other words, does not necessarily lead staff to include such beliefs or practices in their descriptions of how they cope with their work.

Sitting in the MICU on a slow evening, Barbara and I spoke quietly about her background and daily work. Wearing red scrub pants and a blue scrub jacket, Barbara—Irish Catholic and in her thirties—had wanted to be a nurse since she was little, and has worked in this unit for four years. The training period was exhausting, and she finds the work difficult. "You do want to draw some sort of line . . . where I'm not leaving here crying every day, because it is very intense." She tries to draw that line by leaving work at work, and especially by talking with the other nurses. "I think we cope a lot . . . [by talking] with each other, and that makes it a lot easier, because everyone kind of feels the same way. . . . People pull a lot of support from each other." She rarely talks with family or friends about her job, because "They don't understand as well as my peers." She especially looks forward to the days when former patients and family members visit the unit; such visits help her get through the difficult days.

In addition, Barbara describes her personal faith as a "coping mechanism" in the MICU. She grew up Catholic and looks to her faith "for answers to the 'why' questions" that come up in her work. She often goes to Mass with her mom, whom she describes as "extremely religious," and together they "light candles for certain people," including her patients. Barbara says Catholicism helps her in her work because she has "faith" that "everything is happening for a reason" and that "God has a plan for everybody." Not only does she say this helps her at work, but it helps her "sleep better at night" and move more easily through her life.

While Barbara is explicit about how her religious beliefs, memberships, and practices help her cope with her work, other staff members speak of these things more implicitly, especially in terms of prayer. Jamie, for instance, a nurse in her fifties, has worked in the NICU for eight years and has been a nurse for thirty. When we spoke one afternoon in an ICU conference room, she told me that she has gotten used to many parts of this work but not to babies dying. "And it doesn't even matter how long they are here [in the NICU]. One day I had a patient come in at 7:00 a.m., and by 7:00 p.m., we withdrew care. That was just devastating." To get through difficult days and stressful experiences, she talks a lot with other nurses and with her family. "It [the job] is pretty much always stressful. . . . I go home, and I talk to my family about it . . . and vent. It helps." Jamie identifies nominally as Catholic but says she is "not a very good practicing Catholic right now. . . . I don't go to Mass, and there are a lot of things in the Catholic Church that I don't believe in. But I still pray." Among other things, she prays regularly for the babies in her care and believes it helps in her work.

Regardless of their personal religious or spiritual beliefs, many staff members are like Jamie and privately pray for their patients. Neonatal nurse Lisa is Jewish and goes to synagogue once a year. While she does not see herself as conventionally religious or spiritual, she says, "I find myself oftentimes putting a good word in for a certain baby or for all of us that care for the families in the world." Katie, a respiratory therapist, says she is not religious, but adds, "I find myself . . . on my way home sometimes saying, 'God, don't let anything happen to that baby.'" And Penny does not have many religious practices except for those focused on her patients. "When you're driving down the street, you're like, 'Please, dear God, just look at this baby and please watch for the family.'" Sometimes staff members pray for their patients and sometimes, especially in moments of desperation, for themselves. "Even when I'm doing a procedure, sometimes I say—just let me get this right," explained a nurse practitioner. "Everybody knows that you're going to catch people [staff] praying under their breath," explained a neonatologist, pointing to how private these prayers are on the unit. "If you think that it is 3:30 in the morning . . . or I'm overtired, . . . and somebody hasn't gotten a [IV] line in, . . . I say a prayer out of desperation. . . . That has been that way my whole life."

In addition to privately praying, some staff in both units ask their families— especially their mothers and grandmothers—to pray with them, reflecting the centrality of women in lived religious life in families more generally.[17] In the NICU, nurse Kosta keeps her patients in her prayers. When she has a really sick infant, she says, "I've talked to my mom, . . . who seems to have a direct line, like a lot of mom's do, . . . and she'll say a little prayer for them." Lillian in the MICU also "ask[s her] grandmother to put someone [a patient] on her prayer list" when things are not going well, even though she is personally uncertain about her spiritual or religious identity.

Not all staff draw on religious or spiritual practices in their work, however. Some, like Martha, take care of themselves and make sense of their work with no such references. Martha went into nursing looking for secure employment and has worked in ICUs for more than twenty years. She is one of the more senior nurses in the MICU and spends a significant amount of time helping to train newer nurses. Despite her experience, she continues to find ICU work challenging and compares the work to that in combat zones.

On difficult days, she gets support through conversation with coworkers and family members who also work in health care. "How do I deal with it [the work]? I just do it. It's sad. You do the best you can, and again that's a gratification, knowing that you're just doing everything you know how to do, and you are just working 110%." She describes herself as "conventionally anti-religious" and does not include any religious or spiritual practices among those that help her take care of herself in her work. She has learned over time to take care of herself in the ICU by strictly limiting her work hours and having a lot of outside distractions, primarily her family.

ASKING DIRECTLY

In addition to listening for spiritual or religious practices in the ways staff talked about how they take care of themselves in their work, I asked them directly how, if at all, their spiritual or religious backgrounds influenced their work. In addition to helping cope with sickness and death, staff members described several additional connections.

First, several physicians spoke of deriving a sense of vocation from their religious upbringing, a feeling they were called or destined by a higher power to become a physician. Neonatologist Dr. Jooner, a Christian, referred to God in describing being called to medicine, as if "by a magnet, . . . one of those big industrial magnets. . . . This is where I should be." Dr. Brown also used the language of a calling: "I truly was called in medicine. . . . Medicine as a ministry is part of my life." Her focus on ethical issues in medicine also derives from this source, she explained, referring to a famous saying: "'Preach the Gospel and, if you have to, use words,'" as what she is aiming to do. Although he enjoys his children and family, Dr. O'Malley likens his work as a critical-care physician to that of a Catholic priest, saying he likely would have become a priest if he had been born in a different time. "Much of what we do . . . can take on the tenor of a religious vocation. . . . I think with the most dedicated physicians it is a very analogous sort of calling."

Second, a number of physicians and nurses spoke of drawing ethical or moral guidelines from their religious upbringings. Dr. Jackson said he had a "certain set of ethics that are applied across the board that are values from my religious background," and Dr. Waver referenced his religious upbringing in saying that his life "ultimately is made much richer by actually trying to be in service to other people." Dr. Martin described the Jewish concept of *tikkun olam*, meaning "to repair the world" as part of what motivates him in his work. Several nurses, likewise, spoke of learning from their religious or spiritual traditions the importance of being kind to other people and treating them with respect. "I want people to treat me the way I treat them and respect other people. And I think that's part of being a good Christian," a nurse practitioner explained. Similarly, a nurse, Marilyn, described being "brought up . . . to be nice to everybody," and another nurse referenced her faith in trying to be "open and tolerant of everybody."

Finally, several staff members felt their own religious and spiritual backgrounds made it easier for them to connect with patients, both by offering the support of chaplains and by having a better understanding of how religion and spirituality might inform the experiences of patients and families in intensive care. In the MICU, for instance, Laura, a nurse, explained that her sense of spirituality helped her to "recognize that other people are spiritual or religious and think that that's an important quality of life." Mona, a nurse in the MICU, agreed, saying that although she does not currently consider herself especially Catholic, her exposure to religion "may be helpful to some patients." She makes sure "to ask the family if they would like a religious person to come. I think that if you have religion of any kind, you would think of that." Relying less on his awareness of particular religious traditions than on his belief that "we all have a sense of wonderment" that can be tapped into, Dr. Coyle said that his spiritual beliefs influence his work with families by helping them together to tap into that place of wonderment, regardless of its source, in a way that is often relevant in the intense experiences people have in ICUs.

CONCLUSIONS

While rarely publicly evident in the units, religion and spirituality influence how some ICU staff cope with the difficulties and uncertainties of their work. Despite public debates about rights of conscience for health-care providers that are often linked to religion and spirituality, none of the staff members I met at City Hospital pointed to religion or spirituality as reasons they felt uncomfortable with aspects of their work. While many of these influences are invisible on the surface, they are present where they might seem absent here in three distinct ways. First, some influences are present as staff members draw on higher-power and related themes in their hybrid approaches to questions of suffering, death, and illness that are a regular part of their work. Second, they are evident as one part of multiple practices that staff members enact to take care of themselves as they do this work. While some staff explicitly think of patients and families as they attend religious services, others do so more indirectly, and still others do not do so at all. Finally, staff members speak of their senses of vocation and of the kinds of moral and ethical guidance they draw from their religious backgrounds when they are asked directly about how religion and spirituality influences them in their work.

Across these dimensions, variation is evident, primarily among physicians, nurses, and respiratory therapists. While some physicians are quick to speak of vocation and the moral and ethical guidance they draw from their religious traditions, science and randomness play central roles in their talk of suffering and death, and religious or spiritual practices are not so central in the ways they cope with their daily work. Nurses and respiratory therapists are more likely to speak of a higher power in talking about the difficulties they face in their work and in describing how they cope with them in their daily lives. Neonatal nurses are the professional group most likely to draw on religious and spiritual themes in talking about how they make sense of and cope with their daily work, perhaps reflecting their own backgrounds, the tenor of their units, selection into the profession, or their experience in caring for infants.

Staff members' personal religious or spiritual backgrounds and their current beliefs, affiliations, and practices were not predictably connected to the ways they made sense of and took care of themselves in their work. There were no clear patterns, in other words, of personal religious or spiritual affiliation, membership, or attendance, which indicates the complexities of what people mean when they identify as religious or spiritual in interviews.

Learning about the different roles of religion and spirituality in the personal experiences of health-care professionals is important because it points to other ways in which religion and spirituality may be present in hospitals but are not often seen. Perhaps more than in formal chapels or meditation rooms, or in the broadly spiritual work of chaplains, personal perspectives on religion and spirituality shape the experiences not only of staff but of patients and families. They point to the importance of being at least aware of the possibility that the visible evidence of religion and spirituality in these hospitals is but a fraction of their total presence. Where religion and spirituality seem to be absent in hospitals, they may be silently present. Like Shawna and Joy, whose stories began this chapter, some staff members draw on religion and spirituality as they try to make sense of death.[18] It is to the relationship between religion, spirituality, and death that I turn in the next chapter.

CHAPTER 8

Managing Death:
The Personal and Institutional
"Dirty Work" of Chaplains

This Book of Remembrance is presented in loving memory of our baby son, who was born in this hospital but lived for only a few short hours.

Time is a great healer of sorrow.

But memories should be cherished.

—Inscription in the remembrance book located in the Chaplaincy
Department office at Overbrook Hospital

You spent time with me the day before he [my husband] died and listened to who we were and what our life was about. When my husband was conscious, he had prayers with the priest, which gave him comfort. When I needed comfort, I got you. . . . You told me that folks who fought through life sometimes fight against death. When you said that to me, you helped me to know what to say to my husband. . . . It was important for me to tell you that you made a difference on the most significant day of my life.

—Thank you note written to Meg, staff chaplain, Overbrook Hospital

It is not uncommon for ICU staff to equate religion, spirituality, and the work of hospital chaplains with death. At City, Overbrook, and hospitals across the country, chaplains fulfill this stereotype by spending significant amounts of time with dying people and their families. Some families, like the couple who donated the Remembrance Book and the woman who wrote the thank-you note in the epigraphs above, find chaplains helpful in end-of-life situations. Others, like some hospital administrators, have historically worried that by naming and talking of death, chaplains might create the wrong public impression—that hospitals are more places for dying than for living or healing.

This worry was not particularly acute at City or Overbrook Hospitals, but it was in the history of a nearby academic hospital aside from the seventeen described in this book. Nurses, social workers, and psychiatrists at Oak Ridge Hospital asked administrators to hire a staff chaplain in the 1980s to help them care for dying patients.[1] A group of employees had gathered in the 1970s to petition the hospital to build a chapel but were refused. "Some people," Peter, the current director of chaplaincy, remembered, "thought that if we [had] a chapel here, there [would] be funeral services" and other public recognitions of death that hospital administrators thought sent the wrong messages about dying rather than the right messages about living. Nurses and social workers were concerned when patients died, however, and routinely called priests and rabbis not affiliated with the hospital. They called them, Peter remembered, "to come in because a patient was dying, and the family asked for a rabbi, or a priest, or a minister," and the hospital had none to offer. Area clergy visited the hospital when they could, telling administrators over and over again to hire a chaplain to help the staff and even considering a public boycott of the hospital.

In the 1980s, the hospital administrators relented and hired Peter as their first staff chaplain, primarily to help with dying patients. As he recalled, "I came here for my first day, and I was greeted by the chairperson of the Search Committee," who gave him a pager and wished him luck. He had no office, no phone, and his position came with no health-care benefits. Peter quickly realized that the hospital had a "distorted view of spiritual care," seeing the chaplain as someone who was concerned primarily with death, offering last rites to the mostly Catholic patients in the hospital but doing little else. Peter worked for six months to expand their view before submitting his letter of resignation and a short needs assessment outlining the scope of a chaplain's job and the resources required, including an office and a phone. The Search Committee chairperson refused the resignation, and after several weeks and many conversations, Peter returned to the hospital with an office, health insurance, the start of a budget process, and the beginning of a conversation about a chapel. Only after the hospital appointed a new president several years later, who had what Peter describes as a "real ear for spiritual care," did the institution come to see chaplains as people who were concerned not only with death, more through conversation than through last rites alone, but also with, in Peter's words, upholding "the hope that spirituality offers," not just in end-of-life situations but more generally.

This hospital's concern about how publicly it should acknowledge death and the roles that chaplains and chapels play in this process is one example of the ambivalent relationships American hospitals have had with death.[2]

These relationships became more complex in the twentieth century as death moved from the home to medical institutions, and advances in mechanical ventilation and other forms of life support increased the number and ethical complexity of decisions to be made at the end of life.[3] Today, more Americans die in hospitals than anywhere else, and a significant fraction spend time in an ICU before they die.[4] Despite the prevalence of death in hospitals, hospitals are rarely structured to allow for what people want—death that takes place without violence or pain, when someone is at peace, and with at least some control over events.[5] Death is instead seen by some hospital staff, especially surgeons, as a failure that they should almost always avoid.[6] Research describes how hospitals and hospital staff respond to death by avoiding it, distancing themselves from it, focusing on its technical and clinical aspects, and managing it.[7] As anthropologist Sharon Kaufman argues, most deaths are decided upon rather than waited for as in the past. An unproblematic hospital death is rare.[8]

In my conversations with ICU staff and chaplains, death was one of the most common topics. Although I did not ask a single direct question about death in interviews or bring up the topic when shadowing staff, questions about religion and spirituality inevitably lead to talk of death. Some ICU nurses even reinterpreted my research, describing it to each other not as about religion and spirituality or the experiences of ICU staff but as about death in the ICU.[9]

Current research about how people die in hospitals offers only a glimpse into the roles that religion and spirituality play. In a 2009 article in the *Journal of the American Medical Association*, physician Andrea Phelps and colleagues reported that religious cancer patients receive more life-prolonging treatments, such as mechanical ventilation, than do nonreligious patients.[10] They said nothing, however, about the social processes through which this occurs in hospitals. Ethnographic studies of seriously ill and dying people in hospitals occasionally describe them or their families as praying behind privacy curtains or spending time with religious leaders.[11] Researcher Joan Cassell describes an ICU nurse calling a chaplain as a patient dies in *Life and Death in Intensive Care* (2005). Sharon Kaufman similarly describes chaplains standing at bedsides to lead prayer services for patients near death and their families in *And a Time to Die: How American Hospitals Shape the End of Life* (2005). Classic studies of how people die in hospitals conducted in the 1960s by Barney Glaser and Anselm Strauss and by David Sudnow say a bit more about religion and spirituality, mostly showing how, by working with individual patients and families, chaplains also help staff and hospitals as a whole manage death more generally, as Peter did in his first six months at Oak Ridge Hospital.[12]

I build on such research in this chapter by focusing on the relationship between religion, spirituality, and death in large academic hospitals. I move through hospitals—from bedsides to the morgue—exploring how chaplains, whom one chaplaincy director called the "grief folks," describe their work with death.[13] I investigate how ICU staff describe religion and spirituality as relevant in end-of-life situations by asking what chaplains do for dying patients in hospitals, how that is shaped by their institutional contexts, and how they interpret their work with death for themselves. I say less here about how death happens in hospitals—that has been well described by others—than about the multiple ways in which hospital chaplains see themselves acting around death in their daily work and the physical locations in which they do so.[14]

At Overbrook and elsewhere, chaplains describe themselves as working with dying patients and their families as well as with staff members, helping them to make sense of what is happening and to situate the deaths they see in broader contexts and perspectives. This is one of the main sets of tasks that chaplains handle in hospitals, and it is sometimes, but not always, explicitly connected to religion and spirituality. Chaplains challenge frequent medical silences about death by naming death, facilitating conversations about death, and accompanying patients and families through the process. Much as they do in individual cases, they do this for the institution as well, as they work with dead bodies, facilitate trips to the morgue, lead memorial services and other institution-wide death rituals (which never include dead bodies), and act as memory-keepers for families and staff alike. Like much of their other work, the actions of chaplains around death are strongly shaped by their institutional contexts. Those who work in professional and transitional chaplaincy departments are more engaged with death in more ways across hospitals, and especially with staff, than chaplains who work in traditional departments.

Hospital staff and commentators often described dealing with death—with dead bodies, blood and odors, and the grief of families—as "dirty" or low-status work.[15] Barney Glaser and Anselm Strauss, as did several chaplains I interviewed, described doctors quickly delegating families to nurses and chaplains after telling them about a loved one's impending death, leaving it to them to handle the emotions of the families and other "dirty" work.[16] Contemporary chaplains welcome this institutionally low-status work; they do not view it as "dirty" work and do not want to be out from under its shadow. Perhaps to maintain dignity in their work or to honor their personal beliefs, chaplains talk about their work with death in contexts much larger than the status hierarchy of the hospital. They describe working with dying people as a privilege, part of the calling they feel, and as related to how they see God and the sacred in their midst. Regardless of how they personally interpret it, the work chaplains do around death ultimately serves, however, to further solidify and strengthen the connections staff members make between religion, spirituality, chaplains, and death. Chaplains necessarily spend much of their time working around death, leading staff members who watch them to continue to view religion, spirituality, and chaplains as more relevant at the end of life than when healthy children are born, diseases are declared in remission, or in other celebratory hospital contexts.

THE DAILY WORK WITH DEATH AT OVERBROOK HOSPITAL

Unlike the staff at Oak Ridge Hospital in the 1980s, hospital staff at City and Overbrook Hospitals do not equate the work of chaplains exclusively with death, even though chaplains spend significant amounts of their time working with people who are dying and their families. Two to three people die every day at Overbrook, and chaplains aim to attend all of these people, if not at the moment they are dying, then within a few days of their deaths.[17] Chaplains prioritize dying patients when deciding who to visit at Overbrook, and they are called whenever a patient dies. Some deaths happen quietly, but many are complex, involving traumas or complicated family dynamics. "Death is kind of arbitrary," Father William told me. Even in a critical-care hospital, "it doesn't come at normal times, even if it is at the end-of-life."

Chaplains quickly become accustomed not only to seeing dead bodies but also to touching them as they offer blessings and prayers. On the basis of her research with chaplaincy residents, anthropologist Francis Norwood describes how learning to deal with dead bodies is one of many ways chaplains adjust to hospital norms.[18] Judy, a chaplain resident at Overbrook, was not used to touching dead bodies when she started at the hospital. She learned from her CPE supervisor that families often look to the chaplain to see whether it is all right to touch the dead body of a loved one. It generally is, and Judy quickly learned to do so, serving as an example for family members. In addition to touching dead bodies, Judy and fellow chaplain residents quickly learned from their supervisor or staff chaplains how to find the morgue, a stainless-steel room in the basement of the hospital accessible via the service elevators. They learned to check a body out of the morgue, wheel it down the hallway to the viewing room, prepare it for a loved one to see by uncovering the dead person's head, and stay with loved ones as they viewed the body.[19]

In addition to working with dead bodies, which have often been cleaned up before chaplains accompany family members to see them, chaplains at Overbrook are routinely called into messy traumas and codes in the emergency room. Michael, a chaplain resident, was called to the emergency room a few months after he started at Overbrook to pray for a baby delivered there after her mother was in an accident. Both died. The baby's mother, in Michael's words, "had been cut from the chest all the way down, bleeding fiercely," and the doctors were "massaging her heart" as he blessed the blood-covered baby. On another evening, Michael was called to the emergency room to meet a young man hurt in an explosion. "The only thing that wasn't burned on him was his eyes," Michael told me, "and I went up to him, and he reached out his hand, bandages and all. To see things like that," Michael reflected, is "hard." Not only images of injured and dying women and men but the smells of blood, burned flesh, and human excrement, and the sounds of people in pain are intimate parts of the everyday work of chaplains.

In addition to meeting and caring for a dying woman and her baby in the emergency room, Michael and other chaplains offer support at times of death to Overbrook staff, mostly nurses. Pat, the chaplaincy director, told me shortly after this incident that patients do not usually die in the emergency room. Also, because it involved an infant, emergency room staff members were quite upset. In an unrelated meeting I attended with Pat a few days later, news of the event had made its way through the hospital, and staff members present were calling Michael a "very kind man," telling Pat how appreciative they were for the support he provided to everyone—the patient and staff alike—in the ER that night. As conversation about this case continued, Pat offered informal support to a Catholic nurse at the meeting who was present in the ER when the woman who died arrived. She told Pat that she threw some water on the baby before Michael came, as a kind of baptism. She was worried when she did this, though, not about whether the mother would have wanted the child baptized but because the baby was already dead. "What can I do better?" she asked Pat, to care for the soul of the baby in this situation. After a baby dies, Pat explained, a blessing like the one Michael gave is best. The nurse was still worried that she would not know what to say in such a situation, and Pat told her that there were standard things to say that she could get for her. Several other chaplains checked in afterwards with the nurses present at these deaths in the ER to see how they were doing and if they wanted to talk.

Beyond working directly with patients and staff, chaplains at Overbrook

Hospital hold bereavement services in memory of patients and staff members throughout the year. At a meeting of the bereavement committee, the chaplaincy director, social workers, and nurse members spoke about services they organize for families of those who die at the hospital that include readings, poetry, and the names of the deceased. The chaplaincy department also provides a space for and keeps track of the memories of some of these people through a Remembrance Book. A couple whose infant son died at the hospital donated this book to the chaplaincy department many years ago. It is offered to parents whose infants have died in the hospital so they can read what others before them have written and, if they want, write a page about their child when they are ready. Entries include long letters to babies, photos, programs from memorial services, and introductions to children born years later. In this book the department holds the memories of these children, and creates a space for families to visit on death anniversaries and at other times as they work with their grief.

DAILY ACTIONS CONCERNING DEATH MORE BROADLY

As they work around death at Overbrook and elsewhere, chaplains become part of what Barney Glaser and Anselm Strauss call the "trajectory" of dying, or the social processes that individuals go through as they die in hospitals.[20] Depending on the institutional position of chaplains, they may also be part of the trajectory through which the hospital as an institution manages dying patients. Chaplains are probably called more often when patients are dying than at any other time in hospitals, but their positions in the trajectories of individuals and institutions are more varied. They describe their actions as including one or more of the following.

Naming Death

In their work with the dying, chaplains first call death by name. They describe this naming as challenging medical silences around death that come from what a chaplain at Streamside Hospital described as "death-phobic" physicians. It is really difficult to get doctors on board, a chaplain at Creekside Hospital explained, to admit that a patient is dying. Doctors "don't generally pay much attention to the total picture," the director of the chaplaincy department at Center Hospital explained, "the nonmedical factors. And they're particularly dreadful around dying. . . . Generally most physicians see dying as a failure, and they are very difficult to deal with." Despite recent efforts to better train physicians about death and help them work more comfortably with patients and families, chaplains still witness much tension.[21] "I don't think we need to prolong death," Meg at Overbrook said, referring to situations in which it is clear to everyone involved that the patient is going to die soon, but medical interventions continue. Rather than helping families decide to turn off machines and redirect care, physicians often continue aggressive treatment. In Meg's words, "oftentimes the physicians do prolong death."[22]

In *Awareness of Dying*, Barney Glaser and Anselm Strauss describe an elderly patient wanting to talk about his impending death. "The nurses retreated before this prospect," they write, "as did his wife, reproving him, saying he should not think or talk about such morbid matters." It was the hospital chaplain who listened to the patient and then helped the nurses and his wife do the same, "at least to acknowledge more openly that the man was dying."[23] Chaplains spoke of working with people in similar ways. At Overbrook, for example, I attended a support group with Meg for patients and their family members who have a particular health condition. Two members of the group had died the weekend before I attended, and much of the meeting was devoted to helping group members talk through these deaths. The nurse practitioner who leads the group with Meg announced the deaths, and then several group members commented. Meg said this was difficult news for everyone and brought up emotions and concerns that we all have about our health and the health of our loved ones.[24] She encouraged people to listen to and honor their emotions and to share them with each other, which happened through stories in the remainder of the meeting.

The role chaplains play in naming death was particularly evident for one chaplain who, in an extremely uncommon arrangement, had been a physician at the hospital where he now works. There is a small room off the emergency room at this hospital, he explained, where families go when a loved one is brought in by ambulance to be resuscitated. If the person dies, a nurse usually goes to that room to tell the family. When he was a doctor, he thought this should be his responsibility. "I always went in [to this room], and I'd go through my little sequence," letting them know that their loved one had died. After answering their questions, he said, "the grief would come—the howling, the shrieking, the crying, the sobbing, the being stunned, the whatever. And within thirty seconds, I would be so overcome myself, I would just have to quickly excuse myself and get the hell out of that room," sending a nurse in his place. While he did name death as a physician, he then quickly left the situation. Since becoming a chaplain, he is no longer afraid of death or overwhelmed by people's grief. Instead, he voluntarily enters this small waiting room, naming death with families and sitting with them through their early shock and grief.

Facilitating Conversations about Death

In naming death, chaplains create spaces and facilitate conversations about death with people who are dying and their families. According to Glaser and Strauss, these conversations mostly occur between dying people and chaplains. One chaplain, they observe, "could respond to patients' invitations to talk [about death] and indeed draw them into conversation better than could the nursing and medical personnel.[25] The conversations that current chaplains recounted about death more often included the chaplain, the person who was dying, and family members. One man in his early thirties was a bone-marrow transplant patient, one chaplain at City Hospital remembered. Every time the chaplain visited him, the room was full of family. One day when the chaplain looked in, the patient asked his family to leave so he could speak with the chaplain privately. He told the chaplain that he was comfortable with the fact that he was going to die, but he did not want to spend the rest of his time with his family not being comfortable. The chaplain suggested that he invite his family back into the room and begin to have the conversation with the chaplain that he wanted to have with his family. He did, and within a few minutes family members were jumping in with questions that led to the family conversation he had in mind.

In facilitating such conversations, chaplains increase understanding between dying people and their families and routinely teach families and staff members how to talk with others about death. In one case, a woman asked a chaplain at Overbrook how to tell their children about a family member's death. "I was able to talk to them about the different ages," she told me, telling them "that the youngest ones would not understand and would keep asking, 'When is he coming home?'" The parents could help, the chaplain explained, "by talking about how things get broken and don't work anymore. And sometimes our bodies get broken and don't work anymore," which would help children of different ages understand.

In addition to facilitating conversations about death, some chaplains, especially Catholic chaplains, also help families have conversations about end-of-life decisions, more often when there is no conflict between families and medical staff than when there is. At Overbrook, Father William tries to help Catholics understand that it is all right, in his words, "to let nature take its course." "I will say to them—when the machines work, they're miraculous.

When they don't work, they get in God's way." The challenge he finds is getting families to think about what their loved one would want and to see their decisions to stop treatment as potentially justified and as something other than "pulling the plug." Father William and other Catholic chaplains also work regularly with people who are considering terminating pregnancies for medical reasons. Often these families are pro-life, Father William told me, and are now faced with a decision regarding a baby who has anomalies that are not compatible with life. "I've learned over time that what's important," he explained, is that "you don't make any judgments. You try to comfort people, try to reassure them." He tells people, "This is a wanted pregnancy. You have loved this child with all your love, and whatever you believed before you were in this situation, you still believe. . . . Whatever decision you make is the right one." His goal is to eliminate any kind of guilt, he said, and to support whatever decision people determine is right for them.

Accompanying People in Times of Death

As chaplains name death and help dying people and their loved ones talk about it, they accompany people in all stages of the dying process. One chaplain referred to herself as a "spiritual midwife," and all regularly do rituals, such as the Catholic Sacrament of the Sick, for the dying. David Sudnow describes this traditional role at the hospital he studied as the Catholic chaplain made his rounds each day, administering the sacrament. After completing these rounds, Sudnow writes, the chaplain "stamp[ed] the index card of the patient with a rubber stamp that read, 'Last rites administered, date, clergyman.'"[26] After Vatican II, the Catholic Church transitioned from last rites, formally called Extreme Unction and administered at the point of death, to the Sacrament of the Sick, which can be given whenever a person is ill, not just at the end of life. Many Catholics are not aware of this change, however, routinely calling priests to administer last rites, which they do through the Sacrament of the Sick at all of the hospitals I studied.

For this reason, at least among Catholics, chaplains were historically called at the moment of death, and chaplains continue to be called to all deaths at half of the hospitals I studied. By the time the chaplain arrives, the patient has sometimes already died. They are present at the moment of death, in other cases, especially if requested by a family. At one hospital where chaplains are paged for every trauma, a chaplain described standing in the ambulance bay with a patient who had just arrived after being shot. Watching his blood pressure go down on the monitors, she realized the young man was going to die right there. After alerting a nurse, she said, "I stood by him and I prayed [a nondenominational prayer] while his heart finally stopped." At Overbrook, a chaplain resident described several cases in which he was called to sit with people as they died. "I feel glad that there's someone with [them]," he told me. "I'd hate to die alone," he said, and added that he was "happy" to be able to accompany others in the dying process. Chaplains also regularly accompany staff through the processes that follow death in hospitals. They stay with nurses after a physician pronounces death, for example, sometimes accompanying them through postmortem care and to the morgue with the body.

Chaplains also support loved ones in the shock and grief that may follow immediately and in the longer term when a loved one dies.[27] Chaplains stay with families after an unexpected death, sitting with them alone or in the presence of their loved one's body. A chaplain at Overbrook described spending time with a woman whose husband died unexpectedly after cardiac surgery. "She was holding my arm walking into the room to say goodbye to him after he died. . . . I was with them most of the night, and the next morning she said to me that it had made a tremendous difference." "You just hold people while they cry," another chaplain said, "not being afraid to touch people and be physical with them. Just let them experience what they need to experience." Other chaplains speak of helping people begin to acknowledge the death, especially when it is the death of an infant. Father William described spending time with a young father at Overbrook whose son had just died and trying to help him "acknowledge that the raging feelings he had were all appropriate" and eventually to hold the child before he was taken to the morgue.

Sometimes chaplains are present following a death and do little more than listen as the family and friends of the person who died speak about their loved one. Beth, a chaplain resident at Overbrook, was in the emergency room when a young woman died unexpectedly. Her large family assembled, and Beth brought them to the dead woman's side, expecting that she might say a prayer. "Instead, the older sister of the patient and one of the aunts . . . came into the room and then went straight for the head of the bed, . . . and I just stood back. They had their hands on her hands and on her forehead, and they were each sort of praying quietly to themselves. Eventually the prayer got louder, and they started joining together, . . . and it got more and more strong and powerful until they were done." "They knew how to call God into a room," Beth later reflected. "They didn't need me to do it."

When families have difficulty separating themselves from the body of a dead loved one, especially a child, chaplains are also called. A chaplain who works primarily with children estimated that he has held three thousand dead children over the course of his long career as their parents have left the room and the hospital. "I'll normally try to sort of put in their [the parents'] ear," he told me, "that when you've had a chance to hold your child, . . . when you feel you're ready and willing, . . . I'd like for you to hand me your child. I've been doing that for years and years, and it's the most powerful thing. What it does is it helps the mom start to make the transition that her child is dead, . . . which means somewhere in her soul she's getting to the point where she knows she has to do this." Not only does this help the family, but it helps the institution move families out of the hospital so they can prepare the bed and room for the next patient.[28]

Chaplains also help hospitals manage death by accompanying family members who were not at the hospital when their loved one died through hospital basements to the morgue, where they can see the body. One chaplain at Creekside had just come from the morgue when we started to talk, having accompanied a man who wanted to see the body of his wife, who had fallen six stories to her death. Another chaplain had done two morgue visitations the morning we spoke, also with family members wanting to see their loved one's body.[29]

A few chaplains also spoke about ways they support people after the immediate shock of their loved one's death has passed. Several described leading memorial services for families they met at the hospital, weeks and months after an individual died. At Overbrook, Meg described doing a memorial service for a patient who died at the hospital, and Father William similarly described several services he led. In one case, the family contacted him six weeks after their loved one died, asking if he would consider helping them plan a memorial service. He agreed, planning and officiating at the service and joining them at their home afterwards for a small gathering. Other chaplains prefer not to participate in such services or see patients and families outside of the hospital, but they send prayers or readings that families can include.

Rituals for the Institution

In addition to their work with individual patients, families, and staff, chaplains facilitate rituals for hospitals as institutions, planning memorial services for patients and staff and making contributions to public memorial spaces in hospitals.[30] Most hospitals hold services at least annually in honor of patients and staff members who have died that year. These are never funerals (the bodies of the deceased are never present); they are services of remembrance in which names are read and words said, usually in broad spiritual frames that one chaplaincy director described in terms of "American civil religion. . . . It's a benign sort." One hospital has bereavement days as well as bereavement services for different units of the hospital, some of which include the families of patients. Programs for families who lost children before or after birth seem more common than others.

More than the deaths of patients, which are normal parts of hospital life, the deaths of staff members are ritually remembered by other staff, and chaplains are included in the process. Chaplains are frequently called when a staff member dies to name death and spend time with the dead person's colleagues. One chaplain described an informal group he formed with a psychologist and bereavement coordinator at the hospital to take care of the nurses and respond to staff crises. When a prominent surgeon died the day he was to do surgery, this chaplain explained, "he had a staff that was left with a dead surgeon, so our group went into operation." They went to his office and held sessions throughout the hospital naming his death, sharing the shock and sorrow, and supporting his colleagues. At this hospital and others, chaplains help organize individual memorial services for staff when they die. Such services are central to how integrally involved chaplaincy departments are or want to be in their hospitals. "My vision of what institutionally I want to be able to do," the director at Oceanview Hospital explained, is to "gather when you're in grief, or when you had trauma, or when you need to recognize and celebrate the life of an employee that's been here for twenty-five years."

Chaplains also help create seemingly neutral spaces in hospitals where loved ones can share their personal memories of people who have died. While visiting hospitals, I saw memorial quilts and scrapbooks with information families provided about people who died at the hospital. I saw posters in hospital chapels with photos and remembrances of people who died of certain diseases, often cancer, created for or during bereavement services. Describing a yearly memorial service at Creekside Hospital at which these posters are created, the chaplaincy director told me about the two hundred people who attend and are invited, as a part of the service, "to come up to the front and put these things on these boards and then go to the lectern and talk if they want to." "We put these boards in the chapel," he explained, for a month or two following the service, "and then we take them out so they don't get to be too commonplace, because they're not. . . . They are very powerful tributes to people." These displays join the memories people share in remembrance books like the one at Overbrook and in prayer books at other hospitals.

As chaplains help manage death for hospitals by sitting with families in grief, accompanying them to the morgue, organizing institution-wide rituals, and holding the memories of those who died, they do so within a general set of parameters that allow them to recognize death in the hospital while not bringing too much institutional attention to it. Dying patients are frequently put in quieter (David Sudnow would say more socially isolated) areas of hospital units where chaplains can help families manage their grief in ways that do not disturb nurses or loudly bring it to the attention of other patients.[31] Unless gatherings or services are held in the rooms where patients have died or in the morgue, dead bodies are never present at the gatherings and memorial services that chaplains organize—part of the continuing attempts of hospitals to distance themselves from death—if not from the recognition of it, from its overt public display.

Recognizing that chaplains may do memorial services but not funerals with bodies in the hospital chapel, one chaplain at Center Hospital commented on how hospitals continue to "want to hide death.... We don't want to admit to [it]." Imagining the hypothetical situation in which a dead body was present in a hospital chapel, she laughed out loud, "We would have to roll a casket up the street . . . we'd have to admit that people actually die here." While some memory books do contain photos of dead bodies, images on quilts and posters displayed in more public places in hospitals were usually of healthy people—as they were before they were sick and dying, and as family members and hospitals, would prefer to remember them.[32]

Institutional Contexts

Like the other aspects of their work, chaplains' participation in the individual and institutional trajectories of dying in hospitals is strongly influenced by institutional contexts. In professionally oriented chaplaincy departments, chaplains are generally called to all deaths, sit on the palliative care team, are a part of bereavement committees and events, and regularly facilitate rituals concerning death for the institution as a whole. Transitional departments are moving in that direction. In more traditional departments, chaplains are less integrated into hospitals, meaning that they are less likely to be called or to take part in protocols concerning death, less likely to sit on palliative care teams, and less likely to organize or participate in death-related rituals for the institution.

The different ways chaplains work with death are evident, institutionally, in comparing Overbrook and City Hospitals. At Overbrook, a transitional, almost professional department, chaplains are called to all deaths, sit on the palliative care team, and regularly lead memorial services and take families to the viewing room or morgue, managing death for the institution in the process. At City Hospital, a more traditional department, priest-chaplains frequently administer the Sacrament of the Sick, but chaplains are not called to all deaths and have only recently been included in the palliative care team. The few regular bereavement and memorial services that take place were started by nurses and social workers, and I never heard of a chaplain accompanying a family to the morgue. Chaplains who work in the neonatal and medical ICUs at City Hospital also describe more variation in how individual chaplains work with death than do staff chaplains I interviewed at Overbrook.

In comparison to traditional departments, transitional and professional departments often developed systematic, protocol-based ways of ensuring that chaplains were present and available at all deaths. At one such hospital, chaplains had become, the director explained, "the designated requesters for tissue and organ donation," an institutional role that required them to be present at many deaths. At another hospital, they were regularly called to be present when life support was withdrawn or when a family member needed to go to the morgue, roles that enabled them to offer support to dying people and their loved ones. At a third hospital, a chaplain had become responsible for the paperwork involved in releasing dead bodies from the hospital to the mortuary, an institutional role that provides an "official" reason to be present for families after someone dies. Called the "decedent-care" chaplain, this person, according to the director, has "total responsibility for making sure that we [the hospital] know where all the bodies are, [that] we can account for them, that they aren't [going to] stay here longer than. . . . Sometimes we had cases where they were here for eight weeks, and people didn't know about it. . . . It is protecting the hospital." Having a chaplain in this role, the director argued, also helps with Orthodox Jewish, Muslim, and other families who have particular traditions and norms concerning death that require the quick release of the body or other practices a bit outside the hospital's norm. It also establishes a clear, institutionally needed, professional jurisdiction for chaplains, the director said, that "pays off great dividends in terms of caring for patients and families and also in terms of community/hospital relations. The funeral homes really love it. They say, 'We wish every hospital had this. . . . It is so much easier . . . to really coordinate . . . and facilitate . . . so our work gets done, and families aren't waiting and feeling angry.'"

BROADER CONTEXTS AND PERSONAL SENSE-MAKING

In this work with dying people and their families, chaplains do some of what scholars describe as the low-status, "dirty" work of hospitals. Physicians and other high-status employees in hospitals rarely do this work, delegating to nurses, chaplains, and others the tasks of sitting with the dying, managing the emotions of their families, cleaning their dead bodies, and working with the morgue.[33] To the extent that chaplains have clear professional identities and responsibilities in hospitals, the so-called "dirty work" with death is one of the main areas of expertise and primary responsibilities of chaplains in the medical division of labor. As sociologist Everett C. Hughes has pointed out, and as sociologist Charles Bosk confirms in his study of genetic counselors, if status in hospitals is determined by technical prowess and clinical decision making, it is not surprising that chaplains are low in the pecking order, not only because they deal with deaths that physicians often see as failures but because doing so may appear to require little technical skill or clinical decision making.[34]

Chaplains themselves disagree with such characterizations and frame their work with dying people and their families not as "dirty" but as sacred—as about something much bigger than the so-called dirty tasks of the hospital. They recognize this work, and the intense smells, images, and situations that go with it, as among the most difficult things they do—but situate it in frames of meaning much bigger than the hospital. They describe dealing with death and witnessing suffering as the most difficult aspects of their work and part of their vocation. "It is incredibly challenging," a chaplain at Brookfield Hospital stated plainly, "to show up every day for the suffering that you witness at a hospital." "Not only the physical pain," said another at City Hospital, but the "disappointments, heartbreaks." "Death is always painful and difficult," said another. "You don't bond with everybody, but you are diminished by their deaths. You sense it. You feel it. If you're good, you are open to it."

Most chaplains describe their actions concerning death not in terms of work that needs to be done for the benefit of the hospital and its efficient operation, but in broader terms based on their personal beliefs. In their private conversations with me about death, the personal faith perspectives of chaplains became clear. Jean, a Protestant who works as an oncology chaplain at Forest Hills Hospital, described herself as "very proud" to work for her hospital but made clear "that my first loyalty, which transcends the right to the paycheck, . . . is to my understanding of God and divine purposes, . . . which allows me to be in different places yet have a constant." She considered herself "loyal to the institution [hospital]" but said, from a broader view, "always my first loyalty will be to my idea of God and my call."

Many echoed Jean's sentiment, specifically using the language of "calling" to describe their senses of themselves in their work. For some this call is to vocation, in a fairly Christian sense of the term. "As a person of faith," one said, "I would say that it [chaplaincy] is a vocation that I feel called to," and that "this is where God's calling me." For others, this calling was to work with a particular set of patients, often oncology patients. In the words of the oncology chaplain at Streamside Hospital, "I find that most people who've been in oncology for awhile, no matter what their role is, feel a kind of calling to it. . . . They're the ones who don't burn out." Others interpreted the notion of calling more generally, outside of traditional Christian frames. A chaplain at Creekside described the work as "my soul's purpose. . . . I see that what I'm doing is kind of consciously being a channel for divine love and life."

Many also echoed Jean's sense of a broader view that includes God in daily activity, not in a distant or detached way but "very present," one said, "in the mix of things." Reflecting liberal Protestant views common among the disproportionate number of chaplains who are Protestant, chaplains described God as being with them all the time. "Where isn't God in this work?" one laughed. "God is at the center of it all," said another. "Very intricately," a director explained, "I think God is in everybody I talk to, . . . whether their understanding of God is the same as mine or not, . . . in the little things, every conversation, everything." Some replaced the word *God* with *life itself* or *certain qualities of life*, viewing God overall as omnipresent, not as a God that they or others would need to page, because that God is already there with them in their interactions with others.

Chaplains frame their work with the dying, then, in the context of their call to work as chaplains by or with an intimately present God. Rather than seeing death as a failure, as many hospital staff do, or as something to fear, chaplains see spending time with the dying as a special—even sacred—privilege, where the limits of life are stark. Jean, the oncology chaplain quoted above, speaks of the "privilege of being with people who are dying." When they are aware that life is coming to an end, "they are just very honest, and it is so gratifying to get to be sort of a partner in the journey with somebody who is facing that." Jean recognizes that most of the patients she works with will eventually die but says that doesn't "prevent [her from] wanting to be in relationship with them." "Their dying doesn't scare me," she says, but creates possibilities for her work with them. "It seems like a privilege to be paid" for this work, she reflected. For some chaplains, it may be beliefs about the afterlife that cushion their work with dying people. "It is such a privilege to be there, and to know that thin, thin line between this life and another. Another life. And to allow people to breathe and just to be there at that most sacred moment," one reflected.

Despite their broader perspectives and ways of experiencing death, chaplains still find the suffering and death they witness exhausting.[35] Like ICU staff, they have developed sense-making practices—especially around death—to help them take care of themselves and continue to do this often difficult work.[36] At Overbrook, for instance, Father William and Meg are friends and often privately joke about death in the classic tradition of gallows humor that many staff use as a coping mechanism.[37] Sitting down to a meeting one morning, for instance, Father William told Meg of a patient who died the night before. "That SOS [Sacrament of the Sick] worked quickly," she quipped in response. Discussing language in a particular prayer often used with the dying, Meg joked that she wants the word *mansion* not *room* used in the prayer when it is said for her, as she imagines her next life in grand terms. Much like the ICU nurses, other chaplains described getting support from colleagues, family members, and friends. They talk of exercising, crying, gardening, getting outside, and relying on faith communities to help them take care of themselves as they take care of dying people and their families.

Several chaplains spoke also about ways of distancing themselves from the death they see when they are not with the dying or at work.[38] "There are days when I have been with five people who are dying or been at four deaths," one explained. "I have learned to just take a little time out, . . . to go down for coffee, go outside and get some fresh air, go for a little walk." Several spoke of the importance of vacations: "It [all the work] will be waiting for you when you come back. There's a world outside of here too." Another said she writes down words as she goes through difficult days, saying, "By the end of the day, they form a kind of poetry for me, which I like." Others hum or play music. A few have developed private rituals. One said that he washes his hands as soon as he gets home and "just watches the water go down the drain. It's my ritual. I'm not going to carry this." Once a month he does what he calls a "petal ceremony," saying the name of each person who has died that month (that he has "lost," he said) while dropping a flower petal from his balcony at home and doing some writing in a journal. "It is an intense emotional thing. I really have to say that for every person I've lost."[39] Several chaplains commented on how their personal perspectives and ways of being in the world have changed through their work with death. "[I] don't get as perturbed by things, all the little things that drive people nuts each day," said one. "They kind of fade away in terms of importance. . . . A lot of crap just kind of oozes out of your soul and goes away."

CONCLUSIONS

In *The House of God*, a satirical book of fiction published in 1978 and still well known to many medical students and residents, the author, writing under the pen name Samuel Shem, describes a year in the life of a medical intern at a large academic hospital.[40] Religious objects and people appear in the book on only two occasions—both related to death. First, early in the book, one of the main characters, an intern, asks where to find a Bible. When asked why he needs, it he explains, "For pronouncing a patient dead" and then places his hand on the Bible and says, "By the powers vested in me by this great state and nation I hereby pronounce you, Elliot Reginald Needleman, dead."[41] Closer to the end, the interns, concerned that so many patients are dying, page the chaplain. A reform rabbi appears and listens to an intern explain how these deaths could be punishments from God. Puzzled, the rabbi, echoing what most of the chaplains I interviewed would say, replies, "These deaths have to do with physiological fact, not with the whims of Deity. Body, not soul, is what's dying here."[42] Unsatisfied, the intern calls for an Orthodox rabbi, who agrees with his theological interpretation about punishment from God and performs the rituals he wishes.

Shem's attention to religion and spirituality, and especially to chaplains and their work with death, fit conventional ideas that priests and rabbis appear in hospitals only when people are dying and that medical staff see work with death as central to how chaplains spend time. Glaser and Strauss described chaplains mostly as connected to death in their classic *Awareness of Dying*, and more contemporary ethnographies of hospital life often speak of religion and spirituality only when speaking about death. The chaplains and ICU staff I interviewed reinforce these close connections between religion, spirituality, and death, speaking of them as intimately related. As they work with death, however, chaplains at these hospitals do more than just administer last rites; they become a part of the trajectory of dying for individuals and participate in the ways hospitals manage death as institutions.

At Overbrook Hospital, chaplains are integrally involved with death and the hospital's response to death. Chaplains name death, talk with people about death, accompany patients and family members through the process of dying, and help to manage death for the institution as they take families to the morgue, care for staff, and host institution-wide memorial services. They do this within the norms of the institution, not rolling bodies into the chapel for funerals or holding memorial rituals in the center of ICUs or the hospital lobby. They use a range of religious and spiritual languages and shift among them as required by the people whom they are supporting. Chaplains preserve memories of people who die at Overbrook formally in memory books and memorial displays, and informally in their personal rituals and stories.

Beyond Overbrook, a hospital's institutional context influences the extent to which and ways in which chaplains work with death. Like facilitating storytelling and working with ethics, working with death is an essential part of their work. Some chaplains see almost everyone who dies in the hospital and regularly manage death as part of protocols, while others see fewer dying patients, caring for them only when they are called. Directors of professional and transitional chaplaincy departments aiming to confirm the professional jurisdiction of chaplains have frequently found ways to make death a clear part of their jurisdiction—by involving them in palliative care teams or by creating a decedent-care chaplain position. While other hospital staff may see working around death as dirty, low-status work, chaplains situate it in personal frameworks of meaning that transcend hospitals as institutions.

Commentators like bioethicist Nancy Berlinger who are concerned about hospital chaplaincy as a profession have pointed to the death-related work that chaplains do as potentially central to their developing sense of themselves as professionals. In a Hastings Center Report about quality improvement in chaplaincy, she suggests that chaplains begin to focus on patient-centered care by examining how they act around just one issue—death—in ways that might improve palliative care in their own institutions and enable them to contribute to future clinical-practice guidelines, such as those in the 2009 Consensus Report entitled "Improving the Quality of Spiritual Care as a Dimension of Palliative Care."[43]

Given the attention that the chaplains described here focus on death, Berlinger's suggestion is not surprising, but it must be considered in light of the different institutional contexts (and the possibilities they offer) in which chaplains work. Chaplain's greater attention to death may just serve to extend the view of many medical staff that religion and spirituality are most relevant at the end of life and that chaplains do little more than administer last rites. (Recall Father William's noting that he sees the blood pressure of some patients spike when he arrives wearing his clerical collar because they think his presence means they are going to die.) At many institutions they do more than this, though not always in ways that lead them to be consistently present across hospitals, as evident throughout this book and in the concluding chapter.

CHAPTER 9

Conclusion: Looking Forward

It was not unusual to hear nurses refer to some patients as "miracle babies" in the NICU at City Hospital. These babies survived despite poor medical prognoses. Their healings were miraculous, nurses told me, but they differed in what they saw as the source of the miracles. For some, these were miracles of medical science. In Nancy's words, "I don't think it's a miracle like they talk about with the saints and all that stuff. . . . It is a miracle that our doctors and nurses and staff can do. . . . We're a very good hospital with a good reputation, and we can do miraculous things. . . . It's not like somebody came down and put a magical sprinkle on to make the baby go, you know, a certain way."

Other nurses were less sure of the source of miracles, and still others attributed these healings to divine sources. "I guess if anything, it always goes back to God," Tamara said. Another nurse, Hannah, spoke of a miracle that happened in another ICU. "I can't even tell you the whole story because it was a while ago. But some of the nurses actually went to Rome because this person [who facilitated the miracle] was a [Catholic] nun, I guess, and sainted or something."[1]

While nurses in the NICU talked about the source of miracles, pediatric chaplain Elizabeth, like the chaplains at Overbrook, tended to ask broader questions about what a miracle is and what makes something a miracle. When I spoke with Chaplain Meg about the so-called miracle babies, she responded by thinking about what makes something a miracle. "I see miracles here every day," she told me. "Whether others see them as miracles, I don't know. I think it's very subjective. I think a miracle is in the eye of the beholder."

Meg went on to talk about a young woman she had met at Overbrook years earlier who was born with a congenital heart defect. She was not expected to live, but she did for more than twenty years. She had several successful surgeries, Meg remembered, and married and lived a relatively normal life. Meg met her while she was waiting for a heart-lung transplant, which did not come in time. After she died, "her mother felt like . . . it had all been for naught. And you know, I said, well, I'm not so sure I agree with you." When her mother asked why, Meg explained, "I think you had a twenty-five-year miracle. This was a child that you didn't expect to ever come home. You had her for twenty-five years. And not only did you have her for twenty-five years, but she was able to live and have a very functional life. She knew what love was about. She knew what kindness was about. That's a miracle in my mind."

Turning from her story back to me and the miracle babies, Meg said, "I think most people . . . are looking for the big miracle. And I think most miracles are not big, they're small. They come in the minute facts of life. . . . Sometimes they all come together, . . . so that you get a big miracle, but it doesn't happen very often. Usually they're little things that happen. You know, a patient has a good day who has been absolutely miserable and non-communicative with the family, and the family doesn't think they're ever going to have a chance to say goodbye. . . . That's what I think of as miracles."

*

Conversations about miracles with neonatal nurses and staff chaplains illustrated some of the different assumptions and underlying orientations they have regarding religion and spirituality in their work.[2] While neonatal nurses focused on health outcomes for patients and sometimes attributed successes they could not make sense of medically to miracles involving God, medical science, or both, Meg and her chaplain colleagues opened up these questions—not speculating on the source of miracles but thinking with me (and others) about what makes something a miracle. Chaplains rarely described big miracles or medical success stories. Most were what Meg called "small miracles" that happened when patients or family members saw and understood something about their situation in a new and more comforting light.

Individual staff members framed and responded to miracles—like other aspects of religion and spirituality—in a range of ways. While the Joint Commission sets basic guidelines, hospitals respond to them differently. I cannot conclude with a grand synthesis or neat way of explaining the variation I document—the ways religion and spirituality are present in hospitals are too fragmented and inconsistent for that.[3] Rather, I begin to make sense of the messiness by summarizing my main findings, which show how professional training influences how chaplains and staff members understand miracles and religion and spirituality more generally. I then explain what spirituality means in these contexts and how it became the main—what I call strategically vague—frame for talking about religion and spirituality in hospitals. I conclude by considering the implications of these findings for health-care providers and for scholars more broadly. As formally secular organizations where, in the words of sociologist Courtney Bender, "spirituality is produced," these hospitals illustrate the limits of binary approaches to the religious and the secular and to current ways of thinking about religious diversity in contemporary American life.[4]

A BRIEF SUMMARY

Religion and spirituality take different forms in the formal and informal, visible and more invisible ways they are present in large academic hospitals. Some hospitals have seemingly neutral chapel spaces close to main entrances, while others have smaller more distant spaces containing various religious and spiritual symbols. Some have professional chaplaincy departments and assign chaplains to medical teams, while others have traditional departments with few chaplains and page them only occasionally. At hospitals like City Hospital, some medical staff members work closely with chaplains. Others do not understand what chaplains do and wish instead for what one physician in the MICU called a "spiritual social worker." All agree that religion and spirituality are especially relevant in end-of-life situations, but how they bring up the topic and utilize staff chaplains in such situations varies.

While it would be nicely congruent to find that hospitals with particular kinds of chapels hire certain kinds of people as chaplains and have ICU staff who speak and act around spirituality and religion in particular ways, that is rarely the case. Much of the variation evident within and among these hospitals is best understood through the different—professionally informed— languages that chaplains and ICU staff use to think and talk about religion and spirituality. Chaplains, who also influence the design and use of physical chapel spaces, speak broad languages of wholeness, presence, and hope. In the chapels, explicit religious symbols are increasingly replaced with images of nature, water, and art, and chaplains themselves speak in broad terms that they believe will help them connect with a wide range of people and the ways they make meaning. Such approaches function as jurisdictional expansion strategies intended to make the work of chaplains accessible and applicable to as many people as possible. They help chaplains, according to anthropologist Francis Norwood, to make "strategic choices that foster their presence in an otherwise foreign and not entirely welcoming environment."[5] Chaplains utilize these broad languages even as their departments retain specifically religious volunteer programs (e.g., for Catholic Eucharistic ministers) and make items like Bibles and Qur'ans available through their offices.

Physicians and nurses, in comparison, do not always pay attention to spirituality, religion, or other ways people find and make meaning in their lives. When they do, they often speak in terms of specific religious traditions—mostly Catholicism at City Hospital. Nurses pay more attention to such issues than other medical staff, though most everyone is responsive at the end of life, especially when they do not have other medical treatments to recommend. While some medical staff members understand the broad language used by chaplains, neither they nor chaplains recognize the differences in their languages and approaches, nor do they translate easily between them.

Differences in the dominant frames used by chaplains and ICU staff to talk about religion and spirituality lead to a presence of absence and absence of presence. Chaplains are the present, visible, professional carriers of religion and spirituality in hospitals. The broad frames they use to describe their work and their increasingly symbol-free, seemingly neutral chapel spaces leave the images, symbols, and rituals that traditionally transmitted religion among people absent. While chaplains are very present in some hospitals, they are often physically absent as a professional group in others, and there is not a single situation or event that—if it happened simultaneously at all of the hospitals I studied—would lead a chaplain to be present.

It is when religion and spirituality seem to be visibly absent in hospitals that they seem more present. At City Hospital this was evident in the ICUs, where a visitor would rarely see a staff member praying with a patient, but most staff members made space—up to a point—for the religious and spiritual beliefs of their patients. They spoke about those beliefs and practices in terms of specific religious traditions and rituals, though they generally stopped providing space when they came into conflict with medical recommendations. Further, many staff members thought about their patients in the context of their private religious and spiritual practices, or saw religion and spirituality influencing their own work invisibly in the unit.

Without shared understandings of what talk of spirituality and religion is about in hospitals, some chaplains and health-care providers find it challenging to understand one another and work together. Chaplains understand their roles more broadly than do medical staff and more frequently orient to broader frameworks than the health outcomes on which medical staff members focus. Some of the staff in the MICU at City Hospital could not tell the difference between the staff chaplain and hospital volunteers offering communion to Catholic patients and did not have a clear sense of what each did. Such disconnects were reinforced when religiously based conflicts developed around end-of-life situations, and the chaplain was not called to help. Similar disconnects were evident at other hospitals where chaplains spoke of wanting to be more involved with patients earlier in their care and in ways that reflected all that chaplains understand spirituality to encompass. Many medical staff members saw chaplains' roles as more limited and specific to the end of life. These disconnects led to translation problems, as neither chaplains nor medical staff fully understood the other's work and what they were talking about when talking (or acting) in terms of spirituality and religion.[6]

SPIRITUALITY AS A STRATEGICALLY VAGUE FRAME

As attention to spiritual care in health care has grown in recent years, the frame through which it is discussed has shifted from a focus on religion understood within religious institutions to this broader focus on spirituality.[7] In the words of a national leader in hospital chaplaincy, "I've never experienced anything like I've experienced the last ten years. People want to know who I am, what I do, what's going on." Stepping back, he explained, "In the early 1900s, there arose a great hue and cry among medical people that we were not training our doctors and medical people to do a very good job, and what was needed was scientific and structured work. . . . For the twentieth century, that's what we did. And what we got was this wonderful technology, . . . and it sort of leaves us cold. And what we're finding out in the twenty-first century . . . [is that] we're doing a good job technologically, but we need to teach people to be sensitive." "Spiritual care," he continued, "falls very well into that, because when people get sick and come into the hospital, they have anxiety, . . . and they tend to fall back to prayer and seek divine guidance and spirituality, those kinds of things." Leaders in the spirituality in health care movement have encouraged this growth, leading nursing and medical curricula to include spirituality in course offerings and spiritual assessment tools in trainings.

Spirituality has multiple meanings (and histories) in the United States and is increasingly taking on one meaning as it is used in health care, though it is rarely defined as such (or at all). For some individuals (including many nurses), spirituality is set up in contrast to religion. Such individuals will say they are spiritual but not religious because they reject mainstream religions in favor of their own personal beliefs and practices. This meaning was not common among health-care institutions, however. Nor was the spiritual and religious meaning that is common among people who belong to religious organizations and consider the spiritual to be the personal part of the teachings and practices taught in such settings. Rather, health-care institutions favor the meaning of spirituality that is evident in increasingly neutral chapel spaces, in the ways chaplains and chaplaincy directors talk about their work, and in the spirituality in health care movement that I see in these hospitals.[8] Courtney Bender has this sense of the term in mind when she describes "one meaning of *spirituality* as 'more than' religion."[9] This conception suggests that "religious traditions, authorities, and institutions are all second-order expressions of first-order, primary spiritual experiences. This discourse privileges the spiritual over the religious, and likewise often suggests that spirituality is universal, denoting the common experience that lies at the root of every religious tradition."[10] Even people without religious traditions are presumed able to tap into this sense of spirituality because it is conceived as not explicitly connected to religious histories, organizations, or traditions.[11]

This sense of spirituality further assumes that by tapping into it, people can communicate across their differences. Sociologist Don Grant argues, referring to the research of religious studies scholar Wade Clark Roof, that "in today's religiously pluralistic world, individuals tend to view spirituality as a neutral—and perhaps more authentic—language that enables persons from different faith perspectives to exchange ideas on the sacred. Many, therefore, believe that spirituality—as opposed to organized religion—can communicate consensual meanings in a variety of corporate settings, including hospitals."[12] Like neutral chapel spaces and the broadly framed talk of chaplains, this sense of spirituality glosses over rather than engages religious differences.

Despite assumptions to the contrary, this understanding of spirituality is not universally understood or agreed on across differences in hospitals. The Chaplaincy Department at Overbrook, for example, framed its work in this way, but some patients, particularly some Muslim patients, did not understand this broad conception. *Chaplain* is a Christian word, the Muslim chaplain reminded, me saying that when Muslim patients are asked if they would like to see a chaplain, "the first thing that comes to their mind is a priest or a reverend, and maybe they're going to convert me." Such thinking, he explained, leads most Muslims to decline offers to see chaplains, unless an Imam or Muslim chaplain is explicitly offered in those terms. Despite public relations materials that promote chaplains as supporting all of the ways people are spiritual or make meaning, the Muslim chaplain finds, "I don't think they [Muslims] know our policy . . . that chaplains are here to provide a kind of service that's not offensive to any religion."[13]

Not only patients, but also some medical staff members—including those who work in the ICUs at City Hospital—do not understand this meaning of spirituality. At City, for example, Elizabeth the pediatric chaplain, wanted staff members to see her as someone who could provide spiritual support to a wide range of families on multiple issues, not just those that were religious and involved coping with the end of life. She aimed to provide similar spiritual support for staff but in ways that sometimes led to misunderstandings. When she put her hand on the backs of nurses for example and said, "I've got your back," she interpreted the gesture as supporting nurses' spiritually in ways that had little to do with their religious affiliations. Nurses did not reject the gesture but often looked at Elizabeth with a puzzled expression when she passed by, suggesting they did not understand her intent.

This confusion about the meaning and boundaries of spirituality in health care stems from what scholar Nancy Berlinger calls "underlying, perhaps unacknowledged, conceptual paradigms and how they are expressed through language, definitions, and methodological tools, by advocates, critics, and skeptics on all sides of the debate."[14] Spirituality is too small, she argues, when it refers only to praying or going to church, but it is too big when it must stand for ultimate meaning. In a national study, physician Farr Curlin found that even when physicians used the word *spirituality*, they almost always referred to religious communities and traditions rather than to broader meaning-making systems, as chaplains do.[15] Numerous studies report confusion among nurses about what spirituality is, exactly, and how they are to engage with it. Even nurses who personally described their work as spiritual in a study of a large, academic medical centers tended to understand spirituality in ways that differed from its meaning as "more than religious."[16]

Explaining This Approach to Spirituality

The meaning of spirituality as used in hospitals developed through several processes. First, while chaplains likely spoke about religion and spirituality more consistently over time than did physicians or nurses, much of the recent frame comes from the work of physicians like Christina Puchalski and other leaders in the spirituality in health care movement. As physicians and nurses, these individuals needed a standard concept—which religion in its messiness and diversity clearly does not provide—that would fit within their biomedical epistemologies and would be easy to teach their colleagues to utilize in standard ways. Spiritual assessment tools that were easy to remember facilitated this process, as did the rise in research about religion and health that appeared to support their use. Their emphases on a universalistic spirituality that is seen as more than religion made their approach applicable to the widest range of people possible and distanced them from conceptions of religion that were traditionally more controversial and recognized as being more pluralistic in contemporary American medicine.[17]

As this approach to spirituality gained sway and the spirituality in health care movement came together in the 1990s, chaplains adopted this frame as they continued to struggle over their own professional jurisdiction and try to find ways to articulate and regulate that jurisdiction. They did this in the context of their largely mainline Protestant professional history and in light of the increasing religious diversity of the people they interact with in hospitals. A broad notion of spirituality as more than religion enabled chaplains to begin to see beyond their own religious differences and articulate their professional roles and responsibilities in a single professional voice, as is evident in "Professional Chaplaincy: Its Role and Contribution in Healthcare." It also gave chaplains a language that enabled them to connect with a broad range of people whose religious backgrounds were increasingly different from their own.

More broadly, and to the extent that this understanding of spirituality has been adopted by hospital administrators, universalistic notions of spirituality appeal to those seeking to provide care (and public relations) to diverse constituents with wide-ranging beliefs and practices. They also provide a seemingly simple, general way to talk about the different ways in which religion and spirituality are actually present in their institutions. Rarely a central priority in hospitals, broad approaches to spirituality appear—at least on the surface—to include everyone and to emphasize commonalities rather than the differences religions foster.

Defining spirituality as more than religion is a strategic approach, then, for leaders in the spirituality in health care movement, hospital chaplains, and hospital administrators, though they have taken it up for different reasons. For physicians and nursing leaders of the spirituality in health care movement, it fits within their biomedical frames and appears applicable to all patients, regardless of their backgrounds, though it has not been adopted by their nursing and medical colleagues who are not involved in the movement. For chaplains, it is a strategy to expand their professional jurisdictional that may help them to connect to the spirituality in health care movement and to unify and negotiate religious diversity. For health-care administrators, it provides a convenient way to appeal to religiously and spiritually diverse constituents and seems—at least on the surface—to encompass the range of diverse ways in which religion and spirituality are actually present in their institutions. It is not that these groups have made intentional decisions to define and utilize spirituality in this way. Rather, this approach results from their own internal negotiations, which take place for different reasons. Spirituality as more than religion is less an explicit strategy utilized by these groups together, in other words, than the result of each of their individual sets of strategic actions.

Beyond Health Care

Beyond what it suggests about health care, this approach to spirituality shows first that religion and spirituality are indeed present within formally secular organizations in the United States. Rather than a bifurcation between the sacred and the secular, these hospitals suggest how the sacred—increasingly understood as the spiritual—may exist in other formally secular organizations such as schools and universities, prisons, the military, and even some workplaces. Many Americans spend more time in these organizations than in religious ones, leaving open broad questions of how, if at all, they experience religion and spirituality there.[18]

The extent to which this approach to spirituality is present and emerging in other formally secular organizations raises questions about when and how it developed in American religious history and how it compares across sets of organizations. It could be that organizational gatekeepers that adopted what Diana Eck calls pluralistic, exclusionist, or assimilationist approaches played important roles historically, using spirituality as a strategy through which to welcome, minimize, or negotiate increasing religious diversity in organizations in the last fifty years. Differences in the ways such leaders understood spirituality might also help explain—in combination with first amendment jurisprudence, the public or private nature of particular organizations, religious demographics, institutional isomorphism, and the history of chaplaincy—the forms that religion and spirituality take in secular organizations ranging from the military to prisons and private universities.[19]

To the extent that spirituality (meaning more than religion) is evident across secular organizations, it provides further evidence of what Winifred Sullivan calls a broad "areligious secularism"—an emerging "post-Christian space where religion is honored as a human universal and religious pluralism can be creatively negotiated in sites of cultural exchange."[20] Perhaps better termed *spiritual secularism*, it is a broad approach to meaning-making rather than something explicitly connected to religious traditions. These hospitals suggest that broad talk of meaning, symbols of nature and art, and understandings of spirituality as being about more than religion are present in these "post-Christian" spaces. If hospitals are any indication, Christian symbols and rituals continue to be present (at least occasionally), however, suggesting that "areligious secularism" is presently emerging in improvised, creative, and messy ways within sets of organizations—such as hospitals—and even within single organizations, such as City Hospital and Overbrook.

LOOKING FORWARD

In Health Care

Despite the growing national spirituality in health care movement, the question of whether religion and spirituality are relevant in health-care organizations is an open one for some health-care staff. Many do not know how personally religious and spiritual Americans are as a group or that many people draw on such beliefs and practices when they are ill. Some health-care providers are uncomfortable with research about religion and health or skeptical that it might be used in normatively suspect ways, especially by the people conducting it, who are usually assumed to be people of faith.[21] Many of those with whom I spoke—especially physicians—emphasized how religion, not spirituality, caused conflicts in their work and described situations with Jehovah's Witnesses, Orthodox Jews, evangelical Christians, and members of other religious organizations that exist in some tension with biomedicine. They highlighted the problems they had with such patients more often than they spoke of situations in which spirituality or religion was a source of support.

Regardless of how health-care providers personally feel about the appropriate place of religion and spirituality in their organizations, American demographics suggest that large numbers of people who consider themselves religious or spiritual will continue to seek health care in the United States. Many patients experience religion and spirituality as relevant to that care. Studies further show that some patients are not having these needs met. Recent studies of advanced cancer patients, for example, reported that nearly half (47%) had spiritual needs that were minimally or not at all met by religious communities. Close to three-quarters (72%) reported having spiritual needs that were supported minimally or not at all by the medical system. People who had their spiritual needs met experienced higher qualities of life.[22]

Health-Care Providers and Administrators

I encourage health-care providers and administrators to think carefully about how they provide religious and spiritual care, especially to the large fraction of Americans who die in hospitals. To the extent that spiritual or religious support can improve their quality of life or that of their families, I encourage health-care administrators to make that care more fully available.[23] I make this suggestion not based on empirical evidence about the relationship between religion and health—I am as skeptical of much of that research as is Richard Sloan (2006)—or because such care seems likely to reduce costs. Rather, religious and spiritual care should be offered because when it is provided sensitively, optionally, and professionally, it assists people at their most vulnerable. In addition to better health and lower costs—the traditional priorities of health-care organizations—such care highlights an equally important third outcome—compassionate care that is respectful of the experiences of patients and families when offered in professionally appropriate ways.

Health-care staff who want to consider (or reconsider) how religion and spirituality are addressed in their institutions need to recognize that no model fits all situations, and then consider several issues. First, I encourage them to acknowledge the frame that sees the spiritual as more than religious and through which such issues are being discussed nationally, and to ask whether this frame is appropriate for their institution. While many leaders in the spirituality in health care movement encourage attention to spirituality more than to religion, many people in the United States consider themselves spiritual but not religious or both religious and spiritual. Neutral chapel spaces and interfaith chaplain are not necessarily appropriate for every organization. At some hospitals, as at Creekside, multifaith chapel spaces that included symbols from a range of religious traditions seemed well accepted by patients, staff, and families. Providers and administrators might investigate how their chapel spaces are used and whether patients and staff are connecting with chaplains before deciding how neutral or multifaith they should be. More important, health-care administrators need to be aware that, just as some of the Muslim patients at Overbrook do not see themselves included in the institution's conception of spirituality, no one concept will ever include everyone. Rather than assuming it does, administrators and providers need to consider the limits of spirituality as a frame and then decide how to proceed.

Second, health-care staff should consider educational programs that enable a range of staff—rather than just chaplains—to learn a little about religion and spirituality. This takes place at some hospitals today where chaplains guest lecture in medical or nursing school classes, or have students shadow them early in their training.[24] At one hospital, for example, medical students have their first experience on the hospital floors when they spend half a day shadowing a chaplain. While the chaplaincy director says some students enjoy it, and others think it is a waste of time, "The biggest response you get is, 'I never realized how important religion is to people, and I'll definitely be aware of it and ask my patients, . . . seeing if I can help them along.' Most wouldn't feel comfortable praying, but they would be aware of whether there is a chaplaincy program or where local congregations are."

For current hospital staff, continuing education can take place in ethics rounds, lectures, or by including staff in the education of Clinical Pastoral Education students.[25] Such programs need to go beyond generic discussions of spirituality to teach about different kinds of spiritualities and of religions. As physician Daniel Hall and his colleagues argue, spirituality is not a universal language, and it cannot resolve the competing claims of different religions.[26] In addition, hospitals can make reference materials like *The Medical Manual for Religio-Cultural Competence: Caring for Religiously Diverse Populations* available for staff on their units in addition to the pager numbers for the chaplains.[27] I have yet to meet a nurse, doctor, or other medical staff member who physically went to the hospital chaplaincy department office (which usually contains these reference books) looking for such materials. Instead they look on the Internet for answers to questions, sometimes with questionable results.

Third, administrators should work with the director of chaplaincy to decide who is best prepared to offer religious and spiritual care in hospitals. While nurses and physicians can offer some support, staff chaplains, trained and board-certified through one of the professional chaplaincy organizations, are the people with the most specific training. Few hospitals would allow volunteer nurses, and they should think carefully about using volunteer chaplains and others who volunteer through chaplaincy departments. Catholic Eucharistic ministry volunteers I met, who offer communion to Catholic patients, were usually very clear about their roles and limits. Other volunteers who visited patients for longer conversations were less clear and often less informed about patients' different backgrounds and needs. One such volunteer told me about praying with the family of a Buddhist patient who was in surgery. Thinking of the Buddhists I know, I wondered about this, since most do not pray. I became more concerned when the volunteer told me that she asked God in the prayer to take the patient in his hands, only to have family members say that they wanted the patient to be in the doctor's hands! Such misunderstandings are less likely with professionally trained chaplains than with volunteers.

Chaplains

To the extent that chaplains are and wish to remain the religious and spiritual experts in health-care organizations, they need to continue to articulate and clarify their professional roles and responsibilities with others in health care. Chaplains have long struggled with questions of professional jurisdiction. National chaplaincy leaders have promoted standards of practice, participated in efforts to develop national palliative care standards, and begun to develop best-practice guidelines in recent years—all of which help and should continue. As in all professions, however, the vision of chaplaincy promoted by national leaders is not always shared by chaplains on the ground. The directors of many chaplaincy departments want their hospitals to hire more chaplains and want medical staff to take the work of chaplains more seriously, but they cannot explain how their work differs from that of others in the hospital or how hiring more chaplains will help the hospital meet its goals. Department directors who build their departments successfully are those who learn to speak the language of their institutions and make arguments about how chaplains help address larger institutional needs.

As chaplains at the national and local levels continue articulating and clarifying their professional jurisdictions, I encourage them to keep several questions in mind. First, did chaplains expand or change their work as they adopted current meanings of spirituality? Since I completed this research, Pat, the director of chaplaincy at Overbrook, considered changing the department's name to Spiritual Care. She started to think about it after hospital nurses had a two-day conference about spirituality and did not invite any chaplains even to consult. She felt that spiritual care was what the department provided and thought a name change would reflect changes already in motion and facilitate broader connections across the hospital. At some hospitals, such name changes reflect changes in the work of chaplains, while at others, they are primarily public-relations moves intended to better situate chaplains, even as their actual work remains quite consistent.[28]

Second, chaplains need to continue to ask themselves on what or whose authority they do their work in hospitals. Answering this question was easier when chaplains worked in Protestant, Catholic, or Jewish hospitals corresponding to their own backgrounds, when they understood spirituality as operating primarily within religious traditions, and when most of the staff—even in secular hospitals—shared their religious backgrounds and corresponding sources of authority. It is more complicated now, as religiously diverse staff members, including those with no religious or spiritual background, try to make sense of why their hospital has interfaith chaplains, what they do, what they mean in their talk of spirituality, and on whose authority they do this work.

Chaplains are increasingly being asked to provide empirical evidence for their work as part of a transition toward evidence or outcomes-based authority. Some chaplains point to evidence in the scholarship about religion and health, though much of it is controversial. As Nancy Berlinger writes, "Critics of this research argue that these studies are designed to find rather than test causality; that data are selectively interpreted; and that . . . attempts to quantify the Infinite are conceptually flawed. . . . Depending on which article one is reading or which conference one is attending, the connection between spirituality and medicine is clinically proven, unknowable, hazardous, or downright harmful."[29] Such studies tend to focus on traditional measures of religious participation rather than broader understandings of spirituality. Other chaplains point to research that argues that visits from chaplains have positive effects on patients or their families. This body of literature is small, however, and needs further development. [30]

Third, chaplains need to ask themselves what their patients and institutions need and what outcomes are central to their work.[31] I agree with physician and religious studies scholar Margaret Mohrmann that there is a "real need" for chaplains to share language with others in health care—perhaps what she calls a "language of responsibility or accountability"—especially to patients.[32] Such an outcomes-based approach can help chaplains think about how to help their institutions meet their goals. Chaplains at some hospitals, for example, became decedent-care chaplains or family advocates who addressed problems hospitals were having with the treatment of dead bodies and relationships with families. At another hospital, chaplains were staffed not as members of the chaplaincy department but as staff members of the Cancer Center to support staff members, patients, and families in need. Orienting to outcomes for patients and hospitals encourages chaplains to think about their work with reference to the hospitals that employ them rather than the religious organizations that endorse them or professional organizations that certify them. It also challenges them to think of themselves as problem-solvers not only for individuals but also for their institutions.[33]

Orienting to outcomes further challenges chaplains who resist the idea that their work can be measured and that quality-improvement efforts are something other than bureaucratic talk.[34] Chaplains do not need to focus on standard biomedical outcomes related to health or length of stay; they can focus on softer outcomes, such as patient and family satisfaction or emotional adjustments to new health situations.[35] Such a focus on patients not only challenges chaplains to think about outcomes but also requires them to put caring for patients ahead of the education that some provide for CPE students in their hospitals.[36]

Focusing on outcomes for patients and hospitals will be easier for chaplains if their training shifts to include these priorities and to improve their ability to communicate and translate their roles to colleagues on the health-care team. Chaplains have traditionally been trained through a combination of master's-level graduate education and CPE. This education is more humanistic than scientific. Many learn little about what an outcome is or about the standards that administrators refer to when they speak of evidence-based medicine. I encourage chaplains to give priority to educational models that include basic courses about health-care administration, counseling, research methods, and substantive topics such as medical ethics—information that they need in order to function in increasingly complex health-care organizations.[37] Chaplains do not need detailed information about how health-care organizations operate, but they need to know enough about the priorities of the people they work with to communicate with them and translate their work to different audiences.[38]

Chaplaincy educators also need to think carefully about how chaplains learn about religious traditions in addition to their own. The main professional chaplaincy organizations continue to require chaplains to be endorsed by a faith organization in order to be board-certified.[39] While they claim that individuals learn about religious traditions and notions of spirituality beyond their own in this training, the leaders of the profession have been resistant to educational models like that of the Chaplaincy Institute for Arts and Inter-faith Ministry in California, which is based squarely on interfaith models.[40] The Common Standards for Professional Chaplaincy also say little about the substantive knowledge of different religious or spiritual traditions that individuals must have to be certified as chaplains.[41] And while chaplaincy leaders speak about people's spiritualities in terms of their relationships with pets, music, and other things, it is rare to see chaplains training in music or pet therapy, or hospitals with such programs organizing them through chaplaincy departments. On the ground and in their training, in other words, chaplains continue to seem more committed to educational models based on traditional forms of religious education than on interfaith approaches or the broader no-tions of spirituality through which their work is framed nationally.

Interdisciplinary programs that enable future chaplains to learn not only about but with and from students and faculty in public health, hospital ad-ministration, nursing, and other fields are likely to provide the best training for chaplains who will work in hospitals of the future. While chaplains cer-tainly need some of their own religious and spiritual training, they need a wider range of teachers because they will have a wide range of colleagues in their future positions. Situating chaplaincy training programs in universities with strong medical, public health, and divinity schools may capitalize on this interdisciplinary potential and introduce future chaplains to others in health care before they begin their CPE in hospitals. This also might facilitate the development of university-based faculty with expertise in hospital chaplaincy. Historically, educational leaders in chaplaincy have included some faculty at seminaries and divinity schools who specialize in pastoral care, as well as CPE supervisors trained through programs accredited by the Association for Clinical Pastoral Education and employed by hospitals. The lack of univer-sity-based academic leaders—corresponding to faculty in social work and nursing schools for example—is part of the reason why chaplains have not been seen as on par with members of these other professions. This is also why a robust research literature about chaplaincy has not been produced by people motivated to do so by the standards of university tenure and promo-tion committees.[42]

Many people I speak with who are considering careers in health-care chap-laincy are enthusiastic about interdisciplinary professional training programs, though they currently exist in only a few places. Such approaches challenge existing training and professional certification models that are based on less integrated processes of graduate education, CPE , and certification processes controlled by gatekeepers in graduate schools and seminaries, the Associa-tion for Clinical Pastoral Education, and the professional chaplaincy organi-zations, respectively. While chaplaincy leaders and educators in each of these areas could work together to imagine new, more interdisciplinary, and more integrated training models, change is not likely to be easy. Change is impor-tant, however, if chaplains are to become more than "tinkering tradespersons" fulfilling needs seen as peripheral to their organization's main missions.[43]

Given the range of organizations currently involved in training chaplains and the fact that hospitals can continue to hire whomever they want as chap-lains, regardless of their training, chaplains might consider, finally, new ways of regulating their profession. Rather than continuing to lobby the Joint Commission to require hospitals to have chaplains, as they have unsuccessfully for many years, chaplaincy leaders might consider whether the time has come for professional licenses like those required in medicine and nursing. As Raymond DeVries argues, chaplains currently have many credentials but no license to practice, which does not allow them to close the market or prevent competition from local clergy, volunteers, and others who might offer chaplaincy services not only differently but for lower cost.[44] While the politics of licensing chaplains as religious or spiritual workers may be complex, chaplains might at least want to consider whether such efforts could help them regulate the hiring of chaplains by hospitals, how they are trained, and how they provide care. Licensing chaplains might help the profession to regulate not only the hiring of chaplains but the quality of the care they provide.[45]

Beyond Health Care

Beyond health care, these hospitals show how religion and spirituality are framed and how religious diversity is negotiated in American organizations that are formally secular. As microcosms, they show "how spirituality has been promoted by particular people with particular goals," in the words of religious studies scholar Kathleen Garces-Foley.[46] While some hospitals have historically catered to people from single religious traditions, their formal secularization and the increasing diversity of the American population lead to the tensions they face today as many try to create places where religious pluralism can be creatively negotiated. Such negotiation in hospitals raises questions about how other secular organizations negotiate religious diversity as they try (or do not try) to welcome and make space for a range of people.

Hospital chaplaincy directors see themselves as religious pluralists and see spirituality as an umbrella concept under which people of all religious and spiritual backgrounds can fit on their own terms. The question to keep in mind is whether spirituality really functions this way in practice. No concept can include everyone, and in their attempts to welcome all—especially through neutral chapels and the broad talk of chaplains—hospitals are excluding those who do not recognize these spaces or discourses. I encourage chaplains and secular organizations more broadly to interrogate their use of the word *spiritual* to describe people from different religious backgrounds. I encourage them to ask what *spiritual* means, where that meaning comes from, and how the concept actually functions in the daily lives of institutions. At issue is whether the concept of spirituality facilitates multiplicity and diversity or functions to minimize and neutralize them.

To the extent that areligious or spiritual secularism is alive and present in formally secular organizations in the United States, I and others who care about religious diversity encourage organizations to allow differences between people and traditions rather than to minimize them. It is in these emergent spaces in secular organizations that people are often taken by surprise as they attempt to negotiate conflict and cooperation in religious and spiritual multiplicity.

Just as people may be surprised about what emerges from this multiplicity, I was surprised by a phone call near the end of this project. A physician called to tell me that his child was in a coma. His physician colleagues were telling him there was nothing more they could do for the child, and he used Google to look for other ideas and found me. He wanted to know whether I thought some kind of a prayer chain might help save his child. I felt deeply for this man—reaching out to me, a stranger, in a desperate situation—and remembered how the neonatal nurses and Meg spoke about miracles. Thinking that prayers would probably not produce the big miracle this man sought, and that even if they could, I was not the best one to help, I sympathized with him and referred him both to a chaplain and to a physician in the spirituality in health care movement.

Much as this phone call surprised me, the presence of religion and spirituality in hospitals and other secular organizations startles many as it challenges our easy differentiations between the religious and the secular, the visible and the invisible. If we continue to ask better questions about how religion and spirituality are visibly and invisibly produced, consumed, and constructed in formally secular organizations, perhaps we will no longer be taken by surprise.

Research Methods

When I began this project in 2004, research about the relationship between religion and health was booming. Review articles written by scholars across the disciplines asked whether religion influences health, and numerous scholars posited mechanisms to empirically test such relationships.[1] I read these articles and—as a sociologist trained to pay attention to social institutions—was quickly puzzled by their almost exclusive focus on individuals. Study after study analyzed survey data about individuals and attempted to link measures of religion and measures of health without paying much attention to the social institutions—families, religious organizations, and health-care organizations—that might shape such relationships.

Curious, and motivated by the memory of Thai Buddhist monk Taan Čhaokuhn Rattanamēthē dying in a hospital outside of Philadelphia, I continued to read, searching for materials about how religion and spirituality are present and potentially influential not just for individuals but in health-care organizations.[2] I found historical materials and small bodies of literature—often disconnected from one another—that described aspects of religion and spirituality in curricula; among physicians, nurses, and other health-care workers; and in the experiences of some patients and families. Medical sociologists occasionally mentioned the topics in their studies of ICUs or of death but usually in passing and in ways not tied to their central research questions.[3] Chaplains and chaplaincy researchers have also generated a small, mostly applied, research literature published in a separate set of journals not easily accessed by a broad range of researchers.[4] The materials I found suggested that religion and spirituality were present among a range of people in some health-care organizations today. These studies said little that was cohesive, however, about the different forms that religion and spirituality take among the people who move through health-care organizations daily.

Reflecting on what I read in light of my experiences with Taan Čhaokuhn and the questions about hospital chapels, chaplains, and medical staff that I pondered at his bedside, I began to imagine a project that would focus on all of the ways in which religion and spirituality are present in a single health-care institution. Trained as a sociologist of religion having studied religious organizations, I imagined ethnographically investigating one health-care organization, paying attention to the multiple places where religion and spirituality are present and the forms they take among patients, families, and staff. Not only might such a project provide research about religion and health with an awareness of the role of institutions, I thought, but it could also bring together disparate studies about the presence of religion and spirituality in those institutions.

That was the vision. The reality is much less elegant. I outline here the process through which I came to study Overbrook, City Hospital, and the other fifteen academic hospitals described in this book. In so doing, I make an argument about some of the challenges faced by ethnographers in contemporary health-care organizations, especially challenges of access. These challenges led me to gather almost all of the data presented here through interviews and informal shadowing rather than participant observation.[5] The access I could negotiate to a mosaic of health-care organizations allowed me to observe some particular aspects of religion and spirituality in them, especially those pertaining to the institutions and their staff, but not others, particularly those related to patients and families. This access fundamentally shapes the stories I tell and my silences—which I aim to make as transparent as possible in this appendix.

NOTES ON THE ART OF (NOT) GETTING IN

Sociologist Charles Bosk distinguishes between invited guests and uninvited intruders in describing two ways sociologists manage to study medical settings. While he was a guest, invited by the medical staff of a pediatric genetic counseling center to study them, other medical sociologists are uninvited intruders.[6] Many "intruders" seek invitations, or at least permission to conduct research, from medical staff, often attending physicians or other high-status informants. In her study of ethical decision making in NICUs, for example, Renee Anspach (1993) negotiated access through an attending neonatologist.

Robert Zussman (1992) was able to study ethics in ICUs only after the director of the medical service and the president at the hospital he hoped to study intervened with gatekeepers. Before she began research for what became her book *And a Time to Die: How American Hospitals Shape the End of Life*, anthropologist Sharon Kaufman spent a year meeting informally with physicians and nurses at the hospitals she wanted to study to discuss a project on hospital practices surrounding death.[7]

I did not have an invitation to study a hospital when I conceived of this project and began, like any other "uninvited intruder," to try to get permission to study one. I was new to studies of health-care organizations and had a two-year postdoctoral fellowship but no hospital affiliation and no family members, friends, or high-status contacts employed by hospitals that could ease the way.[8] I was also seeking access after Congress had enacted the Health Insurance Portability and Accountability Act (HIPPA)in 1996 to increase the privacy and security of health data. While some researchers like Sharon Kaufman have been able to conduct ethnographic research in health-care organizations that includes attention to patients since HIPPA, this act makes getting permission to do so more difficult. Combined with the requirements of Institutional Review Boards, it has increased the barriers many social scientists face in doing ethnographic research in health-care organizations.

I got permission to study religious organizations in earlier projects by attending services, getting to know lay people, and being introduced to leaders by mutual friends. I doubted such an approach would work in this case, but with the support of several experienced medical sociologists and a number of high-status physicians I met along the way, I began to navigate a path to entry—a path that itself shaped what I was ultimately able to learn in these institutions.

First Steps

Hoping to identify one hospital that would give me permission to investigate inductively the multiple ways in which religion and spirituality were present in the institution, I began by visiting a wide range of hospitals to look around their public areas. I selected hospitals rather than rehabilitation facilities, outpatient clinics, or nursing homes because of the range of people constantly present in them—some of whom stay and some of whom keep moving—and because of the central role they play in the health-care system.[9] I sat in hospital chapels and prayer and meditation rooms, visited gift shops and snack bars, and watched people move through hospital lobbies and parking lots. I quickly realized that I would need the support of medical staff to see more and asked colleagues and friends of friends if I could shadow medical staff members they knew. They agreed to act as intermediaries and made the introductions that allowed me to shadow several attending physicians at large academic medical centers. I attended rounds with one, saw patients in the office with another, and attended staff and patient team meetings with a third.[10] Getting beyond the lobby allowed me to meet some nurses and chaplains, to see when—if ever—medical staff asked patients about spirituality or religion, and to look for evidence of religion and spirituality, which I saw mostly in the offices of staff members and in the jewelry worn by those who worked in street clothes rather than hospital scrubs.

I also started to gather the names of everyone I knew (or might know, through varying degrees of separation) who worked in a hospital, or did research about religion, spirituality, health, or medicine, or had any connection to hospital chaplaincy. During the first six months of this project, I met with as many of these people as possible, explaining my interest in writing a book about religion and spirituality in hospitals. Many were supportive, but few had the combination of status, access, and research experience needed to help me obtain permission to study a single hospital.

A few months into this process, the director of chaplaincy at one hospital— someone an intermediary highly recommended—expressed interest in me and the project. He could not give me a tour of his hospital unless I had a hospital ID badge, so he proposed that we work together to frame a project. We began to draft a proposal for one month of exploratory research that the Institutional Review Board (IRB) at the hospital might approve, which would enable me to get an ID badge and physically enter the nonpublic spaces of the hospital.[11] I communicated informally with a few physicians at this hospital who were interested in my ideas and was surprised, a month later, when the chaplaincy director abruptly informed me that we would neither submit the IRB application nor do the project. Obviously disappointed, he told me that his supervisors did not want me bringing to light how the hospital had handled religion and spirituality in the past. They were also concerned that my work would overlap with the research that nurses and social workers do about these topics.[12] The director of chaplaincy also said he would not have time to work with me on the project. He told me directly to look for another hospital. I only understood this recommendation a few years later, when I learned more about the history of this hospital with regard to religion and spirituality— history that his supervisors did not want brought to light. While much has changed since then, the situation was not stable enough for the leaders of this hospital to risk letting me—someone they hardly knew—poke around.

A New Approach

At this point, on the basis of the relationships I was developing with physicians and chaplains at several different hospitals and because the months of my fellowship period were ticking away, and I was anxious to gather some field data before I returned to full-time teaching, I decided to abandon my search for a single hospital and focus on a mosaic of sites. Because most of the medical staff I was meeting worked in large academic hospitals, I decided for practical reasons to limit my focus to them. It was also increasingly clear from my conversations with informants that even if I got permission to learn about some areas of hospitals, my access would likely be limited to medical staff. I would not have access to patients because of HIPPA regulations and because I was not collaborating with an existing research team that had already obtained permission to gather information from patients. I began reframing the project accordingly.[13]

I am disappointed that the voices of patients and families are not included in this book, because they constitute a large fraction of the people in hospitals, they are the clients whom these institutions are supposed to serve, and they represent a range of spiritualities and religions to which medical personnel do (or do not) respond. Seen as a strength, the absence of patient voices and stories, except as described by hospital staff, enabled me to focus more centrally on what hospitals do concerning religion and spirituality through their physical spaces, decisions about hiring chaplains, and support of hospital staff. As a weakness, the lack of patient and family voices silences the group that is a significant part of the reason hospitals and staff members address religion and spirituality in the first place.

DATA GATHERED

Through a range of mostly disconnected informants, I was able to negotiate access to a series of research sites best described in three main groups. I outline these three groups here thematically rather than in the order in which I obtained permission to study them. The actual data-collection process was messy. I networked repeatedly, attempting to get research permission, and then jumped at opportunities to interview these three sets of people, sometimes conducting interviews on the same day with a chaplain at one hospital and ICU staff member at another. I also sat on a hospital ethics committee while gathering this data but did not have permission to study the committee.

A Formal Cross Section

First, to understand how a cross section of hospitals formally addresses religion and spirituality, I examine seventeen highly ranked, large academic hospitals. These include the complete population of sixteen hospitals that *U.S. News and World Report* designated as having "honor roll" status when this research began and one additional hospital that, while formally part of the same health-care system as one of the sixteen, has its own buildings and chaplaincy department. These hospitals—each with more than five hundred patients—are located across the United States, primarily in large metropolitan areas.[14] Some were founded by religious organizations, but all are currently secular.[15] I also learned about twelve additional teaching hospitals in one state but do not include them in this book in an effort to present a national rather than regional sample.

At each of these hospitals, I focused on how religion and spirituality are formally addressed by the institution, meaning how physical space is set aside for related gatherings or activities, whether chaplains are hired and who they are, and how questions about spirituality and religion are asked at admissions or as part of nursing assessments. To gather this information, I attempted to interview the director of chaplaincy and a staff chaplain at each hospital to understand how each department functions administratively and how chaplains work on a daily basis.[16] Some of these chaplains were CPE supervisors, but I did not intentionally interview CPE supervisors.[17] Prior to beginning any of these interviews, I interviewed eight leaders who hold key positions in hospital chaplaincy nationally to learn about the broad history and current state of the field. I then called or e-mailed the director of chaplaincy at each of these seventeen hospitals, explaining my project and asking them to participate after making clear that the names and identifying details of all individuals and hospitals included would be changed in reports and publications.

Before conducting any interviews, I reviewed all of the information available on the web pages of chaplaincy departments, paying particular attention to the mission statements, services provided, and staff. In interviews, I asked the directors about the history of chaplaincy at the hospitals; their vision and goals for the departments; their missions; their work, including patient and staff demographics; their physical spaces, including chapels; and their successes and failures. I asked staff chaplains about daily life in the hospital, including how they came to work there, how they spend their time, what their good and bad days are like, how often they deal with conflict, how they work with other medical staff, and how they see their work influencing healing—if at all. Individual interviews lasted between thirty minutes and two hours, and were recorded and transcribed. I thanked each individual for his or her time with a thank-you note and small gift certificate to a local coffee shop.

I visited about two-thirds of these hospitals in person, with the research assistance of Jennifer Dillinger, who was then a student in a Master's in Divinity program.[18] We aimed to visit departments with a range of histories and sizes located in diverse geographical areas. On visits, we sat in chapels and in prayer and meditation rooms. We gathered materials for the public that were available in these spaces (paying attention to who prints and pays for them) and toured public areas of each hospital, looking at items in the gift shop, Shabbat elevators, decorations for holidays, donor plaques, and awards on the walls.[19] When possible, we attended formal religious services and gathered handouts about the department that were prepared for patients and families.[20] Some directors invited us to sit in on staff meetings or training sessions or showed us around their offices, though we remained aware that most patients and families spend time with chaplains in hospital rooms or waiting areas, not these offices.[21] Typical offices were small and filled with books, scriptures from a range of religious traditions, religious objects from various traditions, and miscellaneous pamphlets, videos, paintings, reports, hospital policies, and other materials.[22] At the hospitals we did not visit, we asked chaplains to send published materials about their departments, photos of chapels, and other information, which ranged from short pamphlets to extensive organizational charts. We also telephoned all of the departments that had prayer lines to listen to recorded prayers for patients and families.

At all seventeen hospitals, we interviewed—at least briefly—the director of chaplaincy.[23] We interviewed staff chaplains at fourteen hospitals. At the other three hospitals, contact information for staff chaplains was not publicly available, and either the directors would not introduce us to a staff chaplain or told us that they had circulated information about the project, and none of the staff chaplains were interested in participating. We identified staff chaplains to interview through recommendations from directors, information available on the web, and the advice of national chaplaincy leaders. We aimed to interview a mix of staff chaplains across hospitals, including people of different ages, genders, and religious and spiritual backgrounds. At a few hospitals, we interviewed more than one staff chaplain, for a total of twenty-three staff chaplains.

Overall, we interviewed thirty-nine people (sixteen directors and twenty-three staff chaplains). They were older than the U.S. population—on average, between the ages of fifty-five and sixty. Few were younger than forty, and none were younger than thirty. Men comprised two-thirds of the overall sample. The majority were white—close to 80%. Nonwhite chaplains were most frequently Catholic priests from Africa and parts of Asia who, because of U.S. Catholic priest shortages, were recruited from abroad to be chaplains. Most chaplains had master's or doctoral degrees and were ordained or certified as priests, nuns, rabbis, ministers, imams, or otherwise. Two-thirds of the directors were also certified as CPE supervisors through the Association for Clinical Pastoral Education. Most of the staff chaplains had had some CPE, but not all were board-certified or had completed the four units of CPE needed to be board-certified. They had worked in chaplaincy for seventeen years, on average, and at their current hospitals for an average of nine years. The largest fraction were Protestant, mostly mainline Protestant (56%) followed by Catholic (26%) and Jewish (13%). I met only one Buddhist and one Muslim chaplain during this research, along with a few Unitarians and others who consider themselves humanists and agnostics (not all of whom were interviewed).

As described in table A1, the department directors were mostly male (75%) and were older than staff chaplains (average age 65). Most were ordained or certified in their religious traditions. They had worked in chaplaincy for twenty-four years on average (ranging from a few years to more than forty-five years). They had directed their departments for between one and twenty-one years—twelve years on average. Two-thirds were Protestant. About half of the remaining one-third were Catholic, and half were Jewish. Staff chaplains were a bit younger than department directors, and a larger fraction (45%) were women. They have worked in chaplaincy for twelve years on average and been at their current hospitals for seven years on average. The majority were Protestant (52%), followed by Catholic (26%), Jewish (13%), Unitarian (4%), and Buddhist (4%).

It is not possible to approximate how this sample of directors and staff chaplains represents the population in academic hospitals, in hospitals nationally, or in the range of health-care and other institutions in which chaplains work because systematic data about these populations has not been gathered.[24] The Association of Professional Chaplains (APC), National Association of Catholic Chaplains (NACC), and National Association of Jewish

TABLE A1   Descriptive statistics for the cross section of hospitals

Chaplaincy directors ($N = 16$)		Staff chaplains ($N = 23$)	
Gender		*Gender*	
Male	75%	Male	55%
Female	25%	Female	45%
Average age	65 years	*Average age*	53 years
Race		*Race*	
White	75%	White	78%
Unknown	25%	Nonwhite	13%
		Unknown	9%
Ordained		*Ordained*	
Yes	76%	Yes	83%
No	18%	No	17%
Unknown	6%		
Average time working in chaplaincy	24 years	*Average time working in chaplaincy*	12 years
Range	5–46 years	Range	2–38 years
Average time working at this hospital	12 years	*Average time working at this hospital*	7 years
Range	1–21 years	Range	1–20 years
Religion		*Religion*	
Protestant	69%	Protestant	52%
Catholic	19%	Catholic	26%
Jewish	12%	Jewish	13%
Other	0%	Other	8%

Source: Interviews with the directors of chaplaincy and staff chaplains at seventeen highly ranked, large academic hospitals.

Chaplains (NAJC) keep membership lists, but their members work in several types of institutions and sometimes overlap, as individual chaplains belong to more than one association. I roughly approximated the religious distribution of chaplains in these three professional organizations, knowing that many of them work in health care, as described in table 2.3. Based on that approximation, my sample is more Protestant, less Catholic, and slightly more Jewish than national averages. This could represent selection in who works in large academic hospitals, who belongs to one or more of these professional organizations, and who in these health-care organizations was willing to be interviewed. I also estimated a rough age distribution for chaplains nationally, as described in chapter 2, and found that the chaplains interviewed fell relatively representatively within that distribution. Those interviewed are best seen as representative of how chaplaincy is practiced in large academic hospitals but not of who chaplains are and how they do their work beyond those hospitals.

A Case Study of Hospital Chaplaincy: Overbrook Hospital

To learn more about chaplaincy than was possible in interviews and short visits to seventeen hospitals, I also spent one year getting to know the chaplaincy department at the hospital I call Overbrook. After we spent several months getting to know one another, the department director whom I call Pat invited me to interview everyone in her department, attend staff meetings, and occasionally shadow staff chaplains on rounds and at meetings, with the understanding that I would focus on the chaplains and record no information about patients or family members. She saw this invitation as a way to make chaplaincy known to people outside of hospitals, which helps justify their existence, she told me, and educates the broader public about how they support patients, families, and staff. Pat saw my attempts to immerse myself in chaplaincy as a parallel to chaplains trying to immerse themselves in patients as living human documents, and she valued both as experientially focused learning processes.[25]

I shadowed chaplains, attended staff meetings and other departmental events, and interviewed a wide range of staff and volunteers during the year I spent at Overbrook. Guidelines from Pat and the hospital meant that almost all of the data I gathered about Overbrook was collected in interviews. I did not formally conduct any participant observation at events other than public religious services at the hospital. I did shadow chaplains who were attending committee meetings, medical team meetings, orientations for new hospital staff, and organ-donation training, visiting the morgue, and making patient visits, with permission from Pat and individual chaplains. While I watched how chaplains interacted with other staff, patients, and families in these gatherings, my main focus remained squarely on the chaplains and their work. On the few occasions in the text that I mention others in the hospital, I do so only in generic terms, mentioning the position of staff members as nurses, physicians, or social workers, for example, and the gender of patients or family members but nothing more. I also attended chaplaincy staff meetings and educational events, including a retreat, at Pat's invitation, where I took notes with permission.

In addition to this information, Pat gave me access to historical documents about the department, introduced me to former directors, and shared current demographic and statistical reports. I interviewed former directors when possible and, with Pat's permission, spoke with the hospital librarian, who also helped me locate additional historical data. I present little of that information here and intentionally keep what I do present quite vague in an effort not to identify the hospital. In a few instances, I changed minor details about the hospital's history for the same reason.

The majority of the data I present about Overbrook Hospital came through the interviews I conducted with thirty-two staff and volunteers.[26] As described in table A2, this included staff chaplains, hourly chaplains, students enrolled in CPE programs, and volunteers, including many Catholic Eucharistic ministers. Interviews followed an invitation I sent to the whole department by e-mail and posted in the staff room. I interviewed all of the staff chaplains and CPE residents and all of the other staff, students, and volunteers who responded positively to the invitation. Interviews lasted between forty-five and ninety minutes and were conducted in offices, conference rooms, and other private spaces in the hospital. I interviewed several of the hourly chaplains and volunteers in public spaces like coffee shops or in their homes or parishes. As a small thank you, I gave everyone who spent time talking with me two movie tickets or a gift certificate to a local coffee shop. All interviews were recorded and transcribed.

The thirty-two staff, students, and volunteers I interviewed came to this hospital in various ways. About two-thirds were women, including just over half of the staff chaplains, as summarized in table A2. The group was in their mid-fifties on average, with the average age of staff chaplains closer to sixty. Most were white. Staff chaplains either had or were working on master's degrees or doctorates, and half were certified as professional chaplains through one of the professional chaplaincy associations. The majority became staff chaplains by first taking CPE at the hospital, then doing hourly work as chaplains, and eventually becoming staff chaplains. Only a few were hired in searches from outside the hospital. CPE residents and CPE students were of all ages, with very few under the age of thirty. Half of the people I interviewed were Catholic, 25% were Protestant, 9% were Jewish, 9% were Unitarian Universalist, 3% were Pentecostal, and 3% were Muslim. Among the staff chaplains, one-third were Catholic, one-third were Protestant, and the remaining third were Muslim, Jewish, and Unitarian Universalist. The CPE residents and students were primarily Catholic and Protestant.

Staff chaplains had worked in chaplaincy for twelve years on average and at this hospital for ten years. Hourly chaplains had been at the hospital for four years on average, and CPE residents and CPE students had been there for just

TABLE A2   Descriptive statistics for individuals interviewed in the chaplaincy department at Overbrook Hospital

Staff chaplains ($N = 9$)		All staff, students, and volunteers interviewed, including staff chaplains ($N = 32$)	
Gender		*Gender*	
Male	44%	Male	34%
Female	55%	Female	66%
Average age	60 years	*Average age*	55 years
Race		*Race*	
White	89%	White	94%
Nonwhite	11%	Nonwhite	6%
Ordained		*Ordained*	
Yes	55%	Yes	34%
No	44%	No	62%
Average time working in chaplaincy	12 years	*Average time at this hospital*	
		Staff chaplains	10 years
Range	4–25 years	Hourly chaplains	4 years
Average time working at this hospital	10 years	CPE students	<1 year
		Volunteers	10 years
Range	4–25 years		
Religion		*Religion*	
Protestant	33%	Protestant	25%
Catholic	33%	Catholic	50%
Jewish	11%	Jewish	9%
Muslim	11%	Muslim	3%
Other	11%	Other	12%
		Distribution of people interviewed	
		Staff chaplains	29%
		Hourly chaplains	16%
		CPE students	26%
		Volunteers	29%

Source: Interviews with thirty-two staff chaplains, hourly chaplains, CPE students, and volunteers at Overbrook Hospital.

less than a year. Many of the volunteers, in contrast, had been involved with the chaplaincy department for many years—close to eight years on average for the Eucharistic ministers and more than twelve years for the other volunteers. I interviewed approximately two-thirds of all of the staff and volunteers involved with this department, including approximately 90% of the staff.

Since we lack more detailed national data about chaplaincy departments, it is not possible to compare Overbrook's department to others. Among the seventeen departments I learned about, this was one of the larger ones, with more staff chaplains, CPE students, and volunteers than most. I classify it as a transitional department, because, while staff were oriented to professional chaplaincy standards, not all of the chaplains were paid directly by the hospital. The department also had a large volunteer program, and the tasks assigned to volunteers in comparison to staff chaplains were not always clearly differentiated.

The staff and volunteers welcomed me from the start and were generous with their time. As people who spend most of their days listening, several staff chaplains told me that they enjoyed the opportunity to talk in interviews and to reflect on their work. The CPE residents often treated me as a fellow student, and many of the volunteers were excited to talk with someone interested in what they do at the hospital. While it is impossible to know precisely how you are received as a researcher, I felt welcomed by the department during the year I spent there. The challenges I had in getting permission to study a single chaplaincy department, however, led me to walk delicately during my time at Overbrook, just as my agreements with Pat led me to be extremely discreet (and as invisible as possible) when I was in areas of the hospital where I might see patients and families. It was difficult to see ill people and suffering families and emotionally challenging to hear some of the stories staff and volunteers told about their work. Combined with the time I spent in the ICUs, these experiences and conversations led me to adopt some of the emotional coping mechanisms that I describe the staff using and to have even more respect for the work they do daily.

A Case Study of Two Intensive Care Units: City Hospital

In addition to interviewing chaplains who formally engage with religion and spirituality for hospitals, I wanted to understand how religion and spirituality are present in hospitals when chaplains were not around. I knew from shadowing physicians that the topics do come up, and I wanted to focus on one unit or hospital service to see how staff members respond, professionally and personally, to these topics. Rather than focusing on religion and spirituality alone, I decided to try learning about the broader range of ways in which staff see and make meaning in their work. I therefore framed this portion of the project more broadly in terms of the personal beliefs and work experiences of hospital staff.

Over several months, and using intermediaries that bridged three degrees of separation, I developed a working relationship with a senior physician who shared my interest and agreed to collaborate. Through this physician, I got access to and permission to conduct research in one neonatal and one medical ICU at the hospital I call City Hospital, one of the seventeen academic hospitals described earlier. Had my networks and those of my intermediaries, been different, I could just have easily focused these case studies on other units of City Hospital. I intentionally stayed away from palliative care and hospice services in seeking case studies, however, because of the extent to which I knew religion and spirituality were associated with death in Joint Commission policies and in existing research literature. The intensity of birth, possible but not certain death, and uncertainty in these two ICUs made them ideal case studies alone and in comparison to one another, though other units certainly would have encapsulated the meaning-making that takes place in hospitals in other ways. While I would have preferred to study these two units at Overbrook Hospital or the chaplaincy department at City Hospital, the research networks I developed did not make such entry and permission to conduct research possible.

My physician colleague at City Hospital carefully negotiated my access to these units by first introducing me to the medical directors and nurse managers of each and personally endorsing the project from the start.[27] This colleague helped me obtain a hospital ID card as a researcher and receive approval from the hospital's Institutional Review Board. This physician also attended staff meetings of attending physicians (intentionally wearing a white coat) to introduce the project and personally encourage them to participate.[28] The medical director of one of the units encouraged attending physician colleagues to participate, telling them that their patients participated in research studies, and it would be good for them to do the same.

Before interviewing staff, I spent a part of several days a week for one month on each unit shadowing staff—primarily nurses—to get a sense of their work and the rhythms of the unit. I aimed to spend enough time to understand what work was like for staff members but not so much as to be intrusive.[29] As at Overbrook, I focused exclusively on the staff while I was shadowing, not speaking to patients or family members. This time allowed me to adjust slowly to being in the company of severely ill people and to see what it is like for family members and other newcomers to adjust to high-tech medical environments.[30] As I became accustomed to the sounds, smells, lighting, and pace of these units, I frequently felt that I was in the way. I regularly restrained my instinct to help when a nurse had her hands full of supplies and an alarm was going off next to me that I could easily have turned off after she heard it. I shadowed on day and night shifts, getting to know some staff, talking about my project, and gathering their informal feedback. "If you want to know what makes nurses happy" a day nurse told me with a laugh, "it is candy, . . . and when things get really bad, we order out." Another said that "NICU nurses love to talk," when I mentioned hoping to interview some of them.

As I slowly got to know people on both units, I sent an e-mail to all of the attending physicians, staff nurses, respiratory therapists, social workers, and chaplains describing this project and inviting them to be interviewed. I excluded students (including fellows, resident physicians, medical and nursing students) as well as hourly and per diem nurses because most had not spent extensive time in the unit. I also did not interview people who worked in administrative positions because I was primarily focused on those who regularly interact with patients. I posted a description of the project in staff areas, specifying that in exchange for being interviewed, participants would receive two movie tickets or a gift certificate to a local coffee shop.[31] The invitation to participate was signed by me, my physician colleague, the director of the unit, and the nurse manager of the unit, indicating that they all supported the project. It affirmed that only I would know who participated, and that all names would be changed in future reports and publications.[32] Before and during the time I was conducting interviews, I attended ethics rounds on each unit to hear what kinds of issues were being talked about and as a way to continue to meet staff informally.

In addition to staff members who responded to my general invitation to be interviewed, I also contacted others and personally invited them to be interviewed. I e-mailed all of the attending physicians individually, for example, and arranged to interview them in their offices or labs when they were not on a rotation in the ICU. The nurses I got to know while shadowing generally agreed to be interviewed, and I sent personal invitations to them to set up times to talk. They then introduced me to other nurses they thought might participate. I interviewed almost all of the nurses, respiratory therapists, social workers, and chaplains in a conference room near the unit during or immediately before or after a shift. All of their schedules changed with patient needs in the unit, and I frequently rescheduled interviews or spent afternoons at the hospital waiting to see when and if a particular staff member would be free to talk. With the permission of their managers, nurses and respiratory therapists I interviewed during their shifts had colleagues watch their patients while we talked.[33]

Interviews with ICU staff lasted between thirty minutes and one hour and were recorded and transcribed.[34] They began with a set of general questions about how the respondents came to nursing or medicine, how they came to this hospital, and what the best and most difficult aspects of their work were. I then asked about especially memorable patients, how they respond when patients/families ask "Why me" questions, and how they think about suffering. The interviews concluded with questions about whether and when issues related to spirituality and religion come up in their units, how they responded, and how they thought about these issues personally. A few respondents moved through the questions quickly, while others took time to think about them. More than a few—especially nurses and respiratory therapists—held back tears when talking about memorable patients and thanked me at the end of our conversation for the opportunity to reflect on their work. In addition to what I describe in chapters 6 and 7, much of what I learned in these interviews about the ways nurses manage their emotions is described in other articles.[35]

In the NICU, as noted in table A3, I interviewed thirty-five staff. They had worked at this hospital for 11 years on average and in this unit for 10.5 years. The nurses and respiratory therapists had worked there for longer than the attending physicians on average. The majority of staff members were women, though this varied by position; half of the attending physicians were women, as were almost all of the nurses, nurse practitioners, respiratory therapists, social workers, and chaplains. The staff members interviewed were in their fifties on average, and ages did not vary significantly among professional groups. The attending physicians were all MDs or MD/PhDs, while the nurses had first degrees—RN, BA, BS, or some combination—and a quarter had or were working on MAs. Most respiratory therapists had first degrees, and the chaplain had an MA and was professionally certified as a chaplain. As a group, the majority of staff were Catholic (49%), followed by Protestant (19%), Jewish (8%), other (8%), none (11%) and unknown (5%). About half regularly attended a religious or spiritual organization, and 40% had personal religious or spiritual practices. About a third described themselves as spiritual, and close to two-thirds said they prayed at least occasionally for the babies in their care. These thirty-five staff included almost all the attending physicians and about a third of the nurses.

I interviewed thirty-seven staff in the MICU. They had worked at this hospital for 10 years on average and in this unit for 8.4 years. In comparison to nurses in the NICU (who had 13.8 years of experience on average), the nurses in the MICU had half as much experience, 7.5 years. Attending physicians had the longest tenure in this unit, followed by nurses and respiratory therapists. Just over half of the staff were women (54%). The attending physicians were almost exclusively men, and 90% of the nurses were women. Staff

TABLE A3   Descriptive statistics for individuals interviewed in the neonatal and medical ICUs at City Hospital

Neonatal ICU ($N = 35$)		Medical ICU ($N = 37$)	
Position		*Position*	
Attending physician	16%	Attending physician	31%
Nurse	65%	Nurse	53%
Respiratory therapist	16%	Respiratory therapist	11%
Social worker	0%	Social worker	3%
Chaplain	3%	Chaplain	3%
Gender		*Gender*	
Male	11%	Male	46%
Female	89%	Female	54%
Average age	52 years	*Average age*	44 years
Time working in this unit	10.5 years	*Time working in this unit*	8.4 years
Range	1–33 years	Range	1–36 years
Religion		*Religion*	
Protestant	19%	Protestant	11%
Catholic	49%	Catholic	59%
Jewish	8%	Jewish	8%
Other	8%	Other	8%
None	11%	None	11%
Unknown	5%	Unknown	3%
At least occasionally privately pray for patients		*At least occasionally privately pray for patients*	
Yes	65%	Yes	68%
No	22%	No	26%
Unknown	13%	Unknown	6%

Source: Interviews with staff members in the neonatal and medical ICUs at City Hospital.

members in the MICU were younger than those in the NICU, in their 40s on average. This varied by position; the physicians were the oldest—in their 50s—and the nurses were in their 30s. The younger age and fewer years of experience among nurses in the MICU in comparison to the NICU reflects the fact that experience in an MICU is often a path to other jobs in nursing, while experience in an NICU is less likely to be. The physicians and nurses in both the MICU and the NICU had similar educational backgrounds. The social worker had an MA, though the chaplain did not and was not certified as a professional chaplain. As in the NICU, the majority of staff were Catholic (59%), followed by Protestant (11%), Jewish (8%), none (11%), other (8%), and unknown (3%). About half regularly attended a religious or spiritual organization, and three-quarters said they had a personal religious or spiritual practice. Just under one-fifth considered themselves spiritual, and just over two-thirds prayed at least occasionally for the patients and families in their care. These interviews included almost all of the attending physicians and just over a quarter of the nurses. As in the NICU, they may be biased toward those willing to talk with a researcher about their experiences.

I spent more than a year between these units and came to know many staff, especially nurses. I answered questions about myself and my project honestly and was aware of people reinterpreting the topic of the research over time. In talking with each other, several nurses described the project as about end-of-life care, perhaps because of the questions about religion/spirituality—I asked no direct questions about death. Others were less interested in the project and more interested in the coffee gift cards, introducing me to one another as the "free coffee girl." Still others suggested I abandon my topic and do research about something that mattered more in their daily lives, such as the light (not bright enough) and temperature (too cold) of their units. Several used the interviews as opportunities to reflect on ethical conflicts they have with some of the medical procedures they do and their lack of knowledge of long-term outcomes on patients.

Among the approximately one hundred and fifty interviews I conducted between 2004 and 2006, I found those with the ICU staff to be the most difficult. Practically, it took a long time to develop the relationships needed to get permission to study these units. Personally, it was difficult to spend time in the company of ill patients and their family members while shadowing and to sometimes see procedures being done on patients. In interviews, it was not easy to hear some of the stories staff members told, especially about end-of-life situations that did not go well. That said, these interviews did lead me to respect the work these staff members do and the ethical dilemmas that many face quietly on a regular basis.

DATA ANALYSIS AND WRITING

Once I had gathered the data, I put all of the interview transcripts and documents collected during fieldwork into a qualitative analysis program, Atlas-TI, and first coded the data by interview question. I then inductively developed more detailed codes, following the broad principles of grounded theory, coding and recoding as I thought through the material and began to develop an outline for the book and draft chapters.[36] I triangulated sources and read interviews with a careful eye. I was skeptical about what some of the directors of chaplaincy departments told me, for example, as it became clear from my triangulation that the lines between what they actually do in their hospitals and what they would like to do are fuzzy. Often trained as religious leaders in public speaking, they sometimes articulated visions in interviews that were grander than their actions seemed to be in hospitals, judging from their web pages, interviews with staff chaplains, and other materials.

I situated what I learned in all of these interviews historically and contextually based on my reading in history, medicine, sociology, theology, and religious studies. In addition to reading the secondary literature about American religious history, the history of American hospitals, the development of health-care professionals, and religion and spirituality in health and health care more generally, I worked through several sets of historical primary sources, including Joint Commission policies, the annual reports of several hospitals, materials about the American Medical Association's Committee on Medicine and Religion (located through the archives of the American Medical Association), and historical documents about hospital chaplains located through the Association of Professional Chaplains, the National Association of Catholic Chaplains, the National Association of Jewish Chaplains, and the Association for Clinical Pastoral Education (including some through the archives at Pitts Theological Library). I also read many years of the *Journal of Pastoral Care and Counseling* and related chaplaincy publications, and worked with researchers at the American Hospital Association to examine the data they collected about hospital chaplains over time. To situate what I learned about specific hospitals, I interviewed health-care representatives of Catholic diocese and Jewish synagogue councils in some geographic areas to understand how they think about and support hospital chaplaincy financially.

The analytic structure of the book, which is based on the physical locations in hospitals where religion/spirituality is present, became clear only as I analyzed the data and drafted chapters. I frequently described the intensely inductive nature of this project as like doing a jigsaw puzzle without the box top that helps you see what the final product will look like. The ideas presented here have been written about in multiple disciplines that have very different (sometimes competing) orienting assumptions and epistemologies. I aimed to make these ideas as comprehensible to one another and to a broad audience of scholars and the reading public as possible and intentionally put references and notes about more academic matters in footnotes. I tested arguments and gathered feedback at professional meetings of social scientists and religious studies scholars, at meetings of professional chaplains, at talks in chaplaincy departments, in interdisciplinary gatherings of religion and health scholars, and in talks aimed at broader publics.

I also shared the complete manuscript with several of the physicians and chaplains I interviewed at Overbrook and City. They mostly agreed with my analyses and, where they did not, I address our differences in footnotes. Pat, the director at Overbrook, pointed to a number of changes made since I conducted this research but was clear that, in her words, "You can't put in [the book] stuff that is not in your experience," and did not ask me to make specific changes.

I promised my respondents confidentiality and changed the names of all of the individuals and institutions in this book. In some cases I changed or made more general identifiable demographic or institutional details. I have also done my best to protect the internal confidentiality of respondents—especially at Overbrook and City—where people in the chaplaincy department and ICUs might recognize one another.[37] In a few cases I changed the gender or background of respondents. In a very few cases (less than five), I created composite characters to protect people's identifying information.

My experience in getting access to and permission to study these chaplaincy departments and medical staff point to the challenges of learning about religion and spirituality and doing any social science research in hospitals. For the practical reasons outlined, interviews became my central research tool. The silences of patients and families remain, as do the many ways religion and spirituality are likely talked about informally that can only be described through participant observation and research in a wider range of settings than was possible in this project. While informative, the data I gathered are far from perfect. Without information about a broader range of medical staff at City Hospital and the other sixteen hospitals in the sample, for example, it is also impossible to know if the professional and personal approaches to religion and spirituality described in the neonatal and medical ICUs can be generalized beyond those units. Selection is also an issue, as none of these samples were randomly gathered, and more detailed information might have emerged about many of the chaplaincy departments studied had I spent as much time in them as at Overbrook. I also say much more about how chaplains talk about their work than about how they do that work with patients and families. The latter might include more focus on traditionally religious prayers and rituals than is evident here.

Limitations aside, I intend this book as a first look at how religion and spirituality are present in hospitals and try to generalize beyond the data gathered carefully and thoughtfully in the text. Despite how often related topics are spoken of by the media, little is known empirically, and, as I show, many of the ways religion and spirituality are addressed are idiosyncratic and unique to the particular hospitals in question. Hopefully this study will motivate other researchers to think about how religion and spirituality are present in a wide range of hospitals, nursing homes, rehabilitation centers, and other health-care facilities—both religious and secular. Good social science ultimately becomes grist for historians. If nothing more, I hope this book enables historians of the future to better understand how religion and spirituality were present in a specific set of hospitals in the first decade of the twenty-first century.

CHAPTER 1

1. I have changed the names of all of the individuals and hospitals described in this book. In some instances, I concealed identifying details or made them vague to protect people's privacy, as described in the appendix. Quotations come from field notes and interviews, as evident from the context in which they are used in the text.

2. As of 2004 this code of ethics was formally shared by the Association of Professional Chaplains, American Association of Pastoral Counselors, Association for Clinical Pastoral Education, National Association of Catholic Chaplains, National Association of Jewish Chaplains, and Canadian Association for Pastoral Practice and Education: see http://www.spiritual carecollaborative.org/docs/common-code-ethics.pdf.

3. By secular organizations, I mean those without a formal, self-identified, religious mission or identity. For a more nuanced description of these distinctions, see Demerath et al. 1998. Among US hospitals, 12% were religious/church-operated in 2007 (American Hospital Association Annual Survey Database 2007, Chicago: Health Forum, an affiliate of the American Hospital Association, 2009). While there is general agreement that the fraction of all hospitals that are religious or church-sponsored has declined over time, it is impossible to show this precisely because of changes in the way the American Hospital Association codes these hospitals in their aggregate data.

4. In asking these questions, I draw from research and thinking about religion, spirituality, health, and medicine across the disciplines. For overview articles, see Koenig, McCullough, and Larson 2001; Chatters 2000; Chatters, Levin, and Ellison 1998; Ellison and Levin 1998; Sherkat and Ellison 1999; George et al. 2000; Miller and Thoresen 2003; Weaver and Ellison 2004; Cadge 2009a; Cadge and Fair 2010. From anthropologists and religious studies scholars, I draw ideas about healing and examples of how religious traditions, organizations, sites, ideas, and practices shape people's ideas about healing, usually outside of biomedical organizations. From medical research focused on religion and health, I draw evidence of the relationship between these concepts among individuals and the ways they can be measured. From theology,

I draw on the history of Clinical Pastoral Education and various theological approaches to illness and to suffering. And from sociology, I draw from organizational approaches to religion, questions about how religion and spirituality are addressed in secular organizations, and the development of the professions more generally.

5. See Kluger 2009; Kluger 2004; Sheler 2004; Kalb 2003.

6. See Frenk, Foy, and Meador 2010.

7. Funding for related projects through the National Institutes of Health has also increased.

8. Ritter 2005; Kong 1998.

9. Both of these centers and numerous research initiatives related to religion, spirituality, and health, including the now defunct National Institute for Healthcare Research (NIHR), are or have been financially supported by the John Templeton Foundation; see website at http://www.templeton.org/.

10. Some of these courses are supported by grants from the John Templeton Foundation administered through the George Washington Institute for Spirituality and Health. The GWish web page says that forty-nine medical and osteopathic schools have received curricular awards since 1995. For more on the content of these classes, see Sulmasy 1997; Levin, Larson, and Pulchalski 1997; Kelly et al. 1996; Fortin and Barnett 2004; Pelletier and McCall 2005; Barnes 2006; and Berlinger 2004. The John Templeton Foundation also supported a task force of the Association of American Medical Colleges, whose recommendations, entitled "Spirituality, Cultural Issues, and End of Life Care," were included in *Report III. Contemporary Issues in Medicine: Communication in Medicine. Medical School Objectives Project* (1999).

11. Sloan 2006.

12. See, for example, http://www.pbs.org/wnet/religionandethics/episodes/october-23-2009/doctors-patients-and-prayer/4724/. For data about the ways and extent to which patients want their physicians to ask about religion, spirituality, and prayer, see Daaleman and Nease 1994; Ehman et al. 1999; and MacLean et al. 2003. For an exception—a study that does ask how religion and spirituality are present in health-care organizations—see Williams et al. 2011.

13. RI.01.01.01 in JCAHO's 2010 Comprehensive Accreditation Manual for Hospitals. For a summary, see: http://www.uphs.upenn.edu/pastoral/resed/JCAHOspiritrefs2010.pdf.

14. The report is available online at http://www.americanreligionsurvey-aris.org/reports/ARIS_Report_2008.pdf.

15. These surveys are available online at http://pewforum.org/uploadedfiles/Topics/Beliefs_and_Practices/Other_Beliefs_and_Practices/multiplefaiths.pdf.

16. Survey by CBS/*New York Times*, April 29, 1998. Retrieved August 6, 2008, from the iPOLL Databank, The Roper Center for Public Opinion Research, University of Connecticut; available online at <http://www.ropercenter.uconn.edu/ipoll.html>.

17. Survey by *Newsweek*, November 1, 2003. Retrieved February 28, 2006, from the iPOLL Databank, The Roper Center for Public Opinion Research, University of Connecticut; available online at <http://www.ropercenter.uconn.edu/ipoll.html>.

18. Ibid.

19. Jacobs, Burns, and Jacobs 2008.

20. Phelps et al. 2009.

21. See Curlin et al. 2007.

22. See Curlin et al. 2005. For information on pediatric physicians, see Catlin, Cadge, and Ecklund 2008; Ecklund et al. 2007.

23. For studies on the relationship between religion/spirituality and how physicians make decisions, see Seale 2010; Crane 1975; Aiyer et al. 1999; Abdel-Aziz, Arch, and Al-Taher 2004; Imber 1986; Christakis and Asch 1995. For information about how important physicians think religion is in their work with patients, see Greeley 1999; Curlin et al. 2006. For a description of one group of physicians that meets at a large academic hospital to discuss religion in both professional and personal ways, see Messikomer and De Craemer 2002.

24. Grant, O'Neil, and Stephens 2004; Cavendish et al. 2004.

25. I do not include the year in which these rankings were completed to protect the confidentiality of the hospitals included.

26. See Christakis 1999. This is also like sociologist Gary Allen Fine's study of restaurant kitchens, which pays more attention to the workers than to customers (Fine 1996).

27. Glimpses of how religion and spirituality are present in hospitals appear in several recent books, none devoted specifically to the topic. Journalist Julie Salamon's book *Hospital: Man, Women, Birth, Death, Infinity, Plus Red Tape, Bad Behavior, Money, God, and Diversity on Steroids* comprehensively describes the inner workings of Maimonides Medical Center in Brooklyn, including how the hospital and its executives interact with the large Orthodox Jewish population that the hospital serves (Salamon 2008a). Anne Fadiman's *The Spirit Catches You and You Fall Down* focuses not on a hospital but on how medical staff in Merced, California, and a Hmong refugee family view and attempt to treat a child with epilepsy, or what her family calls "a disease where the spirit catches you and you fall down" (Fadiman 1998). Glimpses of chaplains and families' religious beliefs also appear in anthropologist Sharon Kaufmann's *And a Time to Die: How American Hospitals Shape the End of Life* and in sociologist Charles Bosk's *All God's Mistakes: Genetic Counseling in a Pediatric Hospital* (Kaufman 2005; Bosk 1992).

28. I tend to think about religion broadly as what anthropologist Clifford Geertz describes as a "system of symbols which act to establish power, pervasive and long-lasting moods and motivations in men [*sic*] by formulating conceptions of a general order of existence and clothing these conceptions with such an aura of factuality that the moods and motivations seem uniquely realistic" (Geertz 1973, 90). Thinking about this approach to the study of religion in health care and other secular organizations comes up short, however, because it is neither possible nor ideal to learn about the "moods" and "motivations" of everyone in the organization. Lived-religion approaches articulated by religious studies scholars David Hall and Robert Orsi focus on how people live their religions in their daily lives but are also limited because they privilege individuals' experiences over organizational senses of the setting; see Hall 1997; Orsi 1996 and 2003. I build on their approaches by seeing organizations not only as places where people's religious and spiritual experiences are shaped but as groups that themselves act and enact particular conceptions of religion and spirituality that, in turn, influence broader discussions about religion in public life (e.g., in Smith 2003).

29. See Berlinger 2004; Sloan 2006; Sheler 2004.

30. Analyses of the main biomedical research database, PubMed, show a shift away from ar-

ticles using the word *religion* toward articles using the word *spirituality*. Whether the content of these studies has shifted accordingly is a separate question.

31. Bender 2007; Schmidt 2005; Wuthnow 1998; Roof 2003.

32. Bender 2010, 5.

33. Lee 2002, 339.

34. Sullivan 2010.

35. These terms demarcate boundaries as described by Lamont and Molnar 2002; see also Hall 1997.

36. For an excellent discussion, see Fox and Swazey 2008. See also Evans 2002; Bosk 2008, chap. 3.

37. Some are also invited to order kosher, halal, or other foods that fit their religious and dietary guidelines.

38. Many pamphlets are *Care Notes* or *Prayer Notes* supplied by Abbey Press, which is owned and operated by Saint Meinrad Archabbey, a Benedictine monastic community in Indiana (http://www.onecaringplace.com/default.asp).

39. Marking the area with a few boxes of matza, the *eruv* denotes the whole hospital as a communal area within which observant Jews can carry things, the chaplain explained.

40. In addition to staff chaplains, many departments include volunteers such as Catholic Eucharistic ministers, Protestant pastoral volunteers, and Bikur Cholim volunteers who visit Jewish patients. Many also have students enrolled in Clinical Pastoral Education programs.

41. For a study of a similar neonatal ICU, see Catlin et al. 2001.

42. See Chaves 2010 for a discussion of congruence.

43. Sullivan 2009, 230.

44. The first "establishment" case heard by the US Supreme Court was about a hospital, but few subsequent cases focus on health-care organizations. For recent information on a state-level case pertaining to chaplaincy in the Veterans Administration Hospitals, see Sullivan 2009. For broader information on church-state issues, see Hammond 1998; Smith 2003. For recent approaches to secularism, especially as influenced by Charles Taylor, see Warner, Vanantwerpen, and Calhoun 2010.

45. Eck 2001, 47.

46. Ibid.

47. Putnam and Campbell 2010.

48. See Taylor 2007.

CHAPTER 2

1. Chaplains at Overbrook were financially supported by groups outside the hospital until the early 1980s. In the 1980s the hospital began to pay some of the chaplains directly. They started to pay Catholic priest-chaplains directly in the 1990s after negotiating an arrangement with the diocese.

2. I did not interview nursing assistants or "sitters,"—staff or volunteers who sit with patients who may pose a risk to themselves or others. I hope someone else will write about religion and spirituality in their experiences.

3. I am the first, as far as I know, to synthesize this history. For another approach focused on the Netherlands, see Smeets 2006. For comparative perspectives on chaplains in the United Kingdom, see Mowat 2008; Swift 2009.

4. For an overview of these histories see Rosenberg 1987; Stevens 1989; Kauffman 1995; Meier and Tabak 2007. The history outlined here would be different if psychiatric, veterans', and other specialty hospitals were included.

5. See Fox and Swazey 2008.

6. See Wuthnow 1998; Roof 1999; McGuire 2008.

7. See Klassen 2011 for an excellent historical perspective on the changing relationship between medicine and mainline Protestantism.

8. While spirituality became more of a buzzword in medical contexts after 1990, it is important to recognize that it had been becoming more common in broader American culture since the 1960s (Roof 1999; Wuthnow 1998). These different timelines suggest that while some of the same factors help to explain the emergence of spirituality in both contexts, other factors related to the work of chaplains and the advocacy of physicians, nurses, and others in what I call the spirituality in health care movement were responsible for its later emergence in health care. This is further evidence for the argument Courtney Bender makes about spirituality developing and being present differently in different organizational fields (Bender 2010).

9. For histories of hospitals in earlier time periods and locations see Risse 1999; Mollat 1986; Ferngren 2009; Swift 2009; Miller 1997; Meier and Tabak 2007.

10. For more information see Rosenberg 1977; Rosenberg 1987; Starr 1982; Porter 1993.

11. Rosenberg 1987, 48.

12. Rosenberg 1987; Risse 1999.

13. Between 1872 and 1910, the number of Catholic hospitals in the United States increased from 75 to 400, paralleling the growth of general hospitals, which increased from 178 to 4,000 (Kauffman 1995, 130). For more information about the development of Catholic hospitals, see Kauffman 1995; McCauley 2005.

14. For more information on Jewish hospitals, see Kraut and Kraut 2007; Meier and Tabak 2007; Sarna 1987; Levitan 1964.

15. Numbers and Sawyer 1982.

16. Rosenberg 1987; Stevens 1921; Starr 1982.

17. Reverby 1987; Fairman and Lynaugh 1998.

18. Rosenberg 1987, 341.

19. Rosenberg 1987; McCauley 2005.

20. Stevens 1989.

21. Starr 1982.

22. See Rosenberg 1987. The American Hospital Association was founded in 1899 as part of this movement toward modernization and standardization, as was the American College of Surgeons in 1912, which initiated a hospital accreditation process (Stevens 1989). Religious hospitals also began their own associations, including the Catholic Hospital Association (1915) and the American Protestant Hospital Association (1921); see Kauffman 1995; Thomas and LaRocca-Pitts 2006.

23. Additional research is needed about hospital chaplaincy before 1925 with attention to

patterns in public, nonprofit, and other hospitals. For glimpses, see McCauley 2005; Monfalcone 2005. A Jewish geriatric facility in New York had a rabbi as early as 1902 who was primarily responsible for leading worship and providing kosher food (Meier and Tabak 2007; Tabak 2010).

24. Religious services were held in that space (minus the ice) for many years.

25. See McCauley 2005. There were also occasional "hospital missions" such as the one German-born evangelical pastor Julius Varwig started in St. Louis's public institutions for the sick and poor (Berlinger 2008b).

26. The Emmanuel Church in Boston brought some of these ideas together as early as 1905 in what historian E. Brooks Holifield describes as "the first serious effort to transform the cure of souls in light of the new psychology and theology" (1983, 201). See also Gerkin 1997; Holst 1982; Hall 1992; Myers-Shirk 2008.

27. Abbott 1988.

28. White 2009; Myers-Shirk 2008.

29. Holifield 2005; Johnson 1968.

30. See Lemmer 2002; Calabria and Macrae 1994; Meyer 2003; Widerquist 1992.

31. This process developed slightly differently in general hospitals than in psychiatric and mental hospitals. I focus primarily on general hospitals here. See also Holst 1982; Barrows 1993.

32. Hall 1992.

33. See also Asquith 1992; Myers-Shirk 2008; Boisen 1960; Gerkin 1997; Eastman 1951; Leas 2009.

34. Boisen's program began with four students, increasing to twenty by 1930 (Johnson 1968). See also Eastman 1951; Hall 1992; Holifield 1983.

35. Boisen thought CPE should focus on psychiatric hospitals, and he continued to work in them, moving from Massachusetts to Elgin State Hospital in Illinois, where he worked with students from the Chicago Theological Seminary after recovering from another psychotic episode. He also held a faculty position at Chicago Theological Seminary.

36. Thomas 2000, 9. Others, like Charles Hall (1992), describe the CPE movement as an effort to unify conceptual and experiential theological approaches to pastoral care and counseling.

37. See also Allport 1966; Monfalcone 2005; Cabot and Dicks 1936; and MGH annual reports.

38. Holst 1982.

39. Hall 1992; Gerkin 1997.

40. Holifield 1983 and 2005.

41. Hall 1992.

42. Led by Rollin Fairbanks, the Institute of Pastoral Care started the *Journal of Pastoral Care* in 1947, which published more articles on CPE as a form of theological education than on the work of hospital chaplains.

43. The process of forming the ACPE was complex and began in the 1950s formally with the "committee of twelve." For more information, see Hall 1992; Thomas 2000; Gerkin 1997; Hiltner and Ziegler 1961; Johnson 1968. Then, as now, CPE was offered not only in hospitals but in correctional and community settings.

44. The American Protestant Hospital Association was itself formed in 1921 by officials of Protestant hospitals who knew each other through denominational networks and the American Hospital Association, and thought they could benefit from mutual support and conversation (Thomas and LaRocca-Pitts 2006).

45. Dicks 1940, 4.

46. These points were later articulated in "Standards for the Work of the Chaplain in the General Hospital," written by Russell Dicks and adopted by the American Protestant Hospital Association in 1940 and again in 1950.

47. For more on the history and transformations of this association, see Thomas and LaRocca-Pitts 2006; Byrd and Jessen 1988.

48. I focus on these organizations as well as the National Association of Catholic Chaplains and the National Association of Jewish Chaplains in this chapter. Other organizations focused on hospital/health-care chaplaincy have existed, including the Healthcare Chaplaincy described below and what is today known as the Healthcare Chaplaincy Ministry Association (HCMA), which historically placed evangelical Christian chaplains in hospitals on the west coast. For more information on the HCMA, see http://www.hcmachaplains.org/home/history .html. A newer organization with a different approach, not discussed here, is the Chaplaincy Institute for Arts and Interfaith Ministry in Berkeley, CA (http://www.chaplaincyinstitute.org/).

49. The Veterans Administration established a Chaplaincy Service in 1945, though chaplains had been serving in related organizations for almost one hundred years (Monfalcone 2005; see also Sullivan 2010).

50. Some described themselves this way also. See Holst 1982; Holst 1985; Faber 1971.

51. Holifield 2007.

52. At Massachusetts General Hospital, for example, early chaplains were paid by Cabot and then by the Episcopal City Mission, chaired for some years by the same person who was the chairman of the Board of Trustees at the hospital. The Catholic archdiocese of Boston appointed (and paid) the first full-time Catholic chaplain in 1951.

53. For a good description of a Protestant chaplain's daily work in the 1940s, see Burns 1949.

54. For some discussion, see Imber 2008.

55. Risse 1999.

56. Standards for Accreditation of Hospitals Plus Provision Interpretations, Joint Commission on Accreditation of Hospitals, October 1969, 6

57. Brittain and Boozer (1987) argue that holistic models of health care began to be considered more seriously in the 1960s, including attention to spirituality, but that in a survey of nursing programs conducted in the late 1970s, spirituality was addressed only tangentially.

58. Fox and Swazey (2008, 36) quoting the Institute's web page.

59. See also Wolenberg 2011.

60. See Rhoads 1967, 172. For more information on this Committee, see Imber 2008; Wolenberg 2011.

61. This talk was presented at a workshop in Milwaukee, Wisconsin, and published in the *Bulletin of the American Protestant Hospital Association* 29, no. 3 (1965): 10, which published materials about this committee. This talk and these efforts more generally may have been in-

fluenced by developments in psychosomatic medicine at the time. McCleave's biomedical assumptions are clear, however, in his assertion that attention to the "whole person" is new, when many people prior to American physicians conceived of individuals in this way.

62. According to documents in the archives of the Association of Professional Chaplains, the Kansas University Medical School frequently held large events about medicine and religion, one of which attracted four hundred physicians and clergymen in 1971 (Agenda of the Seventh Inter-Organizational Consultation March 30, 1971). While the AMA said the committee ended for financial reasons, Wolenberg (2011) suggests that conflicts over abortion and the emergence of bioethics and hospice—both of which took on some of the responsibilities of the committee—may have played a role.

63. An article by Kepler reported that 40% of medical schools in a small survey conducted in 1966 offered courses about religion, but what those courses included is unknown (Kepler 1968).

64. W. P. L. Myers, "The Care of the Patient with Terminal Illness," in Paul B. Beeson and Walsh McDermott, eds., *Cecil Textbook of Medicine*, vol. 1 (Philadelphia: W. B. Saunders, 1975), 8–12.

65. Maxwell M. Wintrobe et al., eds., *Harrison's Principles of Internal Medicine*, 7th ed. (New York: McGraw-Hill, 1974), 7–8.

66. See Duncombe and Spilman 1971. This group, Ministers in Medical Education, eventually merged with others to form the Society for Health and Human Values, which later merged to form the American Society for Bioethics and Humanities.

67. *Essentials of a Hospital Chaplaincy Program* (Chicago: American Hospital Association, 1961).

68. "Statement on Hospital Chaplaincy" 1967.

69. This specific list of requirements comes from a 1961 document. The requirements were revised during the decade (and beyond) but generally included some version of what is listed here.

70. See Board of Accreditation Minutes, Chaplains Association, American Protestant Hospital Association, September, 1957, available at the Association of Professional Chaplains National Office, Schaumburg, IL. The Association of Mental Health Chaplains created an interfaith certification process in 1968.

71. Harold R. Nelson, "Why Chaplaincies?" Address given to the American Hospital Association, September 1, 1966.

72. Holst 1982; White 2009.

73. See table 2.1 source note for 1954 data.

74. What constituted a "service" was not clearly defined in the survey.

75. Kuby and Begole 1974. The hospitals in this smaller group were mostly federal, state, or local government hospitals, or nongovernmental, not-for-profit facilities.

76. Ibid. While most hospitals arranged for chaplains themselves, some contracted or partnered with others. The Healthcare Chaplaincy, another chaplaincy organization, oversaw some contracting, especially in the greater New York area. It was formed through the merger of the East Midtown Protestant Chaplaincy and the Bible and Fruit Mission in 1978. It started a CPE program and began to provide chaplains for New York area hospitals through a model of out-

sourcing. It has received sizable grants from major foundations and corporate philanthropists in support of its multifaith training, research, and educational mission. For more history, see http://www.healthcarechaplaincy.org/about-us/chronology.html.

77. For a report commissioned by the American Association of Theological Schools on the relationship between CPE and theological schools at this time, see Hiltner and Ziegler 1961.

78. The NACC set up its own training processes shortly after they started and collaborated with the ACPE on training throughout its history. A fair number of Catholics participated in courses run by the ACPE, which certified its first Catholic supervisor, John Allemang, a diocesan priest from Milwaukee, in 1967. See also Gustin and Murray 1985. The NACC did fight a long, ultimately unsuccessful battle with the federal government to have its training programs recognized, as were those of the Association for Clinical Pastoral Education. The federal government refused to grant the accreditation, maintaining Protestant-dominated educational models in CPE by arguing that the (largely Protestant) Association for Clinical Pastoral Education served the educational function (Gustin and Murray 1985, 20).

79. Sources disagree about what year Hollander was certified. Thomas (2000) says he was certified in 1949 by the Council for Clinical Training, a precursor to the ACPE. Tabak (2010) says he was certified in 1958. Regardless, Hollander organized many summer training sessions related to chaplaincy for rabbis across branches of Judaism. The idea of a Jewish chaplaincy organization was discussed in the early 1980s at sessions of the Council of Jewish Federations General Assembly. By the mid-1980s a group of Jewish chaplains working in health care and with geriatric populations approached major rabbinic groups for support in order to organize, without success. About twenty rabbis met before the national chaplaincy meeting, "Dialogue 1988," and in the early 1990s they founded the National Association of Jewish Chaplains (NAJC). Within a few years, the NAJC included chaplains from all branches of Judaism. See also Damon 1985; Meier and Tabak 2007; Tabak 2010; Silberman 1986 and 1992. For information on the challenges that Jewish students have faced in CPE and that Christian supervisors are facing as they try to adapt CPE in Jewish contexts, see Taylor and Zucker 2002; Thiel 2009. Other Protestant and Christian assumptions have been evident in CPE in the language of program goals; the model of education, which is focused largely on personal experience (some of this came from psychology as meditated by Protestant organizations and education); and the experiences of Jewish and other non-Christian students, who see their personal starting points quite differently from what is assumed in CPE.

80. The absence of nurses is noteworthy.

81. John Whitesel, "Report of the Third Inter-Organizational Consultation on Hospital Chaplaincy," *Bulletin of the American Protestant Hospital Association* 31, no. 2 (1967): 15.

82. What ended these collaborations is unclear. Possible factors are the national economic downturn, disagreements among the groups, or the end of the American Medical Association's Department of Medicine and Religion.

83. As outlined by Fred Reid Jr. in an article titled "Chaplaincy in Transition—the Second 25 Years," *Bulletin of the American Protestant Hospital Association* 36, no. 1 (1972): "No longer are we a group of people who reflect only a Protestant point of view. Rather, we are a professional organization which is sensitive to the ecumenical vibrations of our times. Furthermore, I feel that there is evolving within the midst of us a need to relate, a need to cooperatively work

together—for in this unity there is strength and healing for those to whom we minister" (11). The AHA *Manual on Chaplaincy* (1970) similarly had chapters about caring for Catholic, Jewish, and Protestant patients. Discussion of ways to "minister" to patients outside chaplains' own religious traditions was still to come.

84. See John M. Billinsky, "Identity and Power of the Chaplain—Faking It or Facing It," *American Protestant Hospital Association Bulletin*, Post-Convention Issue (Spring 1973): 6–8. This talk was given as the third annual Russell Dicks Memorial Lecture.

85. Risse 1999; Weinberg 2003.

86. Joint Commission, "Rights and Responsibilities of Patients," in *Accreditation Manual for Hospitals* (Oakbrook Terrace, IL: Joint Commission: February 1978).

87. "A comprehensive assessment of the biopsychosocial needs and spiritual orientation of the patient is conducted": see Standard AL.2 in the section entitled "Alcoholism and Other Drug Dependence Services," in *Accreditation Manual for Hospitals* (Oakbrook Terrace, IL: Joint Commission, 1989).

88. On the surface, chaplains seem to be another set of what David Rothman would call "strangers at the bedside," representing an incursion into professional medical authority in the later half of the twentieth century. In reality their presence is more complex, as chaplains were clearly present at the bedside before this time, and their authority rarely actively challenged that of physicians. They best fit the narrative Rothman (1991) presents about the work many did around bioethics as it emerged.

89. Joint Commission, "Patient Rights," in *Accreditation Manual for Hospitals* (Oakbrook Terrace, IL: Joint Commission, 1992). Standard AL.2 pertains to alcohol and drug dependence, and standard RI.1 to broader issues, including dying and grief.

90. Ibid. (Intent of Standard AL.2.4.8).

91. See "Staff Rights Mechanisms," in *Comprehensive Accreditation Manual for Hospitals* (Oakbrook Terrace, IL: Joint Commission, 1995), sec. 2.

92. See "Example of Implementation for RI.1.3.5," in *Comprehensive Accreditation Manual for Hospitals* (Oakbrook Terrace, IL: Joint Commission, 1998).

93. See "Patients Rights and Organization Ethics," in *Comprehensive Accreditation Manual for Hospitals Advanced Core* (Oakbrook Terrace, IL: Joint Commission, January 1999), RI-15. Chaplaincy leaders involved with a liaison group to the Joint Commission challenged the commission in the 1990s to shift their language from "pastoral counseling" to "pastoral care and other spiritual services," in order to better represent what they do.

94. Staten 2003.

95. Fitchett 1993. These tools joined other more traditional ways in which some nurses spoke with patients about spirituality and religion (Wolf 1988; Chambers and Curtis 2001).

96. North American Nursing Diagnosis Association 2007, 208.

97. Gilliat-Ray 2003.

98. Stoll 1979; Fitchett 1993.

99. See Maugans 1996; Puchalski and Romer 2000; Anandarajah and Hight 2001; Mansfield, Mitchell, and King 2002; Fitchett 1993; Hodge 2003; Hodge 2006. Additional spiritual assessments were created for specific areas in health care, such as intensive and cardiac care nursing (Timmins and Kelly 2008); cancer patients (Skalla and McCoy 2006). There is little data about who actually uses these tools and what effects they have.

100. American Association of Medical Colleges 1999.

101. See the *Cecil Textbook of Medicine*, editions 16 through 20. Related themes are mentioned in "Medicine as a Learned Profession," "Ethics in the Practice of Medicine," "Critical Care Medicine," and "Care of Dying Patients and Their Families," in *Harrison's Principles of Internal Medicine*; see similar sections in editions 8 through 14.

102. For representative studies, see Lemmer 2002; Meyer 2003; Narayanasamy and Owens 2001.

103. See Cadge, Freese, and Christakis 2008, which uses data from the American Hospital Association to show that between 54% and 64% of hospitals had chaplains between 1980 and the present, with no significant increasing or decreasing trends during this period. Larger hospitals, those in urban areas, and those that were church-affiliated, were more likely to have chaplaincy services in 1993 and 2003 than were others. See also Flannelly, Handzo, and Weaver 2004.

104. Report to the Executive Committee of the American Protestant Hospital Association from the President of the College of Chaplains, 1981, located in the archives of the Association of Professional Chaplaincy, Schaumburg, IL. See also Gartner et al. 1990; Gleason 1984. The only study that has been conducted about the cost of professional chaplains estimated that chaplains cost between $2.71 and $6.43 per visit in 1994–95 (VandeCreek and Lyon 1994–95). CPE is considered a form of graduate medical education under federal Medicare legislation, allowing hospitals with CPE programs to receive some financial reimbursements from Medicare for care provided by CPE students (Thomas 2000; White 2003).

105. At some hospitals this model was common before the 1980s—see Holst and Kurtz 1973. While many early professional chaplains were religiously liberal, such staffing models likely led more religiously liberal individuals who were comfortable with multiple approaches to the truth to continue to gravitate toward chaplaincy both as an alternative to congregational ministry and as a place where broad approaches to religion and spirituality were welcome.

106. Fitchett 1993.

107. Chaplains devoted significant attention to spiritual assessment in these years, however, as described in Fitchett 1993.

108. "Rationale for Professional Institutional Chaplaincy," *Bulletin of the American Protestant Hospital Association* 45, no. 1 (1982): 13.

109. Some members of each of these organizations did work together through the Association for Clinical Pastoral Education (ACPE) over the years, which also played an important role in joint efforts such as Dialogue 84 and COMISS.

110. See Duvall 1987. Additional groups like the Joint Issues in Pastoral Care Organizations (JIPCO) and the Joint Commission for the Accreditation of Pastoral Services (JCAPS) were also started in the 1980s. JIPCO was to be a forum through which the presidents of professional chaplaincy, pastoral care, and counseling organizations could communicate about issues of common concern. JCAPS intended to set standards and evaluate individual chaplaincy departments, in part because the Joint Commission was not doing so (Thomas and LaRocca-Pitts 2006). For more information about the interfaith meetings held, see Anderson 1987.

111. While data about the religious affiliations of members of the College of Chaplains is not easily accessible, it appears that it has been predominantly Protestant from the start. Documents from 1991 show that less than 10% of members that year were non-Protestants.

112. See http://www.professionalchaplains.org/index.aspx?id=31. Possible names for this new organization included the Association of Professional Chaplains, American Association of Chaplains, American Chaplains Association, American Chaplaincy Association, Association of Pastoral Care Specialists, and Association for Pastoral Care. The following three were put on a ballot, and the membership voted: Association of Professional Chaplains, American Association of Chaplains, and Association for Pastoral Care.

113. In 1988 the ACPE Underground Report was started as a newsletter that critiqued actions of the ACPE. The organization developed into the College of Pastoral Supervision and Psychotherapy in the 1990s, promoting what members see as a different approach to hospital chaplaincy and the training of chaplains. For more information, see http://www.cpsp.org/home.html.

114. July 1991 report from consultants, located in the archives of the Association of Professional Chaplaincy, Schaumburg, IL.

115. Ibid. There were also issues of inclusiveness for women and people of color, as well as for the four different constituencies involved—chaplains; decision makers in specialized settings; leaders and members in the denominations and local churches; and media, policymakers, and the public—who often had different priorities.

116. For more on the development of hospital chaplaincy as a profession, see VandeCreek 1999.

117. Efforts to influence medical education were not without controversy; see Berlinger 2004.

118. RI.01.01.01 in JCAHO's 2010 *Comprehensive Accreditation Manual for Hospitals*. For a summary, see http://www.uphs.upenn.edu/pastoral/resed/JCAHOspiritrefs2010.pdf.

119. Some chaplains report that hospitals have been cited for not following these guidelines, though systematic data has not been gathered.

120. See, for example, McEwen 2004; Lemmer 2002; Meyer 2003; Narayanasamy and Owens 2001; Taylor, Amenta, and Highfield 1995; Cavendish et al. 2004.

121. Flannelly, Weaver, and Handzo 2003; Galek et al. 2007.

122. Grant, O'Neil, and Stephens 2004.

123. In 2005, the American Association of Medical Colleges reported that sixty-six colleges reported teaching religion, spirituality, or related issues at some point during the four-year curriculum (Association of Medical Colleges, AAMC Curriculum Management and Information Tool, online at http://www.aamc.org/currmit [February 10, 2005]; see also Fortin and Barnett 2004; Pelletier and McCall 2005.

124. J. Andrew Billings, "Care of Dying Patients and Their Families," in *Cecil Textbook of Medicine*, 22nd ed., ed. Lee Goldman and Dennis Ausiello (Philadelphia: Saunders, 2004), 10–13.

125. See, for example, Fitchett and Handzo 1998. Some professional associations and standards of practice also address spirituality and religion (Puchalski et al. 2009).

126. See, for example, Chibnall and Brooks 2001; Luckhaupt et al. 2005; MacLean et al. 2003; Post, Puchalski, and Larson 2000; Armbruster, Chibnall, and Legett 2003; Greeley 1999.

127. Cadge, Ecklund, and Short 2009.

128. Professional chaplaincy organizations estimate that there are ten thousand hospital

chaplains. They get this number by combining their membership lists, but it is not known how many people work as chaplains without belonging to a professional organization or how many belong to multiple organizations and are being double- or even triple-counted. For an excellent discussion of the frame through which chaplains work in the UK, see Swift 2009.

129. VandeCreek and Burton 2001.

130. For more information, see http://www.spiritualcarecollaborative.org/mission.asp.

131. This educational approach is being challenged by organizations like the Chaplaincy Institute for Arts and Interfaith Ministry in Berkeley, CA, which develops educational programs around what a leader described to me as "moving around and not having a set faith tradition. . . . It's easier to do in a chaplaincy setting."

132. See Flannelly et al. 2006. For a description of what it is like to work as a chaplain, see Angrosino 2006; Flannelly et al. 2005.

133. See http://www.professionalchaplains.org/index.aspx?id=1210; Autton 1963; Hall 1992.

134. See Berlinger 2008a; Lyndes et al. 2008. In recent years, chaplaincy organizations have worked to develop professional relationships with the American Hospital Association, the American Medical Association, the American Psychiatric Association, the American Hospice Foundation, the American College of Healthcare Executives, and the Red Cross. Chaplains have been more welcomed in some fields than others, especially oncology and palliative care. They have also tried to do some public relations work; for example, the Association of Professional Chaplaincy launched *Healing Spirit*, a glossy magazine, in 2006 and mailed it to fifteen thousand CEOs, administrators, and managers in health-care institutions, hospices, long-term-care facilities, and all APC members.

135. One study that connects the work of chaplains to outcomes for patients and families finds that patients whose emotional and spiritual needs are met are more satisfied with their hospital stays (Clark, Drain, and Malone 2003). Another study suggests that patients suffering from COPD who are regularly visited by chaplains while in the hospital may have better outcome (Iler, Obershain, and Camac 2001). See also Bay et al. 2008; Gibbons, Thomas, and VandeCreek 1991; VandeCreek 2003.

136. These averages are based on information provided to me from the Association of Professional Chaplains (2010) and the National Association of Catholic Chaplains (2009). Age data was missing from about half of the members of the APC.

137. The Association of Professional Chaplains has worked to develop ways for Muslims to be certified as chaplains through their processes in recent years.

138. According to a survey conducted by the Spiritual Care Collaborative, the average staff chaplain made $52,000 in 2011, and about half of them also received housing allowances.

139. Puchalski and Romer 2000.

CHAPTER 3

1. The prayer cards are supplied by the American Bible Society, and the religious texts by organizations in their traditions.

2. The hosts are consecrated by the chaplain-priest in Mass at his home parish before he brings them to the hospital. Some hospitals (not Overbrook) use special hosts, designed to dis-

solve more easily in people's mouths when they are ill. Several Eucharistic ministers at Overbrook told me that the hosts should be stored under a red light: "Any Catholic sacristy [is] supposed to have a red light, denoting that the consecrated body of Christ is in the tabernacle," one explained.

3. Chaplaincy Department, Overbrook Hospital, annual reports.

4. He did not note the potential conflict in hoping the space would welcome everyone but designing it in a way that mostly included objects common in Protestant churches.

5. This stained glass was donated in memory of a family member.

6. As the chapel moved, the main chaplaincy office also moved—as a former director said, to "the other side of the universe" and back again. Office moves were also common at other hospitals when chapels moved. Many chapels initially had offices for chaplains connected to them. Lamenting the separation of her office from the chapel in a recent move, the director at one department told me she "lost something. . . . You could catch a lot of walk-ins, you could identify people that were upset. It doesn't function as well [with the offices at a distance]."

7. The guidelines were set by the director and the CPE supervisor.

8. At a chaplain retreat, the director brought up the topic of the chapel, saying that she wanted to add religious symbols to the space. Two chaplains offered ideas about how to do so.

9. These spaces can be considered what sociologist Wendy Griswold calls a "cultural object" or "part of the broader system we refer to as culture" that we can "hold up" for analysis. As such, the chapels "tell a story," in Griswold's words, pointing to a shift over time as hospitals moved from having tradition-specific chapels to more interfaith spaces (Griswold 1987).

10. In reading this chapter before the book went to press, Pat noted how difficult it is to create a chapel space that does not offend anyone. She spoke of trying to create a "both/and" space—one that *both* welcomes people seeking symbols, prayer rugs, or texts *and* feels comfortable to people made uncomfortable by such religious and spiritual objects. She thinks the people who use the chapel at Overbrook are mostly Christians, Muslims, and those who consider themselves spiritual. She suspects that few Jews use the space because they find the concept of a chapel foreign and might be offended by the Christian symbols.

11. One of the analytic challenges in this chapter was identifying what I mean by spiritual objects, symbols, practices, etc. While someone sitting silently in a meditation room, for example, could be engaged in a spiritual practice, as an observer I would have no way of knowing that. I addressed this issue inductively, asking the directors and staff chaplains I interviewed about both religious and spiritual aspects of their chapel, prayer, and meditation spaces, and relying on them to identify those that they and their institution saw as spiritual. Despite chaplains' emphasis on spirituality described in the next chapter, there was relatively little talk of spirituality in relation to chapel spaces.

12. See Bellah et al. 1985; Roof 1999.

13. Eck 2001, 47. The transitions described here mirror those that Sophie Gilliat-Ray describes in the United Kingdom (Gilliat-Ray 2005a).

14. Despite a large literature about sacred space in religious studies (e.g., Chidester and Linenthal 1995; Nelson 2006; Jones 2000) and literature about hospitals in architectural history (e.g., Adams 2008), little has been written about hospital chapels as sacred spaces.

15. *Oxford English Dictionary*, 1989 edition, s.v. "chapel." A few historical studies describe

specific university, military, and prison chapels in the United States, but none trace chapels historically or compare chapels within or across organizational sectors. In their research in the United Kingdom, sociologists James Beckford and Sophie Gilliat make some contemporary comparisons describing the shrinkage of chapel spaces in UK prisons since the 1950s and movements toward multipurpose and religiously neutral spaces (Beckford and Gilliat 1998). In the United States, they explain, principles of nonestablishment do not allow tax dollars to be used to build separate religious facilities in federal or state prisons. Current policies stipulate that "the space assigned for group prayer and worship should be large enough for the congregation, functional and neutral in design" (quoted in Beckford and Gilliat 1998, 184). This neutrality implies that spaces should not contain permanent symbols from one religious tradition that might be seen as an affront by others. While Veterans Hospitals in the United States have similar guidelines about religiously neutral chapel spaces, private hospitals generally do not.

16. Thompson and Goldin 1973, 24; see also Swift 2009, chap. 1.

17. Some British hospitals in the eighteenth and nineteenth centuries, including the Liverpool General Infirmary (1749), the Edinburgh Royal Infirmary (1778), and the hospital at Kings College London (1839), all had chapels that also served secular purposes as operating theaters and meeting rooms (Thompson and Goldin 1973, 108). In Britain, an article published in the *British Medical Journal* in 1902 recommended that visitors to London stop to see the hospital chapels at Middlesex Hospital and the Great Ormond Street Hospital for Sick Children; "there is not an inch that is not beautiful" ("Hospital Chapels" 2002).

18. The decision to put a statue of Jesus Christ in the Johns Hopkins Hospitals is an interesting wrinkle in this history. See Cadge and Daglian 2008; McCall 1982.

19. This is described in the 1998 annual report from Yale-New Haven Hospital.

20. See Risse 1999, chap. 10 and Fine 2003.

21. Thompson and Goldin 1973, 108.

22. Risse 1999, chap. 10; Joyce 1995, esp. 254–55. See also Fine 2003. Many Jewish hospitals also had a room used for circumcisions.

23. Stevens 1921, 89.

24. Ibid, 216.

25. Quoted in Autton 1969, 65. The circular further stipulated that "the majority of hospital chapels will be 'dedicated' buildings and regulated by the Extra-Parochial Ministry Measure of 1967. In the few cases where the chapels are 'consecrated,' their use is restricted to Church of England services only, except with the sanction of the diocesan bishop."

26. Quoted in Autton 1969, 69.

27. The chaplain I interviewed recently relocated this mortuary chapel in the hospital and reconstructed its history from hospital and other documents. Parts of it were given away when the chapel closed, and the chaplain found its altar in the basement of a financially struggling church in another part of the city.

28. Verderber and Fine 2000, 26. Glimpses of hospital chapels in the 1950s and 1960s are evident in a few articles published in the *Bulletin of the American Protestant Hospital Association*. Two articles in 1955 described architectural renderings of new chapels in Protestant hospitals that looked much like Protestant churches at the time (*APHA Bulletin* 19, no. 3 [1955]: 7; *APHA Bulletin* 19, no. 4 [1955]: 7). In 1966 there was a short article about how to plan a

chapel in the journal *Hospitals* (Mellem 1966). Among other things, the author, Roger Mellem, recommended locating the chapel in a remote or quiet area of the hospital, designing it so that patients could access it, having flexible warm lighting, including symbols so the space could be used by people of multiple faiths, and having flowers and flexible seating.

29. American Hospital Association 1970, 38.

30. Kuby and Begole 1974, table 6.

31. A small study by S. Denton Bassett in 1976 reported that close to two-thirds of the ninety-three hospitals he studied offered Sunday or weekday religious services, often in the chapel (Bassett 1976). See also Jackson 1968.

32. Creager 2000; Dave Jordan, "Groundbreaking for PCMH Interfaith Chapel," September 17, 2009, online at www.witn.com; Joanna Corman, "Hospitals Revamp Chapels Into Interfaith Meditation Rooms," Huffington Post, July 21, 2010; Jennifer Garza, "Hospitals Rethink Spiritual Spaces, Create Meditation Rooms," *Sacramento Bee*, May 13, 2010. Some new spaces seem to be dedicated or blessed by representatives from a range of religious traditions, while others are not. In the UK, Sophie Gilliat-Ray argues that a clear transition from chapels to prayer rooms has taken place not just in hospitals but more generally (Gilliat-Ray 2005a).

33. For its part, the Association of Professional Chaplaincy explained on its website how to prepare an interfaith meditation space: http://www.professionalchaplains.org/index.aspx?id=1088.

34. Of the seventeen hospitals, seven had one chapel/ meditation room, nine had two spaces, and one had three such spaces.

35. These locations are also revealing in their reflection of issues related to pediatrics, cancer, and often end-of-life issues, for which hospital administrators assume religion and spirituality are most relevant.

36. These plaques imply that many chapel renovations are supported by outside donors rather than exclusively by hospital funds. The plaques naming the donors who supported construction and renovation have themselves often changed from stating that the chapel is "Dedicated to the Glory of God" to recognizing generous support for renovations without mentioning God.

37. Neumann 2006.

38. This was also the case at the Millennium Dome in Greenwich, London (Gilliat-Ray 2005b). One exception to this is a hospital that is creating space where Orthodox Jews will be able to store kosher food and spend time together when a loved one is hospitalized. This hospital already has Shabbat elevators and several related accommodations.

39. See Gerlach-Spriggs, Kaufman, and Warner 1998.

40. This is also the case in the United Kingdom; see Swift 2009.

41. The small Catholic chapel, which holds only a few people, is located on the second floor of the chaplain's offices. Behind a door with a printed image of Jesus hanging on it, the space holds flowers and candles on an altar and a few chairs. Statues of Jesus and of Mary holding the baby Jesus hang on the walls.

42. This chapel is most full during Ash Wednesday services, memorial services for staff, and when the hospital holds remembrance services there.

43. Much of the literature in these and other chapel spaces comes from outside organizations. Prayer materials frequently come from the American Bible Society, and psychological materials from Care Notes.

44. See also Cadge 2009b.

45. See also Gilliat-Ray 2005a.

46. See also Gilliat-Ray 2005a.

47. I focus here on formal religious services held in hospitals. A few chaplains mentioned informal prayer services that staff members organized for themselves. "The surgical intensive care unit has started a little prayer service on their own," one chaplaincy director remarked, "and every morning at 9:00 they have a little prayer service, which I think started as a Christian prayer service, and now there is some thought about making it more of an interfaith service." There is some literature about other, informal, religious gatherings amongst staff (e.g., Messikomer and De Craemer 2002).

48. Gilliat-Ray 2005b.

49. O'Reilly 2000, 70. See also Moczynski 1998.

50. Cadge and Daglian 2008.

51. For more on these spaces, see a project in process at http://www.sed.manchester.ac.uk/architecture/research/mfs/.

52. For a related discussion, see Wolfe 2003.

53. See Bellah et al. 1985; Wuthnow 1998; Besecke 2005.

54. Mohrmann 2009.

CHAPTER 4

1. On a random day during this research, the religious demographics of hospitalized inpatients at Overbrook Hospital were 42% Catholic, 20% Christian (not Orthodox), 14% none, 8% unknown, 7% Jewish, 4% unaffiliated, 4% other, and 2% Christian Orthodox. The percentages do not sum to 100 because of rounding.

2. Two smaller masses were also held in the chapel during the day.

3. See also Horsley 2008.

4. In claiming jurisdiction, Andrew Abbot (1988) argues, "a profession asks society to recognize its cognitive structure through excusive rights; jurisdiction has not only a culture but also a social structure" (59). He understands professions as negotiated in relation to one another, which is likely the case for chaplains, but this was difficult to for me to assess empirically without detailed information about all of the other professionals with whom chaplains work in hospitals. I view chaplaincy as a "profession in process," a professional group with many segments in transition. I see them as in the midst of a long transition from the "subjective" to the "official" labor force (Bucher and Strauss 1961).

5. It is not unusual for this to cause tensions in departments, as CPE supervisors trained to instruct CPE students have not necessarily done the work of the staff chaplains they oversee.

6. Evangelical chaplains who do work in hospitals often work through the Healthcare Chaplaincy Ministry Association (HCMA) at community hospitals rather than the large academic

medical centers I studied here. More information about HCMA is online at http://www
.hcmachaplains.org/. I did not meet any chaplains working through HCMA at the hospitals I
studied.

7. Nationally, many people come to occupations related to religion and spirituality as
second careers. See, for example, http://pulpitandpew.org/first-and-second-career-clergy-
some-comparisons-and-questions.

8. The specific requirements have changed over time. In 2004 they were formally agreed
on and issued in a joint statement by the Association of Professional Chaplains, National Association of Catholic Chaplains, National Association of Jewish Chaplains, and several other
organizations.

9. The director strongly encourages individuals completing a one-year residency in chaplaincy to get certified because certification is increasingly necessary to obtain employment as a
chaplain. Current staff chaplains who are not certified mostly did not plan to get certified, saying they were too old or that too much academic work was required to get the master's degree
needed for certification.

10. Although the formal qualifications for certification are the same across the main professional chaplaincy organizations, at least one director claimed that chaplains certified by each
organization do not have equivalent skills—an argument she used for requiring chaplains from
some but not other religious traditions and backgrounds to be board-certified.

11. See Gustin and Murray 1985.

12. Several of the Catholic nuns and priests I met who were either born abroad or born
in the United States but had spent many years working for the church overseas were strongly
encouraged to take CPE when they arrived in or returned to the United States as part of their
adjustment process.

13. *Oxford English Dictionary*, 1989 edition, s.v. "chaplain."

14. Holifield 1983; Gerkin 1997.

15. See Lee 2002 for more on the distinctions between chaplaincy and spiritual care
services.

16. Two of these seventeen departments also include the word *education* in their titles, and
one is a joint department that also includes social work.

17. About a third of these departments also mention educational programs in their mission
statements, generally referring to the CPE programs they run through their departments.

18. For a recent example of outcomes-based chaplaincy, see Richardson, Owens-Pike, and
Bauck 2011.

19. A chaplain working in this model explained that she first goes into a room looking for
what the patient needs right then. She says she wants to get a sense of who the person is and
what his or her resources are. Then, based on the need, she formulates a sense of what she
would like to achieve and what is realistic for the visit. She also thinks about what she needs to
do during the visit to achieve that goal and then begins the process. This includes an intervention, such as dialogue, prayer, counseling, confrontation, supportive presence, or crisis intervention. At the end of the visit, she evaluates. In a situation in which a patient is very anxious
before surgery, she says that her goal is often to decrease anxiety and provide support. To assess
whether her intervention helped to meet that goal, she might ask the patient near the end of the
visit whether she or he is feeling more relaxed.

20. A few also spoke about the lawsuits they think chaplains help hospitals to avoid, though there is no systematic empirical evidence of this.

21. National chaplaincy leaders may articulate the contributions that chaplains make to hospitals differently. Rather than emphasizing wholeness, presence, and relationships, they are more likely to speak of outcomes-oriented chaplaincy and reference spiritual assessment mechanisms, particular skills that chaplains bring to their work, and more of the intellectual history of chaplaincy as a movement. Additional research is needed.

22. See also Monfalcone 2005.

23. The notion of presence likely originated among liberal Protestants in the early twentieth century, when chaplaincy began to develop as a profession, and has spread since then through the profession and across religious and psychological traditions. Research is needed to carefully trace and document this process.

24. For a description of this history, see Myers-Shirk 2008; Rieff 1966.

25. See discussion of the "theology problem" in DeVries, Berlinger, and Cadge 2008.

26. DeVries, Dingwall, and Orfali 2009.

27. Such skepticism is supported by surveys suggesting that chaplains themselves have a range of views about their profession (Barger et al. 1984; Barrows 1993; Holst 1985).

28. For a discussion of the use of the word *spiritual* in this white paper, see Anderson 2001.

CHAPTER 5

1. National professional chaplaincy organizations are making similar arguments about visibility.

2. The hospitals funds three residency positions, and two are funded through donations to the department. One of the nine full-time staff positions is funded by a physician who wants chaplains directly involved with his patients.

3. Nationally, the fraction of all hospitalized patients who see chaplains is unknown. One study estimates it at between 10% and 30% (Flannelly, Galek, and Handzo 2005). Few directors I interviewed could tell me the fraction of patients at their hospitals who are seen by staff chaplains, students, or volunteers—estimates ranged from 20% to 80%. For information on who requests and who needs spiritual care, see Fitchett, Meyer, and Burton 2000.

4. Andrew Abbott would argue that chaplains are challenged because their work is not abstract enough (Abbott 1993).

5. To do so, chaplains "code switch," or alternate between religious languages, symbols, and sometimes rituals in their work with patients and families, as described in Cadge and Sigalow (under review).

6. For individual accounts by chaplains, see Angrosino 2006; Spirn 2000; Mitchell 1972; Holst and Kurtz 1973; Holst 1985.

7. See VandeCreek and Burton 2001.

8. See Burroughs 1998; Fitchett et al., n.d.; Southard 1963. This is roughly consistent with my findings.

9. See Burroughs 1998; Fitchett et al., n.d.; Southard 1963; Flannelly, Galek et al. 2005; Flannelly, Handzo et al. 2005.

10. See Flannelly, Galek et al. 2005.

11. The Catholic Health Initiative's 2002 study, "Measures of Chaplain Performance and Productivity," for example, encouraged directors of departments to clarify and define roles with chaplains, encourage colleagues from outside the department to help articulate outcomes, and create frameworks that define levels of task complexity for each of five to ten areas for chaplains (Catholic Health Initiative 2002).

12. Some evidence suggests that chaplains from various religious backgrounds spend their time in hospitals differently. Catholic chaplains are more likely to provide sacraments, and Jewish chaplains less likely to pray (VandeCreek and Connell 1991; Dworken 2001). Additional research is needed.

13. Even in ritual work, chaplains find ways to facilitate storytelling. A Jewish chaplain who described himself as very liberal told me how much he dislikes delivering Sabbath candles. In his words, "I saw myself as somebody with all these degrees and all this training, and the last thing I wanted to do was deliver electric candles to people." That said, he has found joy in this work through the opportunities such candles present for storytelling, "Some people tell you their stories about their memories growing up lighting candles, or they tell me that everyone adapts the ritual in their own way."

14. Little empirical work has been conducted about these models. Monfalcone describes the major organizational patterns of hospital chaplaincy in terms of full-time chaplains offering direct service and education for ministers through CPE; full-time chaplains offering direct service; part-time chaplains offering direct service or organizing the services of local ministers; or a volunteer program utilizing local ministers. He says these models are supported financially by the hospital, partially funded by the hospital, or funded by outside agencies (Monfalcone 2005).

15. An additional organizational model not present at any of these hospitals is contract pastoral care, through which chaplains are assigned and supervised in hospitals by outside organizations like the Healthcare Chaplaincy in New York City (VandeCreek et al. 2001; Silberman 1986). Proponents argue that this model provides a sense of continuity in the context of an ever-changing health-care system in the United States, in which chaplaincy departments run by hospitals may face downsizing because of budget constraints.

16. Additional research is needed to understand the role of financial resources in this story. It is possible that the professional and transitional departments had more financial resources, either from the hospital, from funds that previous directors developed, or from the community, that enable them to do more and have a broader reach in their hospitals.

17. Despite this fact, some surveys suggest that hospital chaplains are relatively happy with their work. A small survey of mostly Jewish chaplains found low incidence of compassion fatigue and burnout and a high potential for satisfaction from their work (Taylor et al. 2006).

18. Chaplains have different relationships with various groups of medical professionals. Research generally suggests that chaplains work most regularly with nurses (Flannelly, Weaver, and Handzo 2003; Fogg et al. 2004; Koenig et al. 1991). Accounts of the chaplains' relationships with physicians differ. A recent national study of a cross-section of physicians suggests that most have had contact with a chaplain and been satisfied with that contact (Fitchett et al. 2009). An older national survey of physicians in the American Academy of Family Physicians suggests that support for chaplains may be greater in some medical specialties, with more than 80% of

the sampled physicians reportedly making pastoral care referrals (Daaleman and Frey 1998). In a study at Duke Medical Center, 46% of the physicians sampled had made between one and ten referrals to chaplaincy over a six-month period, and 5% had made more than ten (Koenig et al. 1991). Other reports, including an article by chaplains Mary Martha Thiel and Mary Robinson, suggest that physician-chaplain relations are more challenging because the groups work from different worldviews, chaplains are often intimidated by physicians, physicians see the jobs of chaplains as relatively limited, and physicians often call chaplains late in patient/family situations, making it difficult for them to make significant contributions (Flannelly, Handzo et al. 2005; Thiel and Robinson 1997). Physicians who have not worked with chaplains are also reported to worry that chaplains might not listen to patients' concerns. Chaplains and physicians definitely bring different ideas about the work of chaplains to their work together (Cadge, Calle, and Dillinger 2011).

19. At Overbrook and a few other hospitals, chaplains double-document, meaning they write in patient charts and then write in a separate charting system accessible only to people in the chaplaincy department. The latter helps chaplains to know who has been seen and to gather information from previous chaplain visits. These internal systems also help directors document how staff time is spent. In addition to the question of what the note says, as discussed here, is the question of where in the patient's chart the note should go. At some hospitals it goes on a summary sheet, and in others it goes in the nursing notes or elsewhere.

20. Some departments have detailed systems through which they teach CPE students how, in the words of one director, to "chart without getting into trouble."

21. In the words of chaplain Martha Jacobs, "Empirically minded chaplains have called on their colleagues to do more and better research into our patients' spiritual needs so that we can legitimately claim pastoral care as our area of expertise. These researchers remind us that 'chaplains must decide what questions to ask and how to try to answer them.' If we believe—and we do—that the usual patient satisfaction tools have not adequately reflected our work, then we have a professional responsibility to develop tools that allow our contribution to health-care quality improvement to be assessed accurately and thus give us a basis for further improvement. Compared to other health-care professions, however, we do not undertake enough research and we do not write and publish enough. . . . Part of the work of growing into a profession is bringing other professions into conversations" (Jacobs 2008, 3).

22. Ibid., 1.

23. Ibid.

24. Ibid., 3. This lack of standardization is also evident in the UK (Swift 2009).

25. See Bucher and Strauss 1961. Other sociologists might consider chaplaincy a semi-profession, or a profession that does not rest on a body of knowledge beyond what is known by the general public.

CHAPTER 6

1. For similar historical examples in the Catholic tradition, see Orsi 1996.

2. See Kaufman 2005, 338, n. 2. Also, Zier and colleagues (2008) argue that one in five deaths in the United States occurs in an ICU or shortly following discharge from an ICU.

3. Jacobs, Burns, and Jacobs 2008.

4. "Spirituality in Medical Treatment Survey," November 1998, Yankelovich, Roper Center, University of Connecticut. Although relatively few studies ask, one by Richard Wall and colleagues (2007) conducted in Seattle-area hospitals suggests that families who had a loved one die in intensive care or just after discharge were more satisfied with their experience if a pastor or spiritual advisor was involved during their loved one's last twenty-four hours. See also Robinson et al. 2006.

5. For a discussion of how some medical staff think about religion and spirituality, see Cadge, Ecklund, and Short 2009; Catlin et al. 2010; Catlin et al. 2001; Cadge and Catlin 2006. For commentary about whether critical-care physicians should talk with patients about God and how, see Curtis and Rubenfeld 2001; Morrison and Nelson 2007. Existing studies of ICUs say little about how religion or spirituality are present. Anthropologist Sharon Kaufman (2005) describes standing with chaplains at patients' bedsides. Joan Cassell (2005) briefly describes families waiting for miracles and speaks of chaplains mostly in their absence as staff wait for them to show up. Issues related to religion and spirituality are also present in Carol Heimer and Lisa Staffen's ethnography (1998) in three ways: discussion of conflicts about treatment for a patient who is a Jehovah's Witness (151), in terms of parents who think their infants' fates are in "God's hands" (249), and in mention of a mother going to the hospital chapel to pray for her son after he was injured during treatment.

6. See also Curlin et al. 2005.

7. ICUs emerged in the United States in the second half of the twentieth century. Scholars disagree about when the first ICU opened. One study argues that it was a twenty-eight-bed "special intensive care unit" opened by Dr. J. Murray Beardsley in Rhode Island in 1955 (Schecter et al. 1998, cited in Seymour 2001, 8). NICUs began to open more broadly in the 1960s (Anspach 1993; Guillemin and Holmstrom 1986; Heimer and Staffen 1998). The number of hospitals with ICUs and the number of ICUs in individual hospitals expanded quickly, coinciding with improvements in artificial ventilation, cardiopulmonary resuscitation, and the need for care following increasingly sophisticated surgical procedures (Seymour 2001; Luce and Prendergast 2001; Baker 1996). By the mid-1980s, more than 90% of all hospitals had at least one ICU (Luce and Prendergast 2001; Zussman 1992). Early adult ICUs were staffed by physicians trained in a range of specialties. In 1986 the American Board of Medical Specialties began to certify specialists in critical care, who often worked in ICUs in anesthesiology, internal medicine, pediatrics, and surgery; see Zussman 1992; and http://www.sccm.org/About SCCM/History_of_Critical_Care/Pages/default.aspx). Neonatology, the branch of medicine focused on the care of critically ill newborns, evolved as a medical subdiscipline in the 1960s; the first board certifications occurred in 1976 (Guillemin and Holmstrom 1986). Neonatology is distinct from pediatric critical care in its focus on premature and very young infants. Nurses staffed ICUs from the time they emerged, and nurse-to-patient ratios were lower than on general floors. They continually negotiated their responsibilities with physicians, and a group of nurses first began to meet to form the American Association of Critical Care Nurses in the late 1960s (Fairman and Lynaugh 1998).

8. See Anspach 1993.

9. The organization of ICUs, including their finances, is well described in most of the recent ethnographic studies; see, for example, Guillemin 1984; Guillemin and Holmstrom 1986; Anspach 1993; Zussman 1992; Cassell 2005; Heimer and Staffen 1998.

10. For most of their histories, ICUs have had death rates between 10% and 20% (Luce and Prendergast 2001).

11. On a random day during this research, the religious demographics of patients at City Hospital were as follows: 52% Catholic, 17% other Christian (not Orthodox), 16% no preference, 5% unknown, 4% Jewish, 2% other, 2% deferred the question, and 1% Christian Orthodox.

12. For national data, see Curlin et al. 2005.

13. For more discussion of how religion and spirituality come up informally in social service organizations, see Bender 2003.

14. For more on chaplains in ICUs, see Byekwaso 2000; Sharp 1991.

15. Few could take communion by mouth, so Eucharistic ministers prayed the communion prayers with them instead.

16. For a more journalistic account of how issues related to religion and spirituality come up and are addressed in hospitals, see Salamon 2008a and 2008b.

17. Barr et al. 2000.

18. Relatively little is written about medical staff conducting infant baptisms. In one early and one more recent piece, writers describe how to do a baptism in a hospital and why doing one is important (Burns 1947; Campbell and Campbell 2005).

19. Spirituality and religion also likely influence how nurses do postmortem care; see Wolf 1988.

20. After Vatican II, the Catholic Church transitioned from last rites (formally called Extreme Unction) given to people at the point of death to the Sacrament of the Sick, which can be given anytime a person is ill, not just at the end of life. Many Catholics are not aware of this change, however, routinely calling priests to administer last rites, though they use the Sacrament of the Sick at all of the hospitals I studied.

21. For examples of how physicians do or should facilitate end-of-life rituals, see Lo et al. 2002; Lo et al. 2003; Miles 2001.

22. A few other nurses spoke more supportively about Reiki and therapeutic touch. One nurse described a patient who was "into Reiki, crunchy stuff, you know, . . . therapeutic touch, . . . so you [arrange] to have that done here in the ICU." He explained that he is "more than willing to help" patients find things like this, even though "I don't think it will do anything, but it may make them feel more comfortable." At the other end of the spectrum, another nurse actually performs therapeutic touch on patients when they ask. It uses "energy fields," she explained, "to kind of help them get better. . . . I'll throw it out there. Some people really love it, and other people just don't want to do it."

23. This is also evident in Cadge and Ecklund 2009.

24. See also Cadge and Ecklund 2009.

25. See Kaufman 2005, 104–5 and 124.

26. See Heimer and Staffen 1998.

27. See *Newsweek* Survey, Princeton Survey Research Associates, The Roper Center, the University of Connecticut, April 2000.

28. Braude 1997; Orsi 1996; Cadge and Hammonds 2012; Hammonds and Cadge.

29. This research is especially needed because these findings contradict those of sociologist Don Grant and colleagues. In his survey of another large medical center, he reports that 92% of nurses in an adult ICU (like the MICU) say they are comfortable talking about spiritual-

ity, compared to 83% of nurses in a neonatal unit. Similarly, 67% of nurses in an adult ICU say their fellow nurses are comfortable talking about spirituality, compared to 42% of nurses in an NICU (Grant, O'Neil, and Stephens 2004).

CHAPTER 7

1. Fox 1988.

2. See, for example, Anspach 1993; Heimer and Staffen 1998; Guillemin and Holmstrom 1986; Curtis and Rubenfeld 2001.

3. Zussman 1992, 157.

4. For a description of how staff learn detached concern, see Fox 1957. Many who study detached concern focus on how ICU staff use humor, escape into work, use alternative language, and rationalize things on the job to establish and maintain this emotional balance. See also Cadge and Hammonds 2012.

5. See also Hochschild 1983.

6. I draw very loosely from Susan Leigh Star's discussions of the sociology of the invisible, via Anselm Strauss (Star 1991).

7. See also Kaufman 2005.

8. Linda thinks death causes an especially large amount of suffering and pain in the United States because it is so rarely talked about. In her words, there is "so much work to be done around death and dying" here. Someone a long time ago told her that "Americans think it says on their passport they have the right to live forever. Unfortunately it is not true. And I watch people struggle at such a difficult time."

9. See also the discussion of "cheechee" in Zussman 1992, 111–12, and discussions of suffering in Elpern, Covert, and Kleinpell 2006; Kaufman 2005.

10. Many studies have focused on how staff members cope with these challenges publicly by being emotionally detached, using gallows or black humor, having short memories of individual patients, and focusing on the technical aspects of their work, as described above. Additional studies suggest that education; mental health days; staff support groups; and discussions with coworkers, a chaplain, the patient's family, and their own families help ICU nurses cope with patients' deaths (Downey et al. 1995; Heuer et al. 1996).

11. See, for example, Block 2001; Elpern, Covert, and Kleinpell 2006; Foxall et al. 1990; Guillemin and Holmstrom 1986; Guntupalli and Fromm 1996; Oehler and Davidson 1992; Rashotte, Fothergill-Bourbonnais, and Chamberlain 1997; Asch et al. 1997.

12. These are questions about theodicy, but I did not explicitly frame them as such.

13. For a review of how genetic thinking influences public opinion about a range of outcomes, see Freese and Shostak 2009; Shostak et al. 2009.

14. For recent discussion of the religious lives of scientists, see Ecklund 2010. While Ecklund does not include physicians in her study, some of the issues, such as discussion of those whose faith is closeted, may be similar.

15. As Joan Cassell argues in her study of intensive care, "The American intensivists focused primarily on *curing* disordered bodies; the nurses too were interested in cure, but many took a wider focus as well, on *healing* the sick person" (Cassell 2005, 6; see also Guillemin 1984; Anspach 1993 and 1987; Zupancic and Richardson 2002).

16. Hammonds and Cadge (under review).

17. For more on the continued centrality of women in religious practice, especially informally, see Braude 1997.

18. Zussman 1992.

CHAPTER 8

1. Oak Ridge Hospital is not in the sample of seventeen large, academic hospitals analyzed in this book. I spent time at Oak Ridge as a way of understanding how the chaplaincy department at Overbrook Hospital compares to that of hospitals in its geographic vicinity.

2. For discussion of these relationships, see Kubler-Ross 1969; Glaser and Strauss 1965; Sudnow 1967; Seymour 2001.

3. For discussion of these issues, see Kaufman and Morgan 2005; Anspach 1993; Luce and Prendergast 2001; Curtis and Rubenfeld 2001; Rosenberg 1987; Smith 2005.

4. As reported in Kaufman 2005; see also Gruneir et al. 2007.

5. For discussion of this issue, see Seale and van der Geest 2004; Steinhauser et al. 2000a and 2000b; SUPPORT Principal Investigators 1995.

6. Kaufman and Morgan 2005; Cassell 2005; Timmermans 1999.

7. For discussion of these various responses, see Glaser and Strauss 1965; Christakis 1999; Guillemin and Holmstrom 1986; Block 2001; Curtis and Rubenfeld 2001; Luce and Prendergast 2001; Anspach 1993; Zussman 1992.

8. Kaufman 2000. See also Chapple 2010; Kaufman 2005.

9. Some might wonder why chaplains are not present at births—another intense experience that usually takes place in hospitals. They are absent primarily because births are normally not seen as crises in hospitals; many mothers and babies remain in the hospital for only a short time following the birth, and births do not present the same kinds of institutional challenges for hospitals that death and dying do.

10. Phelps et al. 2009.

11. For example, see Fox 1957. In a recent review, Catherine Exley argues that sociologists have tended to overlook religion/spirituality when studying end-of-life and palliative care (Exley 2004).

12. Glaser and Strauss 1965; Sudnow 1967.

13. As Dan Chambliss argues, death in hospitals is an organizational act for which responsibility is diffused across staff (Chambliss 1996). Based on the data I could gather, this chapter is less about how chaplains divide that responsibility with other staff—a good project for a researcher with more ethnographic access—than about how they describe the roles that they play.

14. Others who describe how death happens in hospitals and how staff respond include Johnson et al. 2000; Steinhauser et al. 2000b; Anspach 1993; Chambliss 1996; Zussman 1992. This work builds on quantitative research showing that hospital staff rank the work chaplains do at the end of life and times of grief as among their most important contributions (Flannelly et al. 2006) and that they spend a lot of their time doing this work (Flannelly et al. 2005; Rodrigues, Rodrigues, and Casey 2000). For descriptions of chaplains working with families at such times, see Mitchell 1972; Kudler 2007.

15. See Hughes 1971; Bosk 1992. Chaplains I spoke with about this chapter were ambivalent about the term *dirty work*; some felt that the work was not "dirty" and should not be described as such (Guillemin and Holmstrom 1986).

16. Glaser and Strauss 1965.

17. This estimate comes from data the chaplaincy department gathered, which showed that 85 people died at the hospital in two of the months I was conducting research.

18. Norwood 2006.

19. See chapter 4 for a more detailed description of the viewing room. For an example in Australia, see Horsley 2008.

20. Glaser and Strauss 1965.

21. Some nurses are also uncomfortable with death. Pat, the director of chaplaincy at Overbrook, told me after reading this chapter that when a patient dies, nurses write in the chart that "the patient has gone to ward x" rather than writing "the patient has gone to the morgue." They never write that a patient died. Occasionally they will say a patient "expired."

22. For efforts to try to change this, see Billings and Block 1997; Block 2001.

23. Glaser and Strauss 1965, 70.

24. Not surprisingly, given discussions of how chaplains frame and do their work in earlier chapters, Meg's comments to the group included no mention of God or other religious or spiritual vocabulary or symbols. The broad frame was psychological and emphasized the need to support one another.

25. Glaser and Strauss 1965, 98–99.

26. Sudnow 1967, 73.

27. One study shows that chaplains significantly help next of kin by providing comfort and support, helping with details, acting as surrogate family members, providing a safety net, and serving as a spiritual figure who eases the transition from life to death (Broccolo and Vande-Creek 2004).

28. For a description of how chaplains are involved in pediatric palliative care, see Fitchett et al. 2011.

29. Chaplains report that social workers—the other people who usually accompany families to morgues or viewing rooms—almost always hate the task.

30. Some chaplains also facilitate memorial services for medical schools related to the bodies used as cadavers in gross anatomy labs. As one chaplaincy director explained, "I work with them [medical students] to give a service together, and usually we have some music and poetry they've written, and we light a candle for each of the people that gave their lives [i.e., their bodies to the lab], and they write cards of appreciation that are collected." See also Belgum 1982.

31. Glaser and Strauss 1965; Sudnow 1967.

32. Kaufman and Morgan 2005; Francis, Kellaher, and Neophytou 2005.

33. See Hughes 1971; Glaser and Strauss 1965; Guillemin and Holmstrom 1986. More recently, the idea of "dirty work" has been used to describe aspects of health-care work; see Gansel, Danet, and Rauscher 2010; Brittain and Shaw 2007; Chiappetta-Swanson 2005.

34. Hughes 1971; Bosk 1992.

35. Some chaplains note that it is the intensity of the work that keeps them in it. In the words of one, "There is no bullshit in this work, because people are real when they're that close

to the issues of life and death." Another explains why he stays in chaplaincy, saying, "I'm very good in crisis. I'm awful in chronic care. I can't sustain the emotional involvement." That said, chaplains do struggle with burnout (Taylor et al. 2006; Weaver et al. 2002).

36. See also Dillinger 2008.

37. Coombs and Goldman 1973; Fox 1988; Thorson 1993.

38. For more on how medical staff do this, see Coombs and Goldman 1973; Downey et al. 1995; Fox 1988 and 1957.

39. Some physicians have similar rituals, though few share them publicly; see, for example, Treadway 2007.

40. Shem 1978.

41. Ibid., 58.

42. Ibid., 312–14.

43. See Berlinger 2008a. It is also possible that as palliative care develops as a specialty, the work concerning death is becoming less "dirty" than it was in the past.

CHAPTER 9

1. More nurses in the NICU than in the MICU spoke about miracles. The social worker in the MICU said, "Maybe people on the grown-up side are less willing to admit they're hoping for a miracle."

2. Broader perspectives on what miracles are and how they are understood are evident across the disciplines. See Sulmasy 2007; Widera et al. 2011; Duffin 2009.

3. See Chaves 2010.

4. Bender 2010, 182.

5. Norwood 2006, 21.

6. Studies show that physicians tend to rate the work of chaplains as less important than do nurses and social workers. Directors of medicine, nursing, and social services find the work chaplains do concerning death and grief, prayer, and emotional support to be very to extremely important (Flannelly et al. 2005).

7. This is also the case in the UK, where the term *spirituality* has also become popular in health care because of what Christopher Swift calls its "plasticity" and "its refusal of external authority" (Swift 2009, chap. 6; see also Orton 2008).

8. These three approaches are borrowed from Bender 2007. The spiritual but not religious frame is most evident in Bellah et al. 1985.

9. Bender 2007, 7. There are, of course, ways of understanding spirituality in addition to these three. See for example Besecke 2001; Besecke 2005.

10. Bender 2007, 7.

11. All conceptions of spirituality have some history—see, for example, Schmidt 2005—though it is not unusual for people utilizing such concepts to "forget" their history (Bender 2010).

12. Grant, O'Neil, and Stephens 2004, 270.

13. See also Abu-Ras and Laird 2011. Such misunderstandings between chaplains, patients, and families are further evident in Piderman et al. 2008; Garces-Foley 2006.

14. Berlinger 2004, 687.

15. Curlin, Roach, et al. 2005b.

16. For discussion of these various understandings, see Lemmer 2002; Grant, O'Neil, and Stephens 2004; Meyer 2003; Narayanasamy and Owens 2001.

17. For a similar argument for why researchers focused on prayer in intercessory studies, see Cadge 2009b.

18. Asking such questions requires social scientists to move away from using organized religion as a reference point and to be open to what Don Grant describes as the "twin forces of sacralization and secularization" in secular organizations (Grant, O'Neil, and Stephens 2004, 281). See also Demerath et al. 1998; Ammerman 2007; Bender et al. 2013; Cadge, Levitt, and Smilde 2011; Taylor 2007; Warner, Vanantwerpen, and Calhoun 2010.

19. For information on church-state issues, see Hammond 1998; Smith 2003. While the first Establishment case heard by the U.S. Supreme Court pertained to a hospital, few subsequent cases have. For recent information on a state-level case pertaining to chaplaincy in the Veterans Administration Hospitals, see Sullivan 2009. The national context clearly shapes how religion and spirituality are negotiated in U.S. organizations, as evident in the comparison between prisons in the United States and parts of Great Britain in Beckford and Gilliat 1998; see also Hicks 2008.

20. Sullivan 2009, 230.

21. The policy implications of research about religion and health are also unclear. Few chaplains or health-care administrators are comfortable having health-care providers prescribe or prohibit religious or spiritual beliefs or practices that research studies have found to be conducive or detrimental to people's health. For discussion of these ethical issues, see Berlinger 2004.

22. Balboni et al. 2007; Balboni et al. 2009; Phelps et al. 2009.

23. That this remains an option rather than a requirement for patients is important; not all patients want such support. For a description of one patient who did not, see Berlinger 2004, 692.

24. See for example Graves, Shue, and Arnold 2002.

25. At one hospital, staff members involved in CPE were asked to give CPE students feedback about their work to help them learn how to fit better within the health-care hierarchy. Massachusetts General Hospital took the additional step of starting a CPE program for health-care providers to increase their skills and awareness of religious and spiritual issues and encourage them to share that awareness with colleagues in their units. For more information, see Todres, Catlin, and Thiel 2005; Rimer 2005.

26. Hall, Koenig, and Meador 2004.

27. Tanenbaum Center 2009.

28. In a study of hospital chaplaincy in the United Kingdom, Christopher Swift (2009) found that many Spiritual Care Departments were not providing services that accurately reflected their names.

29. Berlinger 2004, 685–86.

30. See, for example, Clark, Drain, and Malone 2003; Iler, Obershain, and Camac 2001; Bay et al. 2008; Gibbons, Thomas, and VandeCreek 1991; VandeCreek 2003.

31. This argument is also made in VandeCreek 1999.

32. Mohrmann 2009, 6.

33. Excellent examples of innovation in chaplaincy practice are regularly published in *Plain Views*, available online at http://plainviews.healthcarechaplaincy.org/. Thinking of themselves as problem solvers runs against the grain of some chaplains. Many are taught in CPE to be present with patients wherever they are and not to try to solve their problems. As one chaplain told me emphatically in an interview, "As a chaplain, my duty is *not* to fix a problem. The duty is to help people cope with their situations."

34. See Fitchett, Thomason, and Lyndes 2008. Mohrmann 2009 discusses how ways of evaluating CPE students might help chaplains think about measuring and evaluating their own work.

35. See, for example, VandeCreek 2004; VandeCreek et al. 1991. For evidence that a general relationship may exist between religion and patient satisfaction with health care, see Benjamins 2006; Benjamins and Brown 2004.

36. As in the past, some hospitals continue to run CPE programs. The majority of their students go on to work outside of hospitals. Such programs can exist alongside patient-focused chaplaincy care, but when students in these programs are the main people providing chaplaincy care, the priorities of the patients and the students are mixed. Medical students are allowed to take blood pressures and do other simple tasks in academic hospitals when they are well supervised and part of medical teams. CPE students are the equivalent of medical students in chaplaincy departments but often work more individually with patients and not as part of well-supervised teams beyond their CPE supervisor. Just as chaplains would probably not want medical students responsible for their health care, they might more carefully consider how much CPE students can do in one-on-one conversations with patients.

37. National chaplaincy leaders increasingly encourage chaplains to become research literate or conduct such research themselves. I encourage chaplains to become research literate and join collaborative research teams but not do significant amounts of research on their own. Medical and nursing communities will regard research about chaplains as more credible if it is conducted by people trained in standard scientific and social scientific methods who publish their findings in well-known medical and nursing journals. The chaplaincy journals where many chaplains publish their research are not widely read in medical and nursing communities.

38. See also DeVries, Berlinger, and Cadge 2008. For discussion of a collaborative model in which health-care professionals and chaplains work together to provide care, see Sulmasy 2006.

39. Endorsement generally must come from a faith group listed in the Yearbook of American and Canadian Churches or approved by the National Conference of Ministry to the Armed Forces. The point is that a particular faith tradition must endorse those who want to become board-certified, even though many will go on to become interfaith chaplains. See, for example, http://www.professionalchaplains.org/BCCI/index.aspx?id=1862.

40. For details about this model, see http://www.chaplaincyinstitute.org/.

41. These standards are available online at http://www.spiritualcarecollaborative.org/docs /common-standards-professional-chaplaincy.pdf. Leaders often assume that students learn about other traditions as part of their graduate training, but they might investigate whether this

is true while expanding students' knowledge about spiritualities and how people have experienced spirituality in the United States historically and in the present.

42. See VandeCreek 1999.

43. I borrow the phrase "tinkering tradespersons" from Charles Bosk's description of genetic counselors (Bosk 1992).

44. See DeVries, Berlinger, and Cadge 2008; Dingwall 2008. See also the description in Dalzell 1998 of an HMO where trained volunteers provides spiritual assistance to members.

45. See also the discussion of licensing in *PlainViews* that began in vol. 6, no. 9 in 2009, available online at http://plainviews.healthcarechaplaincy.org/.

46. Garces-Foley makes this argument regarding hospice organizations (2006, 130). I contend that it is applicable more broadly.

APPENDIX

1. For overview articles see Koenig, McCullough, and Larson 2001; Chatters 2000; Chatters, Levin, and Ellison 1998; Ellison and Levin 1998; Sherkat and Ellison 1999; George et al. 2000; Miller and Thoresen 2003; Weaver and Ellison 2004; Cadge 2009a; Cadge and Fair 2010.

2. I did find some discussion of the ways religious organizations have sponsored biomedical health programs (e.g., through blood drives, blood-pressure clinics, parish nurse programs, etc.). See, for example, the section entitled "Public Health Practice in Faith-Based Settings" in Chatters 2000, 352.

3. See Anspach 1993; Heimer and Staffen 1998; Zussman 1992; Bosk 1992; Sudnow 1967; Glaser and Strauss 1965. Some medical anthropologists pay attention to the sacred dimensions of health-care organizations but more as devices they use as analytic frames than as the subject of study in Western contexts. See, for example, van der Geest 2005. This use of traditionally religious concepts and languages as analytic frames that ignore their specific religious meanings is also evident among medical sociologists; see, for example, Nicholas Christakis's discussion of "prophecy" (Christakis 1999, 155–59) or the title Charles Bosk gave to his book, *All God's Mistakes* (Bosk 1992); see also van der Geest and Finkler 2004.

4. These journals include the *Journal of Pastoral Care and Counseling* and *the Journal of Healthcare Chaplaincy*, both of which are indexed in PubMed, which does not provide the full text of articles to individuals using PubMed through major research libraries.

5. These challenges are different for journalists who write about hospitals and negotiate their access to them in different ways. See, for example, Fadiman 1998; Salamon 2008a. For a history of hospital ethnography, see Long, Hunter, and van der Geest 2008. Negotiated interactive observation is another approach; see Wind 2008; Casper 1997.

6. See Bosk 1992, chap. 1.

7. See Kaufman 2005. In a few other examples, researchers have gotten permission to conduct ethnographic research about chaplains or CPE students in hospitals—see Norwood 2006; Will 2009; Lee 2002.

8. My status as a newcomer to this field made my task more difficult because I could not

work through existing networks and colleagues, as Sharon Kauffman did, for example, to obtain access to field sites (Kaufman 2005).

9. My approach was similar to that of the organizational ethnographers described by Alan Wolfe (2003), who are informed by new institutionalism and aim to look "behind the generalizations and abstractions of institutional theory to examine how institutions operate in practice" (see Fine 1996, 2; see also Evans 2003; Gorski and Altinordu 2008; Smith 2003).

10. In all the time I shadowed medical staff while working on this book, I wore street clothes. When patients were present, and I was occasionally introduced, it was as a student—a common figure in teaching hospitals. Very occasionally, a chaplain introduced me to a patient or family member as a friend.

11. Technically, the hospital did not see what I was proposing as "research" because it did not involve an "intervention," but by filing the proposal with the Institutional Review Board and having them grant me an exemption, I would have been permitted to enter the hospital for one month.

12. This was ironic, since I had not met any nurses or social workers at this hospital yet and was open to collaboration, given the historically positive relations between them and sociologists in medical institutions.

13. This follows the examples of sociologists Charles Bosk (1979 and 1992) and Nicholas Christakis (1999), both of whom only included the voices of patients and families through observation and interviews with medical staff. As Bosk explains, "The last structured silence in my notes involves the patient's perspective. I did not try to enter the patient's perspective as completely as I did with physicians. . . . It was simply too terrifying for me to try to place myself in their shoes (1992, 168–69).

14. The average hospital in my sample had seven full-time chaplains. The average ratio was one chaplain for every 133 beds at these hospitals. For national ratios, see VandeCreek et al. 2001.

15. Most were formed by one or more mergers of different hospitals and medical organizations.

16. Some of these departments were called Departments of Pastoral Care or Spiritual Care Services, as explained in chapter 4. I describe them as Chaplaincy Departments here for ease of reference.

17. For more on the experience of CPE, see Will 2009.

18. Specifically, Jennifer visited two of these hospitals and interviewed nine people, following the standard interview guides.

19. We also gathered information about prayer books. I have analyzed one in detail (Cadge and Daglian 2008).

20. Services were typically announced on department web pages or on signs close to the chapel.

21. A few oncology chaplains have offices in oncology units or recently constructed oncology buildings. Their offices are close to where patients are cared for, and some meet with patients in their offices. At one hospital, the chaplain's office was one of the first offices you saw when entering the oncology clinic.

22. Chaplains' offices also often had telling images on the walls (e.g., paintings of Jesus, drawings or photographs of clouds, lighthouses, and other nature imagery).

23. Two would only speak briefly by telephone. At one hospital, we interviewed a staff chaplain who described himself as a representative for the director, who was unavailable for an extended period. That person is counted here as a staff chaplain.

24. Slightly less than two-thirds of American hospitals have had chaplaincy services since the early 1980s, but the demographics of those chaplains (whether they are volunteers or are paid by the hospital and other factors) are unknown (Cadge, Freese, and Christakis 2008; Flannelly, Handzo, and Weaver 2004).

25. Pat's graduate training included courses in research, which likely made the research project I described more understandable to her.

26. The director and two staff chaplains are among these thirty-two and are also counted among the thirty-nine people interviewed in the national sample.

27. Reflecting the status of different groups in the hospital, my colleague formally asked the medical and nursing directors of each unit to allow me to conduct this research. E-mails were sent to the director of respiratory therapy asking both for permission and for the names of respiratory therapists who worked in these units. I approached the social workers and chaplains directly. My colleague did not feel it necessary to seek permission from the directors of their departments.

28. Because I was not an employee of this hospital, I was not able to submit an application to their Institutional Review Board as a primary investigator. The physician colleague who negotiated my access served as the primary investigator, and I was a co-primary investigator. Without this colleague, my entry as well as formal permission to do research at this hospital would not have been possible.

29. This time spent shadowing was also about getting access and permission beyond the formal by getting to know staff members and assessing whether they might be interested in talking with me (see Heimer and Staffen 1998). The directors of nursing in each unit were clear that my shadowing and interviews could not get in the way of nurses' work so I was also assessing, in the time I spent shadowing, the best way to ask questions while staying out of the way.

30. See Heimer and Staffen 1998.

31. Almost everyone picked the coffee gift certificate.

32. It also specified that I would not share any identifying information from interviews with anyone else who signed the recruitment letter.

33. This is similar to the approach described in Anspach 1993.

34. Interviews with staff in ICUs were much shorter, overall, than interviews with chaplains, reflecting both how much time each group had in their daily work schedule for interviews and the different norms of conversation that lead physicians and nurses to get right to the point and chaplains to take a less linear path.

35. Cadge and Hammonds 2012; Hammonds and Cadge (under review).

36. For an overview of grounded theory, see Strauss and Corbin 1990.

37. Tolich 2004.

REFERENCES

Abbott, Andrew. 1988. *The System of Professions: An Essay on the Division of Expert Labor*. Chicago: University of Chicago Press.

———. 1993. "The Sociology of Work and Occupations." *Annual Review of Sociology* 19:187–209.

Abdel-Aziz, E., B. N. Arch, and H. Al-Taher. 2004. "The Influence of Religious Beliefs on General Practitioners' Attitudes Towards Termination of Pregnancy—A Pilot Study." *Journal of Obstetrics and Gynaecology* 24, no. 5:557–61.

Abu-Ras, Wahiba, and Lance Laird. 2011. "How Muslim and Non-Muslim Chaplains Serve Muslim Patients? Does the Interfaith Chaplaincy Model Have Room for Muslims' Experiences?" *Journal of Religion and Health* 50, no. 1:46–61.

Adams, Annmarie. 2008. *Medicine by Design: The Architect and the Modern Hospital, 1893–1943*. Minneapolis: University of Minnesota Press.

Aist, Clark S. 1996. "The History of the Association of Mental Health Clergy." *Caregiver Journal* 12, no. 1:35–44.

Aiyer, Aryan N., George Ruiz, Allegra Steinman, and Gloria Y. F. Ho. 1999. "Influence of Physician Attitudes on Willingness to Perform Abortion." *Obstetrics and Gynecology* 93, no. 4:576–80.

Allport, Gordon W. 1966. "The Spirit of Richard Clarke Cabot." *Journal of Pastoral Care* 20, no. 2:102–4.

American Association of Medical Colleges. 1999. *Report III. Contemporary Issues in Medicine: Communication in Medicine. Medical School Objectives Project*. Washington, DC: American Association of Medical Colleges.

American Hospital Association. 1970. *Manual on Hospital Chaplaincy*. Chicago: American Hospital Association.

Ammerman, Nancy. 2007. *Everyday Religion: Observing Modern Religious Lives*. New York: Oxford University Press.

Anandarajah, Gowri, and Ellen Hight. 2001. "Spirituality and Medical Practice: Using the HOPE Questions As a Practical Tool for Spiritual Assessment." *American Family Physician* 63, no. 1:81–89.

Anderson, Herbert. 2001. "Spiritual Care: The Power of an Adjective." *Journal of Pastoral Care* 55, no. 3:233–37.

Anderson, James A. 1987. "Dialogue 88: It's More Than a Lot of Talk." *Journal of Pastoral Care* 41, no. 1:55–57.

Angrosino, Michael. 2006. *Blessed with Enough Foolishness: Pastoral Care in a Modern Hospital*. West Conshohocken: Infinity.

Anspach, Renee R. 1987. "Prognostic Conflict in Life and Death Decisions: The Organization as an Ecology of Knowledge." *Journal of Health and Social Behavior* 28, no. 3:215–31.

———. 1993. *Deciding Who Lives: Fateful Choices in the Intensive-Care Nursery*. Berkeley and Los Angeles: University of California Press.

Armbruster, Christy A., John T. Chibnall, and Sarah Legett. 2003. "Pediatrician Beliefs about Spirituality and Religion in Medicine: Associations with Clinical Practice." *Pediatrics* 111, no. 3:227–35.

Asch, David A., Judy A. Shea, Kathryn M. Jedrziewski, and Charles L. Bosk. 1997. "The Limits of Suffering: Critical Care Nurses' Views of Hospital Care at the End of Life." *Social Science and Medicine* 45, no. 11:1661–68.

Asquith, Glenn H. Jr. 1992. *Vision from a Little Known Country: A Boisen Reader*. Decatur, GA: Journal of Pastoral Care Publications.

Autton, Norman. 1963. "Pastoral Clinical Training in a London Teaching Hospital." *Journal of Pastoral Care* 17, no. 2:106–8.

———. 1969. *Pastoral Care in Hospitals*. London: Free Church Federal Council Hospital Chaplaincy Board.

Baker, Jeffrey P. 1996. *The Machine in the Nursery: Incubator Technology and the Origins of Newborn Intensive Care*. Baltimore, MD: Johns Hopkins University Press.

Balboni, Tracy A., Lauren C. Vanderwerker, Susan D. Block, M. E. Paulk, Christopher S. Lathan, John R. Peteet, and Holly G. Prigerson. 2007. "Religious and Spiritual Support among Advanced Cancer Patients and Associations with End-of-Life Treatment Preferences and Quality of Life." *Journal of Clinical Oncology* 25, no. 5:555–60.

———, Mary E. Paulk, Michael J. Balboni, Andrea C. Phelps, Elizabeth T. Loggers, Alexi A. Wright, Susan D. Block, Eldrin F. Lewis, John R. Peteet, and Holly G. Prigerson. 2009. "Provision of Spiritual Care to Patients with Advanced Cancer: Associations with Medical Care and Quality of Life Near Death." *Journal of Clinical Oncology* 28, no. 3:445–54.

Barger, George W., Brian Austil, John Holbrook, and John Newton. 1984. "The Institutional Chaplain: Constructing a Role Definition." *Journal of Pastoral Care* 38, no. 3:176–86.

Barnes, Linda L. 2006. "A Medical School Curriculum on Religion and Healing." In *Teaching Religion and Healing*, ed. Linda L. Barnes and Ines M. Talamantez, 307–25. New York: Oxford University Press.

Barr, Joseph, Matitiahu Berkovitch, Hagit Matras, Eran Kocer, Revital Greenberg, and Gideon Eshel. 2000. "Talismans and Amulets in the Pediatric Intensive Care Unit: Legendary Powers in Contemporary Medicine." *Israel Medical Association Journal* 2 (April): 278–81.

Barrows, David C. 1993. "'A Whole Different Thing.' The Hospital Chaplaincy: The Emergence of the Occupation and the Work of the Chaplain." PhD diss., University of California, San Francisco.

Bassett, S. D. 1976. *Public Religious Services in the Hospital*. Springfield, IL: Charles C Thomas.

Bay, Paul S., Daniel Beckman, James Trippi, Richard Gunderman, and Colin Terry. 2008. "The Effect of Pastoral Care Services on Anxiety, Depression, Hope, Religious Coping, and Religious Problem Solving Styles: A Randomized Controlled Study." *Journal of Religion and Health* 47, no. 1:57–69.

Beckford, James, and Sophie Gilliat. 1998. *Religion in Prison: Equal Rites in a Multi-Faith Society*. New York: Cambridge University Press.

Belgum, David R. 1982. "Memorial Service as Part of the Deeded Body Program." *Journal of Pastoral Care* 36, no. 1:30–35.

Bellah, Robert, Richard Masden, William M. Sullivan, Ann Swidler, and Steven M. Tipton. 1985. *Habits of the Heart: Individualism and Commitment in American Life*. Berkeley and Los Angeles: University of California Press.

Bender, Courtney. 2003. *Heaven's Kitchen: Living Religion at God's Love We Deliver*. Chicago: University of Chicago Press.

———. 2007. "Religion and Spirituality: History, Discourse, Measurement." *SSRC Forum*. Online at http://religion.ssrc.org/reforum/Bender.pdf.

———. 2010. *The New Metaphysicals: Spirituality and the American Religious Imagination*. Chicago: University of Chicago Press.

———, Wendy Cadge, Peggy Levitt, and David Smilde, eds. 2013. *Religion on the Edge: De-centering and Re-centering the Sociology of Religion*. New York: Oxford University Press.

Benjamins, Maureen R. 2006. "Does Religion Influence Patient Satisfaction?" *American Journal of Health and Behavior* 30, no. 1:85–91.

———, and Carolyn Brown. 2004. "Religion and Preventative Health Care Utilization among the Elderly." *Social Science and Medicine* 58, no. 1:109–18.

Berlinger, Nancy. 2004. "Spirituality and Medicine: Idiot-Proofing the Discourse." *Journal of Medicine and Philosophy* 29, no. 6:681–95.

———. 2008a. "The Nature of Chaplaincy and the Goals of QI: Patient-Centered Care as Professional Responsibility." *Hastings Center Report* 38, no. 6:30–33.

———. 2008b. "From Julius Varwig to Julie Dupree: Professionalizing Hospital Chaplains." *Bioethics Forum*. Available online at http://www.thehastingscenter.org/bioethicsforum/post.aspx?id=704.

Besecke, Kelly. 2001. "Speaking of Meaning in Modernity: Reflexive Spirituality as a Cultural Resource." *Sociology of Religion* 62, no. 3:365–81.

———. 2005. "Seeing Invisible Religion: Religion as a Societal Conversation about Transcendent Meaning." *Sociological Theory* 23, no. 2:179–96.

Billings, J. Andrew. 2004. "Care of Dying Patients and Their Families," in *Cecil Textbook of Medicine*, 22nd ed., ed. Lee Goldman and Dennis Ausiello, 1–13. Philadelphia, PA: Saunders.

———, and Susan D. Block. 1997. "Palliative Care in Undergraduate Medical Education: Status Report and Future Directions." *Journal of the American Medical Association* 278, no. 9:733–38.

Block, Susan D. 2001. "Helping the Clinician Cope with Death in the ICU." In Curtis and Rubenfeld 2001, 183–91.

Boisen, Anton T. 1960. *Out of the Depths: An Autobiographical Study of Mental Disorders and Religious Experience*. New York: Harper & Row.

Bosk, Charles. 1979. *Forgive and Remember: Managing Medical Failure*. Chicago: University of Chicago Press.

———. 1992. *All God's Mistakes: Genetic Counseling in a Pediatric Hospital*. Chicago: University of Chicago Press.

———. 2008. *What Would You Do? Juggling Bioethics and Ethnography*. Chicago: University of Chicago Press.

Braude, Ann. 1997. "Women's History Is American Religious History." In *Retelling U.S. Religious History*, ed. Thomas A. Tweed, 87–107. Berkeley and Los Angeles: University of California Press.

Brittain, John N., and Julie Boozer. 1987. "Spiritual Care: Integration into a Collegiate Nursing Curriculum." *Journal of Nursing Education* 26, no. 4:155–60.

Brittain, Katherine, and Chris Shaw. 2007. "The Social Consequences of Living with and Dealing with Incontinence: A Carer's Perspective." *Social Science and Medicine* 65, no. 6:1274–83.

Broccolo, Gerard T., and Larry VandeCreek. 2004. "How Are Health Care Chaplains Helpful to Bereaved Family Members? Telephone Survey Results." *Journal of Pastoral Care and Counseling* 58, nos. 1–2:31–39.

Bucher, Rue, and Anselm Strauss. 1961. "Professions in Process." *American Journal of Sociology* 66, no. 4:325–34.

Burns, James H. 1947. "Emergency Baptism, with Special Reference to Infants." *Journal of Pastoral Care* 1, no. 2:19–20.

———. 1949. "A Chaplaincy Program in the General Hospital." *Journal of Pastoral Care* 3, nos. 3–4:26–29.

Burroughs, Colleen. 1998. "Peace Be Still." *Journal of Pastoral Care* 52, no. 3:289–90.

Byekwaso, Henry. 2000. "Becoming a Chaplain on the ICU." *Health Progress* 81, no. 3:71–72.

Byrd, Julian L., and Arne K. Jessen. 1988. "The College of Chaplains of the American Protestant Health Association." *Journal of Pastoral Care* 42, no. 3:228–36.

Cabot, Richard, and Russell L. Dicks. 1936. *The Art of Ministering to the Sick*. New York: Macmillan.

Cadge, Wendy. 2009a. "Religion, Spirituality and Health: An Institutional Approach." In *Oxford Handbook of the Sociology of Religion*, ed. Peter Clarke, 836–56. Oxford: Oxford University Press.

———. 2009b. "Saying Your Prayers, Constructing Your Religions: Medical Studies of Intercessory Prayer." *Journal of Religion* 89:299–327.

———, Katherine Calle, and Jennifer Dillinger. 2011. "What Do Chaplains Contribute to Large Academic Hospitals? The Perspectives of Pediatric Physicians and Chaplains." *Journal of Religion and Health* 50, no. 2:300–312.

———, and Elizabeth A. Catlin. 2006. "Making Sense of Suffering and Death: How Health Care Providers Construct Meanings in a Neonatal Intensive Care Unit." *Journal of Religion and Health* 45, no. 2:248–63.

———, and M. Daglian. 2008. "Blessings, Strength, and Guidance: Prayer Frames in a Hospital Prayer Book." *Poetics* 36, nos. 5–6:358–73.

———, and Elaine H. Ecklund. 2009. "Prayers in the Clinic: How Pediatric Physicians Respond." *Southern Medical Journal* 102, no. 12:1218–21.

———, Elaine H. Ecklund, and Nicholas Short. 2009. "Religion and Spirituality: A Barrier and a Bridge in the Everyday Professional Work of Pediatric Physicians." *Social Problems* 56, no. 4:702–21.

———, and Brian Fair. 2010. "Religion, Spirituality, Health and Medicine: Sociological Intersections." In *Handbook of Medical Sociology*, ed. Chloe Byrd, Allan Fremont, Stefan Timmermans, and Peter Conrad, 341–62. Nashville, TN: Vanderbilt University Press.

———, Jeremy Freese, and Nicholas Christakis. 2008. "The Provision of Hospital Chaplaincy in the United States: A National Overview." *Southern Medical Journal* 101, no. 6:626–30.

———, and Clare Hammonds. 2012. "Reconsidering Detached Concern: The Case of Intensive Care Nurses." *Perspectives in Biology and Medicine* 65, no. 2: 266–82.

———, Peggy Levitt, and David Smilde. 2011. "De-Centering and Re-Centering: Rethinking Concepts and Methods in the Sociological Study of Religion." *Journal for the Scientific Study of Religion* 50, no. 3:437–49.

———, and Emily Sigalow. 2012. "Strategies for Negotiating Religious Diversity: The Case of Overbrook Hospital."

Calabria, Michael D., and Janet A. Macrae. 1994. *Suggestions for Thought by Florence Nightingale*. Philadelphia: University of Pennsylvania Press.

Campbell, Anne, and Duncan Campbell. 2005. "Emergency Baptism by Health Professionals." *Paediatric Nursing* 17, no. 2:39–42.

Casper, Monica. 1997. "Feminist Politics and Fetal Surgery: Adventures of a Research Cowgirl on the Reproductive Frontier." *Feminist Studies* 23, no. 2:233–62.

Cassell, Joan. 2005. *Life and Death in Intensive Care*. Philadelphia, PA: Temple University Press.

Catholic Health Initiative. 2002. "Measures of Chaplain Performance and Productivity." Denver: Catholic Health Initiatives Task Force.

Catlin, Elizabeth, Wendy Cadge, and Elaine H. Ecklund. 2008. "The Religious Identities, Beliefs, and Practices of Academic Pediatricians in the United States." *Academic Medicine* 83, no. 12:1146–52.

———, Jeanne H. Guillemin, Julie M. Freedman, Mary Martha Thiel, Sandra McLaughlin, Cheryl D. Stults, and Marvin L. Wang. 2010. "HIV Clinic Caregivers' Spiritual and Religious Attitudes and Behaviors." *Health* 2, no. 7:796–803.

———, Jeanne H. Guillemin, Mary M. Thiel, Shelia Hammond, Marvin Wang, and James O'Donnell. 2001. "Spiritual and Religious Components of Patient Care in the Neonatal

Intensive Care Unit: Sacred Themes in a Secular Setting." *Journal of Perinatology* 21, no.7:426–30.

Cavendish, Roberta, Barbara K. Luise, Donna Russo, Claudia Mitzeliotis, Maria Bauer, Mary A. M. Bajo, Carmen Calvino, Karen Horne, and Judith Medefindt. 2004. "Spiritual Perspectives of Nurses in the United States Relevant for Education and Practice." *Western Journal of Nursing Research* 26, no. 2:196–212.

Chambers, Nancy, and J. Randall Curtis. 2001. "The Interface of Technology and Spirituality in the ICU." In Curtis and Rubenfeld 2001, 193–205.

Chambliss, Daniel F. 1996. *Beyond Caring: Hospitals, Nurses, and the Social Organization of Ethics*. Chicago: University of Chicago Press.

Chapple, Helen S. 2010. *No Place for Dying: Hospitals and the Ideology of Rescue*. Walnut Creek, CA: Left Coast Press.

Chatters, Linda M. 2000. "Religion and Health: Public Health Research and Practice." *Annual Review of Public Health* 21:335–67.

———, Jeffrey S. Levin, and Christopher G. Ellison. 1998. "Public Health and Health Education in Faith Communities." *Health Education and Behavior* 25, no. 6:689–99.

Chaves, Mark. 2010. "SSSR Presidential Address. Rain Dances in the Dry Season: Overcoming the Religious Congruence Fallacy." *Journal for the Scientific Study of Religion* 49, no. 1:1–14.

Chiappetta-Swanson, Catherine. 2005. "Dignity and Dirty Work: Nurses' Experiences in Managing Genetic Termination for Fetal Anomaly." *Qualitative Sociology* 28, no. 1:93–116.

Chibnall, John T., and Christy A. Brooks. 2001. "Religion in the Clinic: The Role of Physician Beliefs." *Southern Medical Journal* 94, no. 4:374–79.

Chidester, David, and Edward T. Linenthal. 1995. *American Sacred Space*. Bloomington: Indiana University Press.

Christakis, Nicholas. 1999. *Death Foretold: Prophecy and Prognosis in Medical Care*. Chicago: University of Chicago Press.

———, and David A. Asch. 1995. "Physician Characteristics Associated with Decisions to Withdraw Life Support." *American Journal of Public Health* 85, no. 3:367–72.

Clark, Paul A., Maxwell Drain, and Mary P. Malone. 2003. "Addressing Patients' Emotional and Spiritual Needs." *Joint Commission Journal on Quality and Safety* 29, no. 12:659–70.

Coombs, Robert H., and Lawrence J. Goldman. 1973. "Maintenance and Discontinuity of Coping Mechanisms in an Intensive Care Unit." *Social Problems* 20, no. 3:342–55.

Crane, Diana. 1975. *The Sanctity of Social Life: Physicians' Treatment of Critically Ill Patients*. New York: Russell Sage Foundation.

Creager, Ellen. 27 May 2000. "Prayer Rooms in Hospitals Acknowledge Power of Faith." *Dayton Daily News*, city ed., May 27, 4C.

Curlin, Farr A., Marshall H. Chin, Sarah A. Sellergren, Chad J. Roach, and John D. Lantos. 2006. "The Association of Physicians' Religious Characteristics with Their Attitudes and Self-Reported Behaviors Regarding Religion and Spirituality in the Clinical Encounter." *Medical Care* 44, no. 5:446–53.

———, John D. Lantos, Chad J. Roach, Sarah A. Sellergren, and Marshall H. Chin. 2005.

"Religious Characteristics of U.S. Physicians: A National Survey." *Journal of General Internal Medicine* 20, no. 7:629–34.

———, Ryan E. Lawrence, Marshall H. Chin, and John D. Lantos. 2007. "Religion, Conscience, and Controversial Clinical Practices." *New England Journal of Medicine* 356, no. 6:593–600.

———, Chad J. Roach, Rita Gorawara-Bhat, John D. Lantos, and Marshall H. Chin. 2005a. "When Patients Choose Faith Over Medicine: Physician Perspectives on Religiously Related Conflict in the Medical Encounter." *Archives of Internal Medicine* 165, no. 1:88–91.

———. 2005b. "How Are Religion and Spirituality Related to Health? A Study of Physicians' Perspectives." *Southern Medical Journal* 98, no. 8:761–66.

Curtis, J. R., and Gordon D. Rubenfeld. 2001. *Managing Death in the ICU: The Transition from Cure to Comfort.* New York: Oxford University Press.

Daaleman, Timothy P., and Bruce Frey. 1998. "Prevalence and Patterns of Physician Referral to Clergy and Pastoral Care." *Archives of Family Medicine* 7, no. 6:548–53.

———, and Donald E. Jr. Nease. 1994. "Patient Attitudes Regarding Physician Inquiry into Spiritual and Religious Issues." *Journal of Family Practice* 39, no. 6:564–68.

Dalzell, Michael. 1998. "Pastoral Service Renews Meaning of Faith in Medicine." *Managed Care Magazine*, March.

Damon, Gladys. "Boston Chaplains: Rabbis Who Serve the 'Invisible' Jews.'" *Jewish Advocate*, September 12, 1985, 2.

Demerath, N. J. I., Peter D. Hall, Terry Schmitt , and Rhys H. Williams. 1998. *Sacred Companies: Organizational Aspects of Religion and Religious Aspects of Organizations.* New York: Oxford University Press.

DeVries, Raymond, Nancy Berlinger, and Wendy Cadge. 2008. "Lost in Translation: The Chaplain's Role in Health Care." *Hastings Center Report* 38, no. 6:2–27.

———, Robert Dingwall, and Kristina Orfali. 2009. "The Moral Organization of the Professions." *Current Sociology* 57, no. 4:555–79.

Dicks, Russell L. 1940. "Standards for the Work of the Chaplain in a General Hospital." *American Protestant Hospital Association Bulletin* 4, no. 7:1–4.

Dillinger, Jennifer. 2008. "Spiritual Care in the United States: A Pilot Study of Hospital Chaplains and Chaplaincy." Master's thesis. Harvard University Divinity School.

Dingwall, Robert. 2008. *Essays on Professions.* Aldershot, UK: Ashgate.

Downey, V., M. Bengiamin, L. Heuer, and N. Juhl. 1995. "Dying Babies and Associated Stress in NICU Nurses." *Neonatal Network* 14, no. 1:41–46.

Duffin, Jacalyn. 2009. *Medical Miracles: Doctors, Saints and Healing in the Modern World.* New York: Oxford University Press.

Duncombe, David C., and Kenneth E. Spilman. 1971. "A New Breed: Ministers in Medical Education." *Journal of Medical Education* 46, no. 12:1064–68.

Duvall, Robert W. 1987. "Dialogue 88: Definitions, Wellspring, and Dream." *Journal of Pastoral Care* 41, no. 1:58–62.

Dworken, Bari S. 2001. "The Prayer Practices of Rabbis During Pastoral Visits." *Journal of Pastoral Care* 55, no. 4:419–24.

Eastman, Fred. 1951. "Father of the Clinical Pastoral Movement." *Journal of Pastoral Care* 5, no. 1:3–7.

Eck, Diana L. 2001. *A New Religious America: How a "Christian Country" Has Become the World's Most Religiously Diverse Nation.* New York: HarperSanFrancisco.

Ecklund, Elaine Howard. 2010. *Science vs. Religion: What Scientists Really Think.* New York: Oxford University Press.

———, Wendy Cadge, Elizabeth A. Gage, and Elizabeth A. Catlin. 2007. "The Religious and Spiritual Beliefs and Practices of Academic Pediatric Oncologists in the United States." *Journal of Pediatric Hematology and Oncology* 29, no. 11:736–42.

Ehman, John W., Barbara B. Ott, Thomas H. Short, Ralph C. Ciampa, and John Hansen-Flaschen. 1999. "Do Patients Want Physicians to Inquire About Their Spiritual or Religious Beliefs If They Become Gravely Ill?" *Archives of Internal Medicine* 159, no. 15:1803–6.

Ellison, Christopher G., and Jeffrey S. Levin. 1998. "The Religion-Health Connection: Evidence, Theory, and Future Directions." *Health Education and Behavior* 25, no. 6:700–720.

Elpern, Ellen H., Barbara Covert, and Ruth Kleinpell. 2006. "Moral Distress of Staff Nurses in a Medical Intensive Care Unit." *American Journal of Critical Care* 14, no. 6: 523–30.

Essentials of a Hospital Chaplaincy Program 1961. Chicago: American Hospital Association.

Evans, John H. 2002. *Playing God? Human Genetic Engineering and the Rationalization of Public Bioethical Debate.* Chicago: University of Chicago Press.

———. 2003. "After the Fall: Attempts to Establish an Explicitly Theological Voice in Debates over Science and Medicine After 1960." In *The Secular Revolution: Power, Interests, and Conflict in the Secularization of American Public Life*, ed. Christian Smith, 434–61. Berkeley and Los Angeles: University of California Press.

Exley, Catherine. 2004. "Review Article: The Sociology of Dying, Death and Bereavement." *Sociology of Health and Illness* 26, no. 1:110–22.

Faber, Heije. 1971. *Pastoral Care in the Modern Hospital.* Philadelphia, PA: Westminister Press.

Fadiman, Anne. 1998. *The Spirit Catches You, and You Fall Down: A Hmong Child, Her American Doctors, and the Collision of Two Cultures.* New York: Noonday Press.

Fairman, Julie, and Joan E. Lynaugh. 1998. *Critical Care Nursing: A History.* Philadelphia: University of Pennsylvania Press.

Ferngren, Gary B. 2009. *Medicine and Health Care in Early Christianity.* Baltimore, MD: Johns Hopkins University Press.

Fine, Gary A. 1996. *Kitchens: The Culture of Restaurant Work.* Berkeley and Los Angeles: University of California Press.

Fine, Steven. 2003. "Arnold Brunner's Henry S. Frank Memorial Synagogue and the Emergence of 'Jewish Art' in Early Twentieth-Century America." *American Jewish Archives Journal* 54, no.2:47–70.

Fitchett, George. 1993. *Assessing Spiritual Needs: A Guideline for Caregivers.* Minneapolis, MN: Augsburg Publications.

———, and George Handzo. 1998. "Spiritual Assessment and Intervention." In *Psycho-Oncology*, ed. Jimmie D. Holland, 790–808. New York: Oxford University Press.

———, Kathryn Lyndes, Wendy Cadge, Nancy Berlinger, Erin Flanagan, and Jennifer Misasi. 2011. "The Role of Professional Chaplains on Pediatric Palliative Care Teams." *Journal of Palliative Medicine* 14, no. 6:704–7.

———, Kathryn A. Lyndes, Marshall Scott, and Larry M. P. E. Wedel. n.d. "The Chaplain's Week: A Study of Chaplain Activities in One-Person Pastoral Care Departments." Unpublished manuscript.

———, Peter M. Meyer, and Laurel A. Burton. 2000. "Spiritual Care in the Hospital: Who Requests It? Who Needs It?" *Journal of Pastoral Care* 54, no. 2:173–86.

———, Kenneth Rasinski, Wendy Cadge, and Farr Curlin. 2009. "Physicians' Experience and Satisfaction with Chaplains: A National Survey." *Archives of Internal Medicine* 169, no. 19:1808–10.

———, Clayton Thomason, and Kathryn A. Lyndes. 2008. "What Health Care Chaplains Think About Quality Improvement." *Hastings Center Report* (November/December): 18.

Flannelly, Kevin, Kathleen Galek, and George F. Handzo. 2005. "To What Extent Are the Spiritual Needs of Hospital Patients Being Met?" *International Journal of Psychiatry in Medicine* 35, no. 3:319–23.

———, George Handzo, Kathleen Galek, Andrew Weaver, and Jon Overvold. 2006. "A National Survey of Hospital Directors' Views about the Importance of Various Chaplain Roles: Differences Among Disciplines and Types of Hospitals." *Journal of Pastoral Care and Counseling* 60, no. 3:213–25.

———, Kathleen Galek, John Bucchino, George F. Handzo, and Helen P. Tannenbaum. 2005. "Department Directors' Perceptions of the Roles and Functions of Hospital Chaplains: A National Survey." *Hospital Topics: Research and Perspectives on Healthcare* 83, no. 4:19–27.

———, George F. Handzo, and Andrew J. Weaver. 2004. "Factors Affecting Healthcare Chaplaincy and the Provision of Pastoral Care in the United States." *Journal of Pastoral Care and Counseling* 58, nos. 1–2:127–30.

———, George F. Handzo, Andrew J. Weaver, and Walter J. Smith. 2005. "A National Survey of Health Care Administrators' Views on the Importance of Various Chaplain Roles.'" *Journal of Pastoral Care and Counseling* 59, nos. 1–2:87–96.

———, Andrew J. Weaver, and George F. Handzo. 2003. "A Three-Year Professional Study of Chaplains' Professional Activities at Memorial Sloan-Kettering Cancer Center in New York City." *Psycho-Oncology* 12, no. 8:760–68.

Fogg, Sarah L., Andrew J. Weaver, Kevin J. Flannelly, and George F. Handzo. 2004. "An Analysis of Referrals to Chaplains in a Community Hospital in New York over a Seven-Year Period." *Journal of Pastoral Care and Counseling* 58, no. 3:225–35.

Fortin, Auguste H. V., and Katherine G. Barnett. 2004. "Medical School Curricula in Spirituality and Medicine." *Journal of the American Medical Association* 291, no. 23:2883.

Fox, Renée. 1957. "Training for Uncertainty." In *The Student-Physician: Introductory Studies in the Sociology of Medical Education*, ed. Robert K. Merton, George G. Reader, and Patricia L. Kendall, 207–41. Cambridge, MA: Harvard University Press.

———. 1988. "The Human Condition of Health Professionals." In *Essays in Medical Sociology: Journeys into the Field*, ed. Renée Fox, 572–87. New Brunswick, NJ: Transaction Books.

———, and Judith P. Swazey. 2008. *Observing Bioethics*. New York: Oxford University Press.

Foxall, Martha J., Lani Zimmerman, Roberta Standley, and Barbara Bene Captain. 2006. "A Comparison of Frequency and Sources of Nursing Job Stress Perceived by Intensive Care, Hospice and Medical-surgical Nurses." *Journal of Advanced Nursing* 15, no. 5:577–84.

Francis, Doris, Leonie Kellaher, and Georgia Neophytou. 2005. *The Secret Cemetery*. New York: Berg.

Freese, Jeremy, and Sara Shostak. 2009. "Genetics and Social Inquiry." *Annual Review of Sociology* 35:107–28.

Frenk, Steven, Steven Foy, and Keith Meador. 2010. "'It's Medically Proven!' Assessing the Dissemination of Religion and Health Research." *Journal of Religion and Health* 50, no.4: 996–1006.

Galek, Kathleen, Kevin J. Flannelly, Harold G. Koenig, and Sarah L. Fogg. 2007. "Referrals to Chaplains: The Role of Religion and Spirituality in Healthcare Settings." *Mental Health, Religion and Culture* 10, no. 4:363–77.

Gansel, Yannis, Francois Danet, and Catherine Rauscher. 2010. "Long-Stay Inpatients in Short-Term Emergency Units in France: A Case Study." *Social Science and Medicine* 70, no. 4:501–8.

Garces-Foley, Kathleen. 2006. "Hospice and the Politics of Spirituality." *Omega* 53, nos. 1–2:117–36.

Gartner, John, John S. Lyons, David B. Larson, John Serkland, and Mark Peyrot. 1990. "Supplier-Induced Demand for Pastoral Care Services in the General Hospital: A Natural Experiment." *Journal of Pastoral Care* 44, no. 3:262–70.

Geertz, Clifford. 1973. *The Interpretation of Cultures: Selected Essays*. New York: Basic Books.

George, Linda K., David B. Larson, Harold G. Koenig, and Michael E. McCullough. 2000. "Spirituality and Health: What We Know, What We Need to Know." *Journal of Social and Clinical Psychology* 19, no. 1:102–16.

Gerkin, Charles V. 1997. *An Introduction to Pastoral Care*. Nashville, TN: Abingdon Press.

Gerlach-Spriggs, Nancy, Richard E. Kaufman, and Sam B. Warner Jr. 1998. *Restorative Gardens: The Healing Landscape*. New Haven, CT: Yale University Press.

Gibbons, James L., John Thomas, and Larry J. A. K. VandeCreek. 1991. "The Value of Hospital Chaplains: Patient Perspectives." *Journal of Pastoral Care* 45, no. 2:.116–25.

Gilliat-Ray, Sophie. 2003. "Nursing, Professionalism, and Spirituality." *Journal of Contemporary Religion* 18, no. 3:335–49.

———. 2005a. "From 'Chapel' to 'Prayer Room': The Production, Use, and Politics of Sacred Space in Public Institutions." *Culture and Religion* 6, no. 2:287–308.

———. 2005b. "'Sacralising' Sacred Space in Public Institutions: A Case Study of the Prayer Space at the Millennium Dome." *Journal of Contemporary Religion* 20, no. 3:357–72.

Glaser, Barney G., and Anselm L. Strauss. 1965. *Awareness of Dying*. Chicago: Aldine

Gleason, John J. 1984. "The Marketing of Pastoral Care and Counseling, Chaplaincy, and Clinical Pastoral Education." *Journal of Pastoral Care* 38, no. 4:264–72.

Gorski, Philip, and Ates Altinordu. 2008. "After Secularization?" *Annual Review of Sociology* 34:55–85.

Grant, Don, Kathleen O'Neil, and Laura Stephens. 2004. "Spirituality in the Workplace: New Empirical Directions in the Study of the Sacred." *Sociology of Religion* 65, no. 3: 265–83.

Graves, Darci L., Carolyn K. Shue, and Louise Arnold. 2002. "The Role of Spirituality in Patient Care: Incorporating Spirituality Training into Medical School Curriculum." *Academic Medicine* 77, no. 11:1167.

Greeley, Andrew. 1999. " Spirituality and Health: A Bubble Burst by *The Lancet?*" *Spirituality and Health* 2, no. 2:10.

Griswold, Wendy. 1987. " A Methodological Framework for the Sociology of Culture." *Sociological Methodology* 17:1–35.

Gruneir, Andrea, Vincent Mor, Sherry Weitzen, Rachael Truchil, Joan Teno, and Jason Roy. 2007. "Where People Die: A Multilevel Approach to Understanding Influences on Site of Death in America." *Medical Care Research Review* 64, no. 4:351–78.

Guillemin, Jeanne. 1984. "Priceless Lives and Medical Costs: The Case of Newborn Intensive Care." *Research in the Sociology of Health Care* 3:115–34.

———, and Lynda L. Holmstrom. 1986. *Mixed Blessings: Intensive Care for Newborns*. New York: Oxford University Press.

Guntupalli, Kalpalatha, and Robert E. Fromm Jr. 1996. "Burnout in the Internist-Intensivist." *Intensive Care Medicine*. 22, no. 7:625–30.

Gustin, Marilyn N., and Harrold A. Murray. 1985. *The National Association of Catholic Chaplains: A Twenty-Year History (1965–1985)*. Milwaukee, WI: National Association of Catholic Chaplains.

Hall, Charles. 1992. *Head and Heart: The Story of the Clinical Pastoral Education Movement*. Decatur, GA: Journal of Pastoral Care Publications.

Hall, Daniel E., Harold G. Koenig, and Keith G. Meador. 2004. "Conceptualizing 'Religion': How Language Shapes and Constrains Knowledge in the Study of Religion and Health." *Perspectives in Biology and Medicine* 47, no. 3:386–401.

Hall, David D., ed. 1997. *Lived Religion in America: Toward a History of Practice*. Princeton, NJ: Princeton University Press.

Hammond, Phillip E. 1998. *With Liberty for All: Freedom of Religion in the United States*. Louisville, KY: Westminster John Knox Press.

Hammonds, Clare, and Wendy Cadge. Under review. "Professional Emotional Management Off the Job: Strategies of Intensive Care Nurses."

Heimer, Carol A., and Lisa R. Staffen. 1998. *For the Sake of the Children: The Social Organization of Responsibility in the Hospital and the Home*. Chicago: University of Chicago Press.

Heuer, Loretta, Marlene Bengiamin, Vicki Wessman Downey, and Nyla Juhl Imler. 1996. "Neonatal Intensive Care Nurse Stressors: An American Study." *British Journal of Nursing* 5, no.18:1126–30.

Hicks, Allison. 2008. "Role Fusion: The Occupational Socialization of Prison Chaplains." *Symbolic Interaction* 31, no. 4:400–421.

Hiltner, Seward and Jesse H. Ziegler. 1961. "The Consultation on Clinical Pastoral Education and the Theological School." *Journal of Pastoral Care*. 15, no. 3:129–143

Hochschild, Arlie Russell. 1983. *The Managed Heart: The Commercialization of Human Feeling*. Berkeley and Los Angeles: University of California Press.

Hodge, David R. 2003. *Spiritual Assessment: A Handbook for Helping Professionals*. Botsford, CT: North American Association of Christians in Social Work.

———. 2006. "A Template for Spiritual Assessment: A Review of the JCAHO Requirements and Guidelines for Implementation." *Social Work* 51, no. 4:317–26.

Holifield, E. Brooks. 1983. *A History of Pastoral Care in America: From Salvation to Self-Realization*. Nashville, TN: Abingdon Press.

———. 2005. "Pastoral Care Movement." In *Dictionary of Pastoral Care and Counseling*, ed. Rodney Hunter, 845–49. Nashville, TN: Abingdon Press.

———. 2007. *God's Ambassadors: A History of the Christian Clergy in America*. Grand Rapids, MI: William B. Eerdmans.

Holst, Lawrence. E. 1982. " The Hospital Chaplain between Worlds." In *Health/Medicine and the Faith Traditions*, ed. Martin E. Marty and Kenneth L. Vaux, 293–309. Philadelphia, PA: Fortress Press.

———. 1985. *Hospital Ministry: The Role of the Chaplain Today*. New York: Crossroad.

———, and Harold P. Kurtz. 1973. *Toward a Creative Chaplaincy*. Springfield, IL: Charles C. Thomas.

Horsley, Philomena A. 2008. "Death Dwells in Spaces: Bodies in the Hospital Mortuary." *Anthropology and Medicine* 15, no. 2:133–46.

"Hospital Chapels (One Hundred Years Ago)." 2002. *British Medical Journal* 324 (March): 722.

Hughes, Everett C. 1971. *The Sociological Eye: Selected Papers*. Chicago: Aldine-Atherton.

Iler, William L., Don Obershain, and Mary Camac. 2001. "The Impact of Daily Visits from Chaplains on Patients with Chronic Obstructive Pulmonary Disease (COPD): A Pilot Study." *Chaplaincy Today* 17, no. 1:5–11.

Imber, Jonathan. 1986. *Abortion and the Private Practice of Medicine*. New Haven, CT: Yale University Press.

———. 2008. *Trusting Doctors: The Decline of Moral Authority in American Medicine*. Princeton, NJ: Princeton University Press.

Jackson, William C. 1968. "Chapel Participation in a Community General Hospital." *Journal of Pastoral Care* 22, no. 1:34–41.

Jacobs, Lenworth M., Karyl Burns, and Barbara B. Jacobs. 2008. "Trauma Death: Views of the Public and Trauma Professionals on Death and Dying from Injuries." *Archives of Surgery* 143, no. 8:730–35.

Jacobs, Martha R. 2008. "What Are We Doing Here? Chaplains in Contemporary Health Care." *Hastings Center Report* 38, no. 6:1–4.

Johnson, Nancy, Deborah Cook, Mita Giacomini, and Dennis Willms. 2000. "Towards a 'Good' Death: End-of-Life Narratives Constructed in an Intensive Care Unit." *Culture, Medicine and Psychiatry* 24, no. 3:275–95.

Johnson, Paul E. 1968. "Fifty Years of Clinical Pastoral Education." *Journal of Pastoral Care* 22, no. 4:223–31.

Jones, Lindsay. 2000. *The Hermeneutics of Sacred Architecture: Experience, Interpretation.* Cambridge, MA: Harvard University Center for the Study of World Religions.

Joyce, Kathleen. 1995. " Science and the Saints: American Catholics and Health Care, 1880–1930." PhD diss., Princeton University.

Kalb, Claudia. 2003. "Faith and Healing." *Newsweek* 142, no. 19:44.

Kauffman, Christopher J. 1995. *Ministry and Meaning: A Religious History of Catholic Health Care in the United States.* New York: Crossroad.

Kaufman, Sharon R. 2000. "In the Shadow of 'Death with Dignity:' Medicine and Cultural Quandaries of the Vegetative State." *American Anthropologist* 102, no. 1:69–83.

———. 2005. *And a Time to Die: How American Hospitals Shape the End of Life.* New York: Scribner.

———, and Lynn M. Morgan. 2005. "The Anthropology of the Beginnings and Ends of Life." *Annual Review of Anthropology* 34:317–41.

Kelly, M. J., K. E. Olive, L. M. Harvill, and H. A. Maddry. 1997. "Spiritual and Religious Issues in Clinical Care: an Elective Course for Medical Students." *Annals of Behavioral Science and Medical Education* 4:29–35.

Kepler, Milton O. 1968. "Medical Schools, Religion, and Human Values." *Journal of Medical Education* 43, no. 9:984–88.

Klassen, Pamela. 2011. *Spirits of Protestantism: Medicine, Healing, and Liberal Christianity.* Berkeley and Los Angeles: University of California Press.

Kluger, J. 2004. "Religion: Is God in Our Genes?" *Time Magazine*, October 25, 62–72.

———. 2009 "Science and Faith: The Biology of Belief" *Time Magazine*, February 23, 62–72.

Koenig, Harold G., Lucille B. Bearon, Margot Hover, and James L. Travis. 1991. "Religious Perspectives of Doctors, Nurses, Patients, and Families." *Journal of Pastoral Care* 45, no. 3:254–67.

———, Michael E. McCullough, and David B. Larson. 2001. *Handbook of Religion and Health.* New York: Oxford University Press.

Kong, Dolores. 1998. "Dose of Religion Tied to Good Health in North Carolina." *Boston Globe*, National/Foreign, August 13, A3.

Kraut, Alan M., and Deborah A. Kraut. 2007. *Covenant of Care: Newark Beth Israel and the Jewish Hospital in America.* New Brunswick, NJ: Rutgers University Press.

Kubler-Ross, Elisabeth. 1969. *On Death and Dying.* New York: Macmillan.

Kuby, Alma M., and Catherine M. Begole. 1974. "AHA Surveys Chaplaincy Programs." *Hospitals: The Journal of the American Hospital Association* 48, no. 1:98–102.

Kudler, Taryn. 2007. "Providing Spiritual Care." *Contexts* 6, no. 4:60–61.

Lamont, Michele, and Virag Molnar. 2002. "The Study of Boundaries in the Social Sciences." *Annual Review of Sociology* 28:167–95.

Leas, Robert D. 2009. *Anton Theophilus Boisen: His Life, Work, Impact, and Theological Legacy.* Decatur, GA: Journal of Pastoral Care Publications.

Lee, Simon J. Craddock. 2002. "In a Secular Spirit: Strategies of Clinical Pastoral Education." *Health Care Analysis* 10, no. 4:339–56.

Lemmer, Corinne. 2002. "Teaching the Spiritual Dimension of Nursing Care: A Survey of U.S. Baccalaureate Nursing Programs." *Journal of Nursing Education* 41, no. 11:482–90.

Levin, Jeffrey S., David B. Larson, and Christina M. Pulchalski. 1997. "Religion and Spirituality in Medicine: Research and Education." *Journal of the American Medical Association* 278, no. 9:782–83.

Levitan, Tina. 1964. *Islands of Compassion: A History of the Jewish Hospitals of New York.* New York: Twayne.

Lo, Bernard, Delaney Ruston, Laura W. Kates, Robert M. Arnold, Cynthia B. Cohen, K. Faber-Langendoen, Steven Z. Pantilat, Christina M. Puchalski, Timothy R. Quill, Michael W. Rabow, Simeon Schreiber, Daniel P. Sulmasy, James A. Tulsky, and Working Group on Religious and Spiritual Issues at the End of Life. 2002. "Discussing Religious and Spiritual Issues at the End of Life: A Practical Guide for Physicians." *Journal of the American Medical Association* 287, no. 6:749–54.

———, Laura W. Kates, Delaney Ruston, Robert M. Arnold, Cynthia B. Cohen, Christina M. Puchalski, Steven Z. Pantilat, Michael W. Rabow, Simeon Schreiber, and James A. Tulsky. 2003. "Responding to Requests Regarding Prayer and Religious Ceremonies by Patients Near the End of Life and Their Families." *Journal of Palliative Medicine* 6, no. 3:409–15.

Long, Debbi, Cynthia L. Hunter, and Sjaak van der Geest. 2008. "When the Field Is a Ward or a Clinic: Hospital Ethnography." *Anthropology and Medicine* 15, no. 2:71–78.

Luce, John M., and Thomas J. Prendergast. 2001. "The Changing Nature of Death in the ICU." In Curtis and Rubenfeld 2001, 19–29.

Luckhaupt, Sara E., Michael S. Yi, Caroline V. Mueller, Joseph M. Mrus, Amy H. Peterman, Christina M. Puchalski, and Joel Tsevat. 2005. "Beliefs of Primary Care Residents Regarding Spirituality and Religion in Clinical Encounters with Patients: A Study at a Midwestern U.S. Teaching Institution." *Academic Medicine* 80, no. 6:560–70.

Lyndes, Kathryn A., George Fitchett, Clayton L. Thomason, Nancy Berlinger, and Martha R. Jacobs. 2008. "Chaplains and Quality Improvement: Can We Make Our Case by Improving Our Care?" *Journal of Health Care Chaplaincy* 15, no. 2:65–79.

MacLean, Charles, Beth Susi, Nancy Phifer, Linda Schultz, Deborah Bynum, Mark Franco, Andria Klioze, Michael Monroe, Joanne Garrett, and Sam Cyert. 2003. "Patient Preference for Physician Discussion and Practice of Spirituality." *Journal of General Internal Medicine* 18, no. 1:38–43.

Mansfield, Christopher J., Jim Mitchell, and Dana E. King. 2002. "The Doctor as God's Mechanic? Beliefs in the Southeastern United States." *Social Science and Medicine* 54, no. 3:399–409.

Maugans, Todd A. 1996. " The SPIRITual History." *Archives of Family Medicine* 5, no. 1: 11–16.

McCall, Nancy. 1982. "The Statue of the Christus Consolator at The Johns Hopkins Hospital: Its Acquisition and Historic Origins." *Johns Hopkins Medical Journal* 151, no. 1:11–19.

McCauley, Bernadette. 2005. *Who Shall Take Care of Our Sick? Roman Catholic Sisters and the Development of Catholic Hospitals in New York City.* Baltimore, MD: Johns Hopkins University Press.

McEwen, Melanie. 2004. "Analysis of Spirituality Content in Nursing Textbooks." *Journal of Nursing Education* 43, no. 1:20–30.

McGuire, Meredith. 2008. *Lived Religion: Faith and Practice in Everyday Life*. New York: Oxford University Press.

Meier, Levi, and Robert P. Tabak. 2007. "Hospitals." In *Encyclopaedia Judaica*, vol. 9, ed. Michael Berenbaum and Fred Skolnik, 562–65. Detroit, MI: Macmillan.

Mellem, Roger C. 1966. "Chapel Design." *Hospitals* 40:36.

Messikomer, Carla M., and Willy De Craemer. 2002. "The Spirituality of Academic Physicians: An Ethnography of a Scripture-Based Group in an Academic Medical Center." *Academic Medicine* 77, no. 6:562–73.

Meyer, Cleda. 2003. "How Effectively Are Nurse Educators Preparing to Provide Spiritual Care?" *Nurse Educator* 28, no. 4:185–90.

Miles, Steven H. 2001. "The Role of the Physician in Sacred End-of-Life Rituals in the ICU." In Curtis and Rubenfeld 2001, 207–11.

Miller, Timothy S. 1997. *The Birth of the Hospital in the Byzantine Empire*. Baltimore, MD: Johns Hopkins University Press.

Miller, William R., and Carl E. Thoresen. 2003. "Spirituality, Religion, and Health: An Emerging Research Field." *American Psychologist* 58, no. 1:24–35.

Mitchell, Kenneth R. 1972. *Hospital Chaplain*. Philadelphia, PA: Westminster Press.

Moczynski, Walter V. 1998. "The Prayer Box." *Journal of Pastoral Care* 52, no. 3:283–85.

Mohrmann, Margaret E. 2009. "Ethical Grounding for a Profession of Hospital Chaplaincy." *Hastings Center Report* 38, no. 6:18–23.

Mollat, Michel. 1986. *The Poor in the Middle Ages: An Essay in Social History*. Trans. Arthur Goldhammer. New Haven, CT: Yale University Press.

Monfalcone, Wesley R. 2005. "General Hospital Chaplain." In *Dictionary of Pastoral Care and Counseling*, ed. Rodney J. Hunter, 456–57. Nashville, TN: Abingdon Press.

Morrison, Wynne, and Robert M. Nelson. 2007. "Should We Talk to Patients (and Their Families) About God?" *Critical Care Medicine* 35, no. 4:1208–9.

Mowat, Harriet. 2008. *The Potential for Efficacy of Healthcare Chaplaincy and Spiritual Care Provisions in the NHS (UK): A Scoping Review of Recent Research*. Aberdeen: Mowat Research.

Myers-Shirk, Susan E. 2008. *Helping the Good Shepherd: Pastoral Counselors in a Psychotherapeutic Culture, 1925–1975*. Baltimore, MD: Johns Hopkins University Press.

Myers, W. P. L. 1975. "The Care of the Patient with Terminal Illness," in *Cecil Textbook of Medicine*, vol. 1, ed. Paul B. Beeson and Walsh McDermott, 8–12. Philadelphia, PA: W. B. Saunders.

Narayanasamy, Aru, and Jan Owens. 2001. "A Critical Incident Study of Nurses' Responses to the Spiritual Needs of Their Patients." *Journal of Advanced Nursing* 33, no. 4:446–55.

Nelson, Louis P., ed. 2006. *American Sanctuary: Understanding Sacred Spaces*. Bloomington: Indiana University Press.

Neumann, Janice. 2006. "Hospitals Set Aside Space for Muslim Prayer Rooms; Patients, Families, Staff Seek Privacy for Rituals." *Washington Post*, Metro ed., August 26, B07.

North American Nursing Diagnosis Association. 2007. *Nursing Diagnoses: Definitions and Classifications, 2007–2008*. Philadelphia, PA: NANDA International.

Norwood, Frances. 2006. "The Ambivalent Chaplain: Negotiating Structural and Ideological

Difference on the Margins of Modern-Day Hospital Medicine." *Medical Anthropology* 25, no. 1:1–29.

Numbers, Ronald L., and Ronald C. Sawyer. 1982. "Medicine and Christianity in the Modern World." In *Health/Medicine and the Faith Traditions*, ed. Martin E. Marty and Kenneth L. Vaux, 133–60. Philadelphia, PA: Fortress Press.

Oehler, Jerri M., and M. G. Davidson. 1992. "Job Stress and Burnout in Acute and Nonacute Pediatric Nurses." *American Journal of Critical Care* 1, no. 2:81–90.

O'Reilly, JoAnn. 2000. "The Hospital Prayer Book: A Partner for Healing." *Literature and Medicine* 19, no. 1:61–83.

Orsi, Robert A. 1996. *Thank You, St. Jude: Women's Devotion to the Patron Saint of Hopeless Causes*. New Haven, CT: Yale University Press.

———. 2003. "Is the Study of Lived Religion Irrelevant to the World We Live In? Special Presidential Plenary Address, Society for the Scientific Study of Religion." *Journal for the Scientific Study of Religion* 42, no. 2:169–74.

Orton, Meg. 2008. "Emerging Best Practice Pastoral Care in the UK, USA and Australia." *Australian Journal of Pastoral Care and Health* 2, no. 2:1–28.

Pelletier, Allen L., and John W. McCall. 2005. "A Modular Curriculum for Integrating Spirituality and Health Care." *New Directions for Teaching and Learning* 104:51–8.

Phelps, Andrea C., Paul K. Maciejewski, Matthew Nilsson, Tracy A. Balboni, Alexi A. Wright, M. E. Paulk, Elizabeth Trice, Deborah Schrag, John R. Peteet, Susan D. Block, and Holly G. Prigerson. 2009. "Religious Coping and Use of Intensive Life-Prolonging Care Near Death in Patients with Advanced Cancer." *Journal of the American Medical Association* 301, no. 11:1140–47.

Piderman, Katherine M., Dean V. Marek, Sarah M. Jenkins, Mary E. Johnson, James F. Buryska, and Paul S. Mueller. 2008. "Patients' Expectations of Hospital Chaplains." *Mayo Clinic Proceedings* 83, no. 1:58–65.

Porter, Roy. 1993. "Religion and Medicine." In *Companion Encyclopedia of the History of Medicine*, ed. William F. Bynum and Roy Porter, 1449–68. New York: Routledge.

Post, Stephen, Christina Puchalski, and David B. Larson. 2000. "Physicians and Patient Spirituality: Professional Boundaries, Competency, and Ethics." *Annals of Internal Medicine* 132, no. 7:578–83.

Puchalski, Christina, Betty Ferrell, Rose Virani , Shirley Otis-Green, Pamela Baird, Janet Bull, Harvey Chochinov, George Handzo, Holly Nelson-Becker, Maryjo Prince-Paul, Karen Pugliese, and Daniel Sulmasy. 2009. "Improving the Quality of Spiritual Care as a Dimension of Palliative Care: The Report of the Consensus Conference." *Journal of Palliative Medicine* 12, no. 10:885–904.

———, and Anna L. Romer. 2000. "Taking a Spiritual History Allows Clinicians to Understand Patients More Fully." *Journal of Palliative Medicine* 3, no. 1:129–37.

Putnam, Robert D., and David E. Campbell. 2010. *American Grace: How Religion Divides and Unites Us*. New York: Simon & Schuster.

Rashotte, Judy, Frances Fothergill-Bourbonnais, and Marie Chamberlain. 1997. "Pediatric Intensive Care Nurses and Their Grief Experiences: A Phenomenological Study." *Heart and Lung* 26, no.5: 372–86.

Reverby, Susan M. 1987. *Ordered to Care: The Dilemma of American Nursing, 1850–1945.* Cambridge: Cambridge University Press.

Rhoads, Paul. 1967. "Medicine and Religion A New Journal Department." *Journal of the American Medical Association* 200, no. 2:162.

Richardson, Margaret, Suzanne Owens-Pike, and Peter Bauck. 2011. "The Bottom Line Challenge: Demonstrating Effectiveness Beyond Press Ganey." *Chaplaincy Today* 27, no. 1:22–31.

Rieff, Philip. 1966. *The Triumph of the Therapeutic: Uses of Faith After Freud.* New York: Harper & Row.

Rimer, Kathleen P. 2005. "Spiritual Care and Transformative Learning in Biomedicine: Clinical Pastoral Education for Healthcare Providers." Ph.D. diss., Graduate School of Education, Harvard University.

Risse, Guenter B. 1999. *Mending Bodies, Saving Souls: A History of Hospitals.* New York: Oxford University Press.

Ritter, Jim. 2005. "Is Religion Good for Health? Researchers Say Amen; African American Believers Less Likely to Be Depressed." *Chicago Sun Times*, April 14, 4.

Robinson, Mary R., Mary M. Thiel, Meghan M. Backus, and Elaine C. Meyer. 2006. "Matters of Spirituality at the End of Life in the Pediatric Intensive Care Unit." *Pediatrics* 118, no. 3:719–29.

Rodrigues, Bartholomew, Deanne Rodrigues, and D. L. Casey. 2000. *Spiritual Needs and Chaplaincy Services: A National Empirical Study on Chaplaincy Encounters in Health Care Settings.* Medford, OR: Providence Health System.

Roof, Wade C. 1999. *Spiritual Marketplace: Baby Boomers and the Remaking of American Religion.* Princeton, NJ: Princeton University Press.

———. 2003. "Religion and Spirituality: Toward an Integrated Analysis." In *Handbook of the Sociology of Religion*, ed. Michele Dillon, 137–50. Cambridge: Cambridge University Press.

Rosenberg, Charles E. 1977. "And Heal the Sick: The Hospital and Patient in Nineteenth-Century America." *Journal of Social History* 10, no. 4:428–47.

———. 1987. *The Care of Strangers: The Rise of America's Hospital System.* New York: Basic Books.

Rothman, David J. 1991. *Strangers at the Bedside: A History of How Law and Bioethics Transformed Medical Decision Making.* New York: Basic Books.

Salamon, Julie. 2008a. *Hospital: Man, Women, Birth, Death, Infinity, Plus Red Tape, Bad Behavior, Money, God, and Diversity on Steroids.* New York: Penguin Press.

———. 2008b. "Hospital or Holy Ground?" *Search Magazine*, July/August.

Sarna, Jonathan D. 1987. "The Impact of Nineteenth-Century Christian Missions on American Jews." In *Jewish Apostasy in the Modern World*, ed. Todd M. Endelman, 232–54. New York: Holmes and Meier.

Schecter, S., C. J. Capalbo, J. R. Bowen, and T. Perry. 1998. "On the Development of the Surgical Intensive Care Unit: The Rhode Island Experience." *Medicine and Health Rhode Island* 81, no. 1:318–20.

Schmidt, Leigh E. 2005. *Restless Souls: The Making of American Spirituality.* New York: HarperSanFrancisco.

Seale, Clive. 2010. "The Role of Doctors' Religious Faith and Ethnicity in Taking Ethically Controversial Decisions During End-of-Life Care." *Journal of Medical Ethics* 36,
no. 11:883–85.

———, and Sjaak van der Geest. 2004. "Good and Bad Death: Introduction." *Social Science
and Medicine* 58, no. 5:883–85.

Seymour, Jane E. 2001. *Critical Moments: Death and Dying in Intensive Care*. Philadelphia,
PA: Open University Press.

Sharp, Cecil G. 1991. "Use of Chaplaincy in the Neonatal Intensive Care Unit." *Southern
Medical Journal* 84, no. 12:1482–86.

Sheler, J. L. 2004. "The Power of Prayer." *U.S. News and World Report*, December 20, 52–54.

Shem, Samuel. 1978. *The House of God*. New York: Random House.

Sherkat, Darren E., and Christopher G. Ellison. 1999. "Recent Developments and Current
Controversies in the Sociology of Religion." *Annual Review of Sociology* 25:363–94.

Shostak, Sara, Jeremy Freese, Bruce G. Link, and Jo C. Phelan. 2009. "The Politics of the
Gene: Social Status and Beliefs about Genetics for Individual Outcomes." *Social Psychology Quarterly* 72, no. 1: 77–93.

Silberman, Jeffery M. 1986. "A Jewish Experience of Clinical Pastoral Education." *Journal of
Pastoral Care* 40, no. 4:354–57.

———. 1992. "The National Association of Jewish Chaplains." *Journal of Pastoral Care* 46,
no. 1:1–2.

Skalla, Karen A., and J. Patrick McCoy. 2006. "Spiritual Assessment of Patients with Cancer:
The Moral Authority, Vocational, Aesthetic, Social, and Transcendent Model." *Oncology
Nursing Forum* 33, no. 4:745–51.

Sloan, Richard. 2006. *Blind Faith: The Unholy Alliance of Religion and Medicine*. New York:
St. Martin's Press.

Smeets, William. 2006. *Spiritual Care in a Hospital Setting: An Empirical-Theological Explo-
ration*. Trans. M. Manley. Boston: Brill.

Smith, Christian. 2003. *The Secular Revolution: Power, Interests, and Conflict in the
Secularization of American Public Life*. Berkeley and Los Angeles: University of California
Press.

Smith, David H. 2005. *Partnership with the Dying: Where Medicine and Ministry Should
Meet*. Lanham, MD: Rowman and Littlefield.

Southard, Samuel. 1963. "Criteria for Evaluating Supervisors-in-Training." *Journal of Pastoral Care* 17, no. 4:193–202.

Spirn, Charles A. 2000. *My Life As a Chaplain: How a Hospital Chaplain Helps Patients*.
Rockville, MD: Shengold.

Star, Susan L. 1991. "The Sociology of the Invisible: The Primacy of Work in the Writings of
Anselm Strauss." In *Social Organization and Social Process: Essays in Honor of Anselm
Strauss*, ed. David R. Maines, 265–83. New York: Aldine De Gruyter.

Starr, Paul L. 1982. *The Social Transformation of American Medicine*. New York: Basic
Books.

"Statement on Hospital Chaplaincy." 1967. *Bulletin of the American Protestant Hospital Association* 31, no. 2:14.

Staten, Pat. 2003. "Spiritual Assessment Required in All Settings." *Hospital Peer Review* 28, no. 4:55–56.

Steinhauser, Karen E., Nicholas A. Christakis, Elizabeth C. Clipp, Maya McNeilly, Lauren McIntyre, and James Tulsky. 2000a. "Factors Considered Important at the End of Life by Patients, Family, Physicians, and Other Care Providers." *Journal of the American Medical Association* 284, no. 19:2476–82.

———, Elizabeth C. Clipp, Maya McNeilly, Nicholas A. Christakis, Lauren M. McIntyre, and James A. Tulsky. 2000b. "In Search of a Good Death: Observations of Patients, Families and Providers." *Annals of Internal Medicine* 13, no. 10:825–32.

Stevens, Edward F. 1921. *The American Hospital of the Twentieth Century: A Treatise on the Development of Medical Institutions, Both in Europe and in America, Since the Beginning of the Present Century.* New York: Architectural Record Company.

Stevens, Rosemary. 1989. *In Sickness and in Wealth: American Hospitals in the Twentieth Century.* Baltimore, MD: Johns Hopkins University Press.

Stoll, Ruth I. 1979. "Guidelines for Spiritual Assessment." *American Journal of Nursing* 79, no. 9:1574–77.

Strauss, Anselm, and Juliet Corbin. 1990. *Basics of Qualitative Research: Grounded Theory Procedures and Techniques.* Newbury Park, CA: Sage.

Sudnow, David. 1967. *Passing On: The Social Organization of Death.* Englewood Cliffs, NJ: Prentice-Hall.

Sullivan, Winnifred F. 2009. *Prison Religion: Faith-Based Reform and the Constitution.* Princeton, NJ: Princeton University Press.

———. 2010. "Religion Naturalized: The New Establishment." In *After Pluralism,* ed. Pamela Klassen and Courtney Bender, 82–97. New York: Columbia University Press.

Sulmasy, Daniel P. 1997. *The Healer's Calling: A Spirituality for Physicians and Other Health Care Professionals.* New York: Paulist Press.

———. 2006. *The Rebirth of the Clinic: An Introduction to Spirituality in Health Care.* Washington DC: Georgetown University Press.

———. 2007. "What Is a Miracle?" *Southern Medical Journal* 100, no. 12:1223–28.

SUPPORT Principal Investigators. 1995. "A Controlled Trial to Improve Care for Seriously Ill Hospitalized Patients: The Study to Understand Prognoses and Preferences for Outcomes and Risks of Treatment (SUPPORT)." *Journal of the American Medical Association* 274, no. 20:1591–98.

Swift, Christopher. 2009. *Hospital Chaplaincy in the Twenty-first Century: The Crisis of Spiritual Care on the NHS.* Burlington, UK: Ashgate.

Tabak, Robert. 2010. "The Emergence of Jewish Health-Care Chaplaincy: The Professionalization of Spiritual Care." *American Jewish Archives Journal* 62, no. 2:89–109

Tanenbaum Center for Interreligious Understanding. 2009. *The Medical Manual for Religio-Cultural Competence: Caring for Religiously Diverse Populations.* 2009. New York: Tanenbaum Center for Interreligious Understanding.

Taylor, Bonita E., Kevin J. Flannelly, Andrew J. Weaver, and David J. Zucker. 2006. "Compassion Fatigue and Burnout Among Rabbis Working As Chaplains." *Journal of Pastoral Care and Counseling* 60, nos. 1–2:35–42.

———, and David J. Zucker. 2002. "Nearly Everything We Wish Our Non-Jewish Supervisors Had Known about Us as Jewish Supervisees." *Journal of Pastoral Care and Counseling* 56, no. 4:327–38.

Taylor, Charles. 2007. *A Secular Age*. Cambridge, MA: Harvard University Press.

Taylor, Elizabeth, Madalon Amenta, and Martha Highfield. 1995. "Spiritual Care Practices of Oncology Nurses." *Oncology Nursing Forum* 22, no. 1:31–39.

Thiel, Mary M. 2009. "Contextualizing CPE: Developing a Jewish Geriatric CPE Program." In *Expanding the Circle: Essays in Honor of Joan E. Hemenway*, ed. Catherine F. Garlid, Angelika A. Zollfrank, and George Fitchett, 245–62. Decatur, GA: Journal of Pastoral Care Publications.

———, and Mary R. Robinson. 1997. "Physicians' Collaborations with Chaplains: Difficulties and Benefits." *Journal of Clinical Ethics* 8, no. 1:94–103.

Thomas, John R. 2000. *A "Snap Shot" History (1975–2000) of the Association for Clinical Pastoral Education, Inc.: A Celebration of the 75th Anniversary of CPE*. Association for Clinical Pastoral Education. Decatur, GA.

———, and Mark LaRocca-Pitts. 2006. *Compassion, Commitment and Conscience: The Rise of Professional Chaplaincy*. Schaumburg, IL: Association of Professional Chaplains.

Thompson, John D., and Grace Goldin. 1973. *The Hospital: A Social and Architectural History*. New Haven, CT: Yale University Press.

Thorson, James A. 1993. "Did You Ever See a Hearse Go By? Some Thoughts on Gallows Humor." *Journal of American Culture* 16, no. 2:17–24.

Timmermans, Stefan. 1999. *Sudden Death and the Myth of CPR*. Philadelphia, PA: Temple University Press.

Timmins, Fiona, and Jacinta Kelly. 2008. "Spiritual Assessment in Intensive and Cardiac Care Nursing." *Nursing in Critical Care* 13, no. 3:124–31.

Todres, I. D., Elizabeth A. Catlin, and Mary M. Thiel. 2005. "The Intensivist in a Spiritual Care Training Program Adapted for Clinicians." *Critical Care Medicine* 33, no. 12:2733–36.

Tolich, Martin. 2004. "Internal Confidentiality: When Confidentiality Assurances Fail Relational Informants." *Qualitative Sociology* 27, no. 1:101–6.

Treadway, Katherine. 2007. "The Code." *New England Journal of Medicine* 357, no. 13:1273–75.

VandeCreek, Larry. 1999. "Professional Chaplaincy: An Absent Profession?" *Journal of Pastoral Care* 53, no. 4:417–32.

———. 2003. *Professional Chaplaincy and Clinical Pastoral Education Should Become More Scientific: Yes and No*. New York: Haworth Pastoral Press.

———. 2004. "How Satisfied Are Patients with the Ministry of Chaplains?" *Journal of Pastoral Care and Counseling* 58, no. 4:335–42.

———, and Laurel Burton. 2001. "Professional Chaplaincy: Its Role and Importance in Healthcare." *Journal of Pastoral Care* 55, no. 1:81–97.

———, and Loren Connell. 1991. "Evaluation of the Hospital Chaplain's Pastoral Care: Catholic and Protestant Differences." *Journal of Pastoral Care* 45, no. 3:289–95.

———, Arne Jessen, John Thomas, James Gibbons, and Stephen Strausser. 1991. "Patient and

Family Perceptions of Hospital Chaplains." *Hospital and Health Services Administration* 36, no. 3:455–67.

——, and Marjorie A. Lyon. 1994–95. "The General Hospital Chaplain's Ministry: Analysis of Productivity, Quality and Cost." *Caregiver Journal* 11, no. 2:3–13.

——, Karolynn Siegel, Eileen Gorey , Sharon Brown, and Rhoda Toperzer. 2001. "How Many Chaplains Per 100 Inpatients? Benchmarks of Health Care Chaplaincy Departments." *Journal of Pastoral Care* 55, no. 3:289–301.

van der Geest, Sjaak. 2005. "'Sacraments' in the Hospital: Exploring the Magic and Religion of Recovery." *Anthropology and Medicine* 12, no. 2:135–50.

——, and Kaja Finkler. 2004. "Hospital Ethnography: Introduction." *Social Science and Medicine* 59, no. 10:1995–2001.

Verderber, Stephen, and David J. Fine. 2000. *Healthcare Architecture in an Era of Radical Transformation.* New Haven, CT: Yale University Press.

Wall, Richard J., Ruth A. Engelberg, Cynthia J. Gries, Bradford Glavan, and J. R. Curtis. 2007. "Spiritual Care of Families in the Intensive Care Unit." *Critical Care Medicine* 35, no. 4:1084–90.

Warner, Michael, Jonathan Vanantwerpen, and Craig Calhoun. 2010. *Varieties of Secularism in a Secular Age.* Cambridge, MA: Harvard University Press.

Weaver, Andrew J., and Christopher G. Ellison. 2004. "Featured CME Topic: Spirituality 'Introduction.'" *Southern Medical Journal* 97, no. 12:1191–93.

——, Kevin. J. Flannelly, David B. Larson, Carolyn L. Stapleton, and Harold G. Koenig. 2002. "Mental Health Issues Among Clergy and Other Religious Professionals: A Review of Research." *Journal of Pastoral Care and Counseling* 56, no. 4:393–403.

Weinberg, Dana B. 2003. *Code Green: Money-Driven Hospitals and the Dismantling of Nursing.* Ithaca, NY: Cornell University Press.

White, Christopher. 2009. *Unsettled Minds: Psychology and the American Search for Spiritual Assurance, 1830–1940.* Berkeley and Los Angeles: University of California Press.

White, Lerrill. 2003. "Federal Funding Preserved for CPE Programs." ACPE Web page at http://www.acpe.edu/AdminMedicare.html.

Whitesel, John. 1967. "Report of the Third Inter-Organizational Consultation on Hospital Chaplaincy." *Bulletin of the American Protestant Hospital Association* 31, no. 2:15.

Widera, Eric W., Kenneth E. Rosenfeld, Erik K. Fromme, Daniel P. Sulmasy, and Robert M. Arnold. 2011. "Approach Patients and Family Members Who Hope for a Miracle." *Journal of Pain and Symptom Management* 42, no. 1:119–25.

Widerquist, Joann G. 1992. "The Spirituality of Florence Nightingale." *Nursing Research* 41, no. 1:49–55.

Will, Willard W. I. 2009. "Making Hospital Chaplains in an Age of Biomedicine." PhD diss., Department of Anthropology, McGill University, Montreal.

Williams, Joshua A., David Meltzer, Vineet Arora , Grace Chung, and Farr A. Curlin. 2011. "Attention to Inpatients' Religious and Spiritual Concerns: Predictors and Association with Patient Satisfaction." *Journal of General Internal Medicine.* 26, no. 11:1265–71.

Wind, Gitte. 2008. "Negotiated Interactive Observation: Doing Fieldwork in Hospital Settings." *Anthropology and Medicine* 15, no. 2:79–89.

Wintrobe, Maxwell M., et al, eds. 1974. *Harrison's Principles of Internal Medicine*. 7th ed., 7–8. New York: McGraw-Hill.

Wolenberg, Kelly. 2011. "American Interest in Medicine and Religion in the Twentieth Century." Unpublished paper, University of Chicago Divinity School.

Wolf, Zane R. 1988. *Nurses' Work, the Sacred and the Profane*. Philadelphia: University of Pennsylvania Press.

Wolfe, Alan. 2003. *The Transformation of American Religion: How We Actually Live Our Faith*. New York: Free Press.

Wuthnow, Robert. 1998. *After Heaven: Spirituality in America Since the 1950s*. Berkeley and Los Angeles: University of California Press.

Zier, Lucas S., Jeffrey H. Burack, Guy Micco, Anne K. Chipman, James A. Frank, James M. Luce, and Douglas B. White. 2008. "Doubt and Belief in Physicians' Ability to Prognosticate During Critical Illness: The Perspective of Surrogate Decision Makers." *Critical Care Medicine* 36, no. 8:2341–47.

Zupancic, John A., and Douglas K. Richardson. 2002. "Characterization of Neonatal Personnel Time Inputs and Prediction from Clinical Variables: A Time and Motion Study." *Journal of Perinatology* 22, no. 8:658–63.

Zussman, Robert. 1992. *Intensive Care: Medical Ethics and the Medical Profession*. Chicago: University of Chicago Press.

INDEX

Italicized page numbers refer to figures and tables.